Endometriosis

Endometriosis

Understand your symptoms
Get the right treatment
Reclaim your life

JEN MOORE

GREEN TREE
LONDON · OXFORD · NEW YORK · NEW DELHI · SYDNEY

GREEN TREE
Bloomsbury Publishing Plc
50 Bedford Square, London, WC1B 3DP, UK
Bloomsbury Publishing Ireland Limited
29 Earlsfort Terrace, Dublin 2, D02 AY28, Ireland

BLOOMSBURY, GREEN TREE and the Green Tree logo are trademarks of Bloomsbury Publishing Plc

First published in Great Britain 2025

Copyright © Jen Moore, 2025

Jen Moore has asserted her right under the Copyright, Designs and Patents Act, 1988, to be identified as Author of this work

For legal purposes the Acknowledgements on p. 291 constitute an extension of this copyright page

All rights reserved. No part of this publication may be: i) reproduced or transmitted in any form, electronic or mechanical, including photocopying, recording or by means of any information storage or retrieval system without prior permission in writing from the publishers; or ii) used or reproduced in any way for the training, development or operation of artificial intelligence (AI) technologies, including generative AI technologies. The rights holders expressly reserve this publication from the text and data mining exception as per Article 4(3) of the Digital Single Market Directive (EU) 2019/790

Bloomsbury Publishing Plc does not have any control over, or responsibility for, any third-party websites referred to or in this book. All internet addresses given in this book were correct at the time of going to press. The author and publisher regret any inconvenience caused if addresses have changed or sites have ceased to exist, but can accept no responsibility for any such changes

A catalogue record for this book is available from the British Library

Library of Congress Cataloguing-in-Publication data has been applied for

ISBN: TPB: 978-1-3994-2448-6; eBook: 978-1-3994-2444-8

2 4 6 8 10 9 7 5 3 1

All inside illustrations by Barking Dog Art with the exception of page 98

Typeset in Minion Pro by Deanta Global Publishing Services, Chennai, India
Printed and bound in Great Britain by CPI Group (UK) Ltd, Croydon CR0 4YY

To find out more about our authors and books visit www.bloomsbury.com
and sign up for our newsletters
For product safety related questions contact productsafety@bloomsbury.com

The information contained in this book is provided by way of general guidance in relation to the specific subject matters addressed herein, but it is not a substitute for specialist advice. It should not be relied on for medical, healthcare, pharmaceutical or other professional advice on specific health needs. This book is sold with the understanding that the author and publisher are not engaged in rendering medical, health or any other kind of personal or professional services. The reader should consult a competent medical or health professional before adopting any of the suggestions in this book or drawing inferences from it

The author and publisher specifically disclaim, as far as the law allows, any responsibility from any liability, loss or risk (personal or otherwise) which is incurred as a consequence, directly or indirectly, of the use and applications of any of the contents of this book

CONTENTS

Introduction	1
Chapter 1: What is endometriosis?	9
Chapter 2: Dealing with the system – how to get help	63
Chapter 3: Understanding endometriosis care and surgery	109
Chapter 4: The evil step-sisters – associated conditions	147
Chapter 5: Living with endometriosis – the art and the science	169
Chapter 6: Not all endometriosis pain is physical	201
Chapter 7: Endometriosis doesn't discriminate – why do we?	223
Chapter 8: This is not the end	247
Appendices	263
References	267
Resources	288
Acknowledgements	291
Index	293

Before we get stuck in, just a quick note to say that I am not a doctor or a medical professional of any kind. I am purely an 'expert by experience'. This book is about my own lived experiences, conversations with other patients, research and insights from global endometriosis experts. It is intended to give you a comprehensive and holistic understanding of endometriosis, to arm you with the information to make the best choices for yourself, your body and your future. It does not constitute or replace individualised, expert medical advice.

Up-to-date and accurate information about endometriosis is frighteningly hard to come by due to an historic lack of prioritisation, funding and research. The following chapters are packed with references to papers, reports, studies, and expert observations and opinions. These may not be perfect, and their inclusion does not necessarily mean that I endorse or recommend them. Likewise, I make no recommendations for individual surgeons or endometriosis centres.

For every single one of us who has ever been told our pain is normal.
I believe you.

INTRODUCTION

Endometriosis
(en-doe-mee-tree-oh-sis)

You might think it would be difficult to write an entire book about a disease we don't know much about. We don't even know what causes endometriosis – and we don't know how to cure it either. A lot of what we think we know is outdated or simply incorrect, perpetuated by myths and a deeply patriarchal medical system. But this makes it even more important to share what we do know, bringing both patients and clinicians alike up to date with our current knowledge of this disease.

In an ideal world, this book wouldn't exist. It wouldn't need to, because we would simply go to the doctor's when we started experiencing symptoms. We wouldn't feel embarrassed talking about those symptoms after years of being told to keep them to ourselves. We would be able to get an appointment with our doctor and tell them what we were struggling with. They would listen; they would believe us. Our doctor would have received up-to-date, accurate education and training about endometriosis and would recognise the symptoms that can indicate its presence. They would know that endometriosis is a complex condition that requires expert intervention, and they would refer us straight away to an endometriosis expert who had dedicated their career to understanding the disease. This referral would be prompt because there would be plenty of experts, reflecting just how common the disease is. The expert would diagnose us, talk us through the options and start assembling the multi-disciplinary team (MDT) that it takes to support an endometriosis patient for the long term. If surgery was agreed upon by us and the surgeon, the waiting list would be short. Surgery would be undertaken only by specialists who would be experienced enough to spot all of the disease and remove it using complete excision (where the whole area is surgically removed) – currently the most effective method. Support would not end after surgery. Instead, the MDT would continue to monitor and check in on us. Physiotherapy, mental health, nutrition – all of these would play a role.

Unfortunately, we do not live in this utopia. In fact, if you are reading this, you have probably had the opposite experience to the one detailed above. Despite considerable medical advances in recent decades, endometriosis has arguably fallen through the gaps. Endometriosis care is still riddled with misinformation, myths and accusations of overly emotional women. It impacts at least one in 10 women, and those assigned female at birth, a comparable statistic to that for asthma or diabetes. Yet, unlike those very familiar conditions, general awareness and understanding of endometriosis is pitifully low. And that is why this book exists. Let's bust the myths, share what we do know, push for change and research to fill in the gaps and find ways to feel less alone. I don't have all the answers (mainly because lots of people still are not asking or researching the right questions), but I have brought everything we do know together to help you push for the right treatment for you.

While this book undeniably focuses on endometriosis, it also touches on two very common 'sister' conditions: adenomyosis and fibroids. These two conditions often occur alongside endometriosis but could also occur on their own and be confused for endometriosis. It's important to understand them, the symptoms they cause, and the options for management and treatment. You can find out more about adenomyosis and fibroids in chapter 4.

This book might be challenging in parts, maybe uncomfortable or even difficult reading. It is not meant to frighten you, but to educate you on the realities and just how debilitating endometriosis can be. When I and other campaigners are trying to raise awareness and push for change in endometriosis care, we often talk about extreme cases. We do that to highlight just how damaging this disease can be. But remember, an endometriosis diagnosis is not an instant sentence to these extremes. Endometriosis is a spectrum disease, and many people are able to find a way to live with their symptoms without it becoming debilitating. There is always hope. There are ways to manage your symptoms, access expert help and support yourself. And you're never alone. I will be here, throughout the following chapters, metaphorically holding your hand through it all.

The best place to start is with a definition of what endometriosis is. I have lost count of the number of doctors, organisations and media outlets that simply have the definition of endometriosis wrong. They call it a period condition or a uterine disease, or they talk about the lining of the womb gone rogue. None of these are correct. And if we can't get the definition right, everything that follows is going to be wrong too. If your doctor has been

Introduction

taught that endometriosis is a uterine condition, then of course they will think that a hysterectomy will cure the issue (even though current research shows us that this is clearly not the answer). A hysterectomy does not cure endometriosis; I am living proof, writing this just over a year after my hysterectomy but with endometriosis throughout my pelvic cavity and on some of my vital organs. We will be going into the who, what, where, when and why of endometriosis in much more detail later in the book, but let's get this sorted right from the start:

> Endometriosis is a systemic, inflammatory disease characterised by the presence of endometrium-like tissue found outside the uterine cavity.

We will break down what that means in much more detail soon, but the key parts are as follows:

- 'Systemic' means we are talking about the whole body rather than an individual part of it. In other words, endometriosis is a disease that affects the entire body. It is not a 'uterine' condition, meaning of the uterus. In fact, it has been found on every organ and in every system of the human body.
- 'Inflammatory' refers to some of the mechanisms driving endometriosis. Inflammation, a response to an illness or injury (or the perception of one), is an important part of our body's defence system. But when there is excess inflammation, or inflammation for a prolonged period, issues can arise. As we will see, inflammation is a key driver of endometriosis and underpins why this disease can cause so much pain.
- 'Endometrium-like' is where the definition gets a little sticky. Truthfully, we know so much more about what endometriosis *isn't* than what it actually *is*. Endometriosis cells are similar to those that line the womb, aka the endometrium, but they are fundamentally different in appearance, behaviour and structure. Why we are still referring to these cells as 'endometrium-like' rather than as something in their own right, I really can't tell you. Addressing this point would be a relatively simple switch that could help avoid some of the prolonged confusion around this disease.

But endometriosis is so much more than the biological mechanisms that cause it to grow, spread and recur. Why? Because we are so much more than a bundle of organs and bones. We are people. People with lives, hopes, dreams, goals and plans. And endometriosis invades all of these.

Endometriosis has profoundly changed me. It has taken so much from me that sometimes, when I stop and think about it all, I struggle to breathe. Beyond the physical symptoms, the pain, the surgeries and the loss of organs, this disease has impacted every single aspect of my life. My independence, my freedom, my spontaneity, my career, my financial stability, my faith in so many things, my dreams for a future that I'll never have – it's a pain that is next to impossible to describe. Despite having suffered broken bones, an illness that left me with scarred lungs, multiple surgeries and a near-fatal car accident, endometriosis eclipses them all. Combined. Yet I am still told that I am exaggerating or making it up. Believe me, I am far more likely to downplay my symptoms than overstate them.

Despite affecting (at a conservative estimate) one in 10 women worldwide, endometriosis is not taken seriously. It is, increasingly, talked about, which is a good start, but it is still not prioritised enough to do something about it. Generations of us, all over the world, have the same story. Recent research in the UK shows that endometriosis care has not changed in 24 years. That's a quarter of a century where nothing has improved. And considering that in 2024 it was also revealed that the average diagnosis time for endometriosis in the UK had *increased* from seven years and six months (2021) to eight years and 10 months (2024), an argument could be made that not only are things not changing, but they are actually getting worse.

Endometriosis has been pushed aside, dismissed, ignored and even mocked for far too long. The same is true for conditions that often accompany endo, such as adenomyosis and fibroids – both of which we'll explore. We sufferers have been called hysterical, dramatic, weak and attention seekers. Enough is enough. It is time for us to have our say. It is time for the true endometriosis experts who have dedicated their entire careers to this disease to be heard. And it is time for the medical system and policy makers to understand that endometriosis is a public health crisis that desperately needs attention and action. The time has passed for simply raising awareness. We know the problem exists. It is now time to do something about it.

It infuriates me when policy makers and advocacy organisations recommend that we teach young people more about their bodies – apparently

Introduction

the answer is to increase menstrual education and encourage girls and women to speak up when something is wrong. And it *is* absolutely vital, especially in certain communities and groups where stigma is still a huge issue when it comes to discussing female anatomy and bodily processes. But, by and large, we *have* been speaking up. For decades. It means absolutely nothing if we are also not addressing the next step in the chain: the education of all GPs to recognise that endometriosis is a full-body disease and that symptoms can present throughout the entire cycle. Those GPs then need the knowledge to refer patients on to endometriosis specialists for diagnosis and treatment. And those specialists need to be plentiful in number to rebalance the significant gap between demand and supply that currently exists. Speaking up means nothing without someone believing us and then knowing how to provide the best possible outcomes. Without that, we are just screaming into a void.

This book is my contribution to that push for change. It contains as much as information as I could fit into a single book, and is designed to plug some of the huge gaps left by a medical system that is still playing catch-up (and not very well) with what we know about this disease. I don't have all the answers; no one does. This book won't be able to give you a silver bullet that will destroy endometriosis, because there isn't one. But it will give you the tools you need to understand the disease, navigate the healthcare system and make the best choices for you, your body and your future. Dip in and out as you need. Just been diagnosed and want to understand what on earth endometriosis is? Head to chapter 1. Struggling to get your GP to listen? Chapter 2 has some tips for advocating for yourself in the doctor's surgery. Trying to navigate the minefield of hormonal options for symptom management? Chapter 2 will be your guide. Thinking about surgery? Chapter 3 is the one you need. Looking to support your body and manage symptoms through lifestyle changes? Read chapter 5 to see what options are working for others. Just been told you might adenomyosis or fibroids as well, or even of instead of endometriosis? Chapter 4 will walk you through what you need to know.

Each case of endometriosis is different and each of us has different goals and life plans. Your experiences and choices may differ from mine and the other case studies in this book, and that is okay. Your body is yours, and you know it best.

I hope this book becomes an invaluable resource in your journey with endometriosis. If you are a sufferer of this cruel disease, I hope it becomes your guide, teaching you what is happening inside your body, encouraging you to powerfully advocate for your health and comforting you and validating your experiences along the way.

If you are someone supporting a loved one with endometriosis, I hope this book helps you to understand what they are going through. I hope it also provides you with tools to navigate this new role in your own life, because you matter too. Let me take this opportunity right now to say thank you. You are appreciated more than you know.

And if you are a healthcare professional of any kind, I hope it opens your eyes to how complex endometriosis truly is. I hope it enables you to empathise with your patients and the struggles they are facing. I hope it inspires you to call out misinformation when you come across it and, above all, to believe in your patients' pain.

The enigma that is endometriosis

Unfortunately, the jury is still out when it comes to most aspects of endometriosis. Almost everything is unresolved, with findings from different research studies often contradicting each other. Even expert surgeons meeting at global conferences will fiercely debate certain topics based on their own understanding and clinical observations.

The human brain loves to simplify things. It loves to break things down into the most basic forms it can, label them and file them away securely in a neat little box. The brain then likes to create a type of algorithm, a process it can follow to access that information and repeat it. But endometriosis, and its endless complexities, does not allow for this process of oversimplification. The desire to create a formulaic path for the disease that can be applied to every patient has a clear appeal. But it is simply not possible. Very rarely are things black and white; life exists in the shades of grey in between. And endometriosis certainly follows this pattern. It is a fundamentally complicated disease that has nuance baked into every single facet.

Introduction

> While this book seeks to provide a comprehensive and up-to-date look at what we know about endometriosis and how to live with it, it cannot tell you what to do. It is entirely up to you, at every stage of your journey with endometriosis, which paths you choose. Some options may work fantastically for you; others may not, but they might work for someone else. This disease and how it affects you will be as unique as your fingerprint.

Before we get stuck in, a quick note on language. Endometriosis is a disease that almost exclusively affects those assigned female at birth (AFAB). Overwhelmingly, this means cis women, but AFAB individuals also include trans men and non-binary individuals. But the story doesn't end there, as there are also documented cases of endometriosis in cis men. Not many – compared to those in women, the number is miniscule – but their very existence throws up interesting questions that we will address later in the book. However, despite its presence across the gender spectrum, endometriosis is still considered a 'women's disease', relegated to the neglected corner of 'women's health' that's so underfunded and under-researched. As such, this book uses the words 'women' and 'women's health', along with 'endometriosis patients' and 'people with endometriosis'.

Endometriosis patients have often been dismissed and ignored for years, even decades. The layers of racism, classism, homophobia, transphobia and fatphobia add further obstacles to inclusion. I am very aware that I am a straight White woman with undeniable privilege, and I have tried to amplify the experiences of people who truly understand these additional barriers to care that I have never even had to consider. I want all of you to feel seen and heard when reading this book, and I have tried to be as inclusive as possible throughout. That said, I am human and, despite my best efforts, my language may not always be perfect. I humbly ask for kindness. This book is for all endometriosis sufferers.

Chapter 1

What is endometriosis?

'I know endometriosis has become very trendy, but women need to realise it isn't as common as they think.' – GP

To kick off the book, we are going to deep-dive in to endometriosis: what it is, what causes it, who it affects. By the end of this chapter, you will likely know more about endometriosis than many clinicians. I know that sounds flippant, but, sadly, it's true. The contents of this chapter will cover more than is currently being taught in our medical schools about endometriosis.

If you are anything like me, when you were first diagnosed with endometriosis, you googled it. Maybe you looked on social media for some accounts to follow. Maybe you bought a book on the subject. Or maybe, like me, you did all those things. Pretty quickly, you will have started to notice that each website, charity leaflet, NHS webpage, social media post or book more often than not contains contradictory information. Unfortunately, a lot of it is also outdated or just plain wrong. So, what do you believe? Which advice do you act upon? On which information do you base your decisions over potentially life-altering treatments? For a community that is exhausted, in debilitating pain and in desperate need of relief, this overwhelmingly incorrect information is the last thing they need.

In this chapter, we are going to be smashing the myths and misinformation that stubbornly persist around endometriosis. Think of it as your endometriosis roadmap: it is loaded with up-to-date, research-backed information that you can arm yourself with. So, grab your highlighters, get ready to make some notes and let's get to work.

What is endometriosis?

As we saw in the Introduction, endometriosis is a whole-body disease characterised by inflammation and the presence of endometrial-like tissue outside the uterus. These endometriosis cells create lesions that penetrate or grow on the surface of tissues, including organs, *anywhere in the body*. Endometriosis cells can also create adhesions, which 'stick' tissues together or pull them out of place, and cysts known as endometriomas (also referred to as chocolate cysts). We will cover the different types of endometriosis later in the chapter (*see* pages 15–18).

While a lot of sufferers, myself included, first suspect that something is wrong due to heavy, painful periods, endometriosis is not a period disease; nor is it a uterine or a menstrual condition. Your symptoms may increase during your period as endometriosis responds to your hormonal cycle, but stopping your periods will not halt or slow the progress of the disease. This means any treatment to stop your periods or ovarian function, such as the pill, the coil, chemical menopause or even a hysterectomy, may help provide symptom relief but will not treat or cure endometriosis itself (*see* pages 30–32).

A huge but persistent falsehood about this disease is that endometriosis acts like a mini-period each month: that endometriosis cells build up, shed and bleed (like the lining of the womb) each cycle, but then have nowhere to exit the body so become trapped and cause pain. This is entirely wrong. Endometriosis lesions themselves do not build up, bleed and try to shed with your cycle. Unfortunately, this 'bleed and shed' narrative is one of the most stubborn pieces of misinformation that we need to address. Endometriosis lesions do not act like the endometrium because they are fundamentally different in structure and behaviour. Endometriosis creates its own oestrogen and has glands that secrete an inflammatory substance, which can irritate the surrounding tissue and destabilise blood vessels, causing localised bleeding. However, there is no mini-period getting trapped somewhere in your body.

Why is this so important? You might think I am being a bit pedantic. Surely, saying 'endometrial-like cells' isn't wildly different to saying 'endometrial cells'? It's only four little letters after all. Does it matter if someone thinks endometriosis lesions basically have mini-periods inside our bodies every month? However, if we don't fight against these myths, we end up in a situation where the following scenarios will persist:

- Researchers and drug companies will continue to look at hormonal management only, which we know does not treat endometriosis.

What is endometriosis?

- Doctors will continue to promote hormonal treatments and dismiss extra-pelvic symptoms (occurring outside the pelvis; *see* pages 22–27).
- Those without periods (e.g., post-menopausal people, trans men and those who are pregnant or on hormonal contraception) will continue to be excluded from care.
- Endometriosis will continue to be dismissed as 'women's troubles' and something we should all just deal with.
- An additional, unnecessary barrier to endometriosis care will persist in cultures and societies where periods are taboo.
- Life-changing but ineffective 'cures' (e.g. hysterectomies, chemical menopause and pregnancy) will continue to be pushed to vulnerable, desperate patients.

I completely understand how overwhelming all the conflicting information can be. And it comes from all sides. Social media, yes, but also media articles, charities, doctors themselves, even those referring to themselves as 'endometriosis specialists'. Knowing what information to trust and how to make the right choice for you and your body adds another unnecessary layer of stress to living with endometriosis.

You are in pain and you are suffering, and you have been taught to trust medical professionals and institutions to understand what is happening and give you answers. However, this disease is incredibly complex, and sadly the lack of investment and education regarding endometriosis has resulted in a perpetual cycle of outdated information being passed from generation to generation. During my research for this book, Mr Mikey Adamczyk, consultant gynaecologist and endometriosis surgeon, explained to me how he has witnessed this among his colleagues. 'In obstetrics and gynaecology, endometriosis has long been underfunded and neglected in both research and education. Because of this, a lot of clinicians are simply repeating what they were told by their mentors years ago. I've seen it first-hand – how common myths and misinformation persist, like advising patients to get pregnant as a treatment or recommending hysterectomy for deep endometriosis (*see* pages 60–61), even when these approaches don't align with what we know now . . . Only by improving education and awareness can we give patients the informed, effective treatment they should be receiving.'

If you only read and absorb one thing in this book, please let it be this: getting the definition right must be the foundation of changing the landscape of endometriosis care. Without this most simple of things in place, everything that follows falls apart. If we do not use the correct language to describe this disease, we are ignored, dismissed and left with ineffective, often harmful treatment options – if we can access care at all. If your consultant uses the wrong definition, please find a new one. If they are not even getting the basic understanding of the disease right, and are not even able to tell patients what it is, they have no business operating on your body. When I spoke to Heather Guidone, Board Certified Patient Advocate and member of the team at the Center for Endometriosis Care in the USA, she summed it up perfectly: 'If you can't define it correctly, you definitely shouldn't be treating it'.

Did you know?

German physician Karl Freiherr von Rokitansky is credited with 'discovering' endometriosis in 1860, although at that stage it was referred to as adenomyoma. Reading between the lines, the disease seems to have been documented in medical literature for centuries, and they were describing it pretty accurately, all things considered. Even in the 17th century, a physician called Thomas Sydenham noted an endometriosis-like disease causing 'hysterical lumps … throughout the body, pain in the bladder, vomiting, diarrhoea, and back pain'. Hundreds of years ago we were (unknowingly) referencing endometriosis as a full body disease, not the uterine condition that it is often mistakenly referred to as today.

I know how exhausting it is to constantly have to analyse and question the information you are being given, but an endometriosis diagnosis is not simply a label for your symptoms. It also initiates you into a community and a movement for change. Bet you weren't expecting that, were you?

What is endometriosis?

Table 1.1: Endometriosis versus endometrium

Endometriosis (outside of the uterus)	Endometrium (lining of the uterus)
Tissue similar to the endometrium ('endometrium-like')	The uterine lining
Found anywhere in the body	Found in the uterus
Changes and behaves *separately to* the menstrual cycle	Predictable and regular pattern of behaviour *in line with* the menstrual cycle
Lesions *do not* shed and bleed during a period	Lining breaks down, bleeds and exits the body during a period
Activity *does not cease* post-menopause	Activity *ceases* post-menopause
Endometriosis tissue and the endometrium have different reactions to the hormones oestrogen and progesterone	
Oestrogen receptors (proteins found in cells) do not change during the menstrual cycle	Oestrogen receptors change during the menstrual cycle
Expresses aromatase (an enzyme that is responsible for the production of oestrogen in the body, in a process called biosynthesis)	No aromatase enzyme activity
Visual appearance varies – can be black, dark brown, red, white, multi-coloured or even clear	(Normal) endometrium is smooth and pale red
Histology (under microscope) does not show spiral arteries	Histology shows the presence of spiral arteries, which supply blood to the functional zone of the endometrium (the part that sheds during menstruation)
Histology shows fibrotic tissue (scarring) inside and around lesions (another reason endometriosis is so painful!)	No fibrosis on histology in healthy endometrium
Produces its own oestrogen – does not require ovarian oestrogen	Requires oestrogen from the ovaries to function

As you can see from Table 1.1, the differences between endometriosis and the endometrium are numerous and significant. Controlling the menstrual cycle does not treat endometriosis as endometriosis is not endometrium that has implanted elsewhere in the body. We know this, and have done for a while. However, for some reason this information is not being routinely disseminated and reflected in patient care. So, you can hopefully begin to see how tricky this all is as you start to navigate your endometriosis care.

How common is endometriosis?

The accepted statistic is that endometriosis affects one in 10 women. This equates to approximately 190 million people worldwide. To put that into context, if you put all diagnosed endometriosis sufferers into one location, we would constitute the eighth largest country in the world by population size. Endometriosis is as common as diabetes or asthma yet receives a fraction of the interest, research, funding or prioritisation.

Truthfully, however, one in 10 is likely to be a vast underestimate of those who have the disease. This conservative number only considers women and girls of reproductive age, but we know that endometriosis starts before the onset of your period (a girl aged six recently underwent surgery to remove endometriosis) and continues post-menopause. Dr José Eugenio-Colón, an endometriosis specialist at the Center for Endometriosis Care, told me that he once operated on a 65-year-old woman, 15 years post-menopause, who still very much had active endometriosis. So, if we take the accepted one in 10 statistic and apply it to the number of women, girls and those assigned female at birth currently on the Earth, we get a number closer to 400 million.

Research is slowly catching up and recognising that one in 10 is likely too conservative. A 2023 study by the Australian Institute of Health and Welfare shows that the incidence is more likely to be one in seven, or 14 per cent. Also, bear in mind that these figures reflect only *diagnosed* cases. It is thought that 20–25 per cent of endometriosis patients are asymptomatic (do not experience any symptoms) – these individuals are known as having 'silent endometriosis' and often do not know they have the disease at all (*see* page 36). That is a large chunk of people who are not included in the statistics. Next, what about all those suffering with endometriosis but who have been unable to find someone to listen? Or those who do not know what it is that is happening inside their bodies?

We also know that endometriosis has been found, albeit rarely, in cis men, not just in women. These men have also been excluded from the one in 10 data. You can see how the number keeps increasing. One thing is for sure, the doctor who told 21-year-old me, 'Listen, you do not have endometriosis. It is really quite rare; it is just becoming fashionable to think you have it' was very, very wrong.

The three types of endometriosis

When we talk about endometriosis, we are discussing one or a combination of three distinct categories of disease:

1. Superficial peritoneal endometriosis (SPE)
2. Deep infiltrating endometriosis (DIE)
3. Ovarian endometriomas (OMAs)

Superficial peritoneal endometriosis

SPE is defined as endometriosis lesions that are less than 5mm deep. The peritoneum is a thin membrane covering the organs in the abdomen and pelvic cavity. While SPE is commonly found here, it can also be found elsewhere in the body. And don't let the word 'superficial' fool you: SPE can cause severe symptoms.

These lesions are often missed on imaging – both ultrasound and magnetic resonance imaging (MRI), a technique used to produce detailed images of the body's internal organs and structures (*see* page 49) – so it is important to remember that if you do get offered a scan and it is 'clear', it does not mean there is no endometriosis. An absence of evidence is not evidence of absence. A 2024 Endometriosis UK report found that only 18 per cent of those with confirmed endometriosis were diagnosed by scan. My first ultrasound was 'clear'. A few months later mild-moderate endometriosis was confirmed on MRI. A few more months later and severe endometriosis was diagnosed at surgery. Scans are only as reliable as those performing and reading them.

Deep infiltrating endometriosis

DIE is defined as endometriosis lesions that are more than 5mm deep, where disease is found deep within a tissue or organ. More common than previously thought, DIE lesions, or nodules, represent 15–30 per cent of cases.

By embedding more deeply in tissues, DIE reaches closer to other structures such as blood vessels, nerves, the bladder, the bowel and other organs. For this reason, DIE is more likely to cause significant symptoms, but not always. Some people with DIE can be completely asymptomatic.

Ovarian endometriomas

OMAs are dark, blood-filled cysts also known, completely unappetisingly, as 'chocolate cysts' due to the texture and colour of the contents. They are most commonly found inside the ovaries and can grow to a tremendous size. These cysts affect 17–44 per cent of patients with endometriosis and are often indicators of DIE also being present.

Endometriomas are a very complicated and distinct category of endometriosis. They behave differently from lesions and have a higher recurrence rate. The entire cyst wall needs to be removed, as opposed to simply draining the contents, potentially followed by medication to reduce the risk of recurrence. Hormonal treatment may help manage this specific type of endometriosis, but we desperately need more in-depth research into this complicated aspect of the disease.

You may have one or a combination of these types of endometriosis. I was found to have all three in various areas of my body. No matter which type or types you are diagnosed with, the gold standard remains complete excision surgery, where disease is removed entirely, not just destroyed at the surface, by a skilled and experienced endometriosis specialist. But, as we will see in chapter 3, surgery is not a silver bullet and may not be accessible, desirable or even an option for some people.

There is also a fourth element of the disease that is highly relevant to our discussion and that you will likely come across in your endometriosis journey, and that is adhesions.

Adhesions

Although they are not specifically a type of endometriosis, adhesions absolutely must be part of our education around the disease. Endometriosis can create adhesions, and surgery – especially repeated, poor surgeries – can lead to adhesions too. Adhesions can be a huge source of pain and other problems. No one explained adhesions to me during my journey to diagnosis or before or after surgery, despite them wreaking havoc on my insides, and I know I'm not the only one. Let's have a look at what they are.

Our organs and other tissues are usually protected from 'sticking' together by thin surfaces. However, when there is irritation, injury or inflammation in the body, a repair mechanism kicks in and creates bands of fibrous scar tissue

What is endometriosis?

known as adhesions. Endometriosis, as if it did not already cause enough problems, can also cause adhesions to form. These adhesions can stick or fuse our organs and other tissues together, particularly in the pelvis, where things are already pretty crowded.

Over time, these adhesions can become tighter and harder, pulling and trapping organs and tissues that should normally be flexible. This can cause a significant amount of pain, often characterised by a pulling, tugging, ripping or tearing sensation. Sound familiar? I know these descriptions absolutely resonate with me: I would often tell my husband it felt like something had just ripped apart inside me. Often I would experience sharp tugging, twisting and ripping pains. Even turning over in bed could cause intense pain. Turns out those feelings were caused by some pretty hefty adhesions. In extreme cases, this build-up and tightening of adhesions can lead to what is called a 'frozen pelvis', where the organs and structures of the pelvis are densely stuck together, causing a distorted anatomy, pain and other symptoms such as those affecting the bowels or bladder.

The best way to describe adhesions is to imagine a pumpkin at Halloween. You're ready to carve it, so you cut off the top, and inside there is a packed network of stringy, fibrous material criss-crossing the cavity. That is what you need to picture when you think of adhesions.

Some symptoms of adhesions to be mindful of are as follows:

- Tight, pulling pain
- Constipation and/or rectal bleeding
- Urinary issues
- Fertility issues
- Cramps

Adhesions can be surgically removed, although this should ideally be done at the same time as excision surgery because, as noted above, surgery itself is known to be a causal factor in the creation of adhesions. So, we want to minimise how many times we go under the knife.

This is yet another reason why something called ablation surgery is not ideal. Ablation surgery is a superficial treatment where the surgeon burns, or 'destroys', visible endometriosis lesions. However, this only destroys disease on the surface, leaving the deeper 'roots' intact (*see* page 115 for further discussion of ablation surgery). Patients who have had numerous ablation surgeries have reported a higher incidence of adhesions and the associated problems.

Can we avoid adhesions? Sadly, there is no magic wand to prevent them. What we do know is that both endometriosis and adhesions thrive in an inflammatory environment. Add in to the mix the fact that endometriosis itself creates both inflammatory conditions and adhesions, and the odds are not looking too favourable. There are, however, some options to hopefully lessen the chance of them occurring and worsening.

You can help your body create a less inflammatory environment through lifestyle changes such as diet, movement, physiotherapy and stress reduction (easy to say, I know). If you think adhesions are contributing to your pain, speak to a doctor about relief options, which we also explore in chapter 3. Finally, avoid surgery where at all possible. In the context of endometriosis, this means opting for expert excision surgery over ablation and avoiding any surgeon who is not a true endometriosis specialist. I know that may be hard to hear when there are shockingly few of these surgeons, they are difficult to access and we are so desperate for relief, but no surgery truly is better than a bad surgery. You will find more on how to pick a surgeon and what to look out for in chapter 3.

The four stages of endometriosis

I am including this section for the sake of completeness because you will very likely hear these phrases mentioned or see them in your medical records at some point. But, and this is super important, please do not worry about or set too much store by the 'stages' of endometriosis.

Endometriosis is classified into four stages, as defined by the American Society for Reproductive Medicine:

- Stage 1: minimal
- Stage 2: mild
- Stage 3: moderate
- Stage 4: severe

Originally, the stages were created to predict fertility outcomes, with the criteria for each stage based on disease location, depth and extent, the

What is endometriosis?

presence and size of endometriomas and the presence and severity of adhesions, as follows:

- Stage 1: Few superficial implants
- Stage 2: More and deeper implants
- Stage 3: Many deep implants, small cysts on one or both ovaries and the presence of filmy adhesions
- Stage 4: Many deep implants, large cysts on one or both ovaries and many dense adhesions

The thing to understand is that these stages do not correlate to pain levels, any other symptoms or the *impact those symptoms have on your quality of life*. For example, one patient can have stage 4 endometriosis and have no symptoms whatsoever, while another patient can have stage 1 endometriosis and suffer from completely debilitating pain and other symptoms.

For example, Sarah, a 49-year-old endometriosis patient I spoke to when researching this book, has stage 1 endometriosis. It was causing her excruciating pain, often leaving her bedbound. She was diagnosed after 14 years of presenting to the GP with her symptoms. During her surgery, she was diagnosed with stage 1 endometriosis. She didn't think much of the staging, as she was 'so relieved that someone was actually telling me there was a real reason for my pain!' But later, when she went back to the GP for help with the return of her symptoms, the staging of endometriosis was used to dismiss her. 'You're only stage 1; that's barely worth worrying about, let alone taking up the specialist's time,' the GP told her. Once she heard this, Sarah started to question herself, much as she had when she was first trying to get answers for her pain. 'Is it really that bad? So many women have stage 4 and seem to cope so much better than I do – am I being weak?' Spoiler alert: she was not being weak, and it really was that bad. Any pain is certainly worth 'taking up the specialist's time'.

So, please do not get hung up on the numbers and terminology of staging. It can lead to us dismissing our own symptoms or comparing ourselves to others when we just don't know the reality.

I understand why we like knowing which stage we are. The simple labelling of such a complex disease can help us feel validated and can make sense of our suffering and the world into which we have been plunged.

But sometimes, we, as patients and as a community, can attach too much significance to the number that sits before our diagnosis – a number that, in reality, has no bearing on our symptoms and was formulated only with our fertility in mind, not our quality of life.

As with anything to do with endometriosis care, the staging system has a lot of flaws. Numerous new systems have been proposed – more descriptive ones that accurately reflect the patient experience and surgical findings. As with absolutely every single part of endometriosis care, the current scale is only really relevant in the hands of skilled specialists who can recognise and find all disease. My first surgeon wildly miscategorised my endometriosis as stage 2, because a lot of disease was missed. Fewer than four months later, a specialist changed that to stage 4.

My preferred way to describe endometriosis is by location and type (SPE, DIE, OMAs). I do sometimes refer to my diagnosis as stage 4, but, especially when talking to other endometriosis patients, I try to avoid doing so. It invites comparison, which is not helpful to anyone processing and navigating this already incredibly isolating and difficult journey. Instead, let's focus on you as the individual human you are. Let's focus on your symptoms, your goals and, most importantly, your quality of life.

Where does endometriosis grow?

Endometriosis is a full-body disease in every sense of the word. While it is most commonly found around the pelvic cavity, it is by no means restricted to that area of the body. There is not an organ or bodily system where endometriosis has not been found. To give you an idea, here is a quick list of some of those locations:

- Brain
- Eyelids
- Skin
- Sciatic nerve
- Clitoris
- Scars
- Muscles
- Liver

- Diaphragm
- Heart
- Nose
- Liver
- Ovaries
- Fallopian tubes
- Uterosacral ligaments
- Cervix

What is endometriosis?

- Vagina
- Pouch of Douglas (*see* below)
- Bladder
- Bowel
- Ureter
- Navel
- Appendix
- Kidneys

We can have lesions in multiple locations, so making sure you have a specialist who both knows what to look out for and knows to look *everywhere* is so important.

Endometriosis can and does invade and even, in some cases, destroy organs. If you have any concerns about symptoms anywhere in your body, please seek medical advice and *keep asking questions* until someone is able to give you an answer.

The pouch of Douglas

This peculiarly named part of the body is a common site for endometriosis, yet it is never really explained to patients what or where it is. A regular mention on our medical notes can be an 'obliterated Pouch of Douglas (POD)' – something I receive monthly messages about from mystified patients due to its rather ominous wording. So, what is it? Also known as the rectouterine pouch or cul-de-sac, the POD is a small area deep in the pelvis between the uterus and rectum (*see* Figure 1.1). 'Obliteration of the pouch' is a consequence of inflammation in the pelvis, often seen in endometriosis patients, and refers to the POD no longer being visible, perhaps due to adhesions or endometriosis. Obliteration can be partial or complete depending on how much the organs are stuck together.

POD obliteration can be seen if you have the right kind of scan, performed and interpreted by an expert, and can suggest that endometriosis is present. Some studies suggest that POD obliteration may be suggestive of bowel endometriosis also being present, but more research is needed in this area (as usual).

And yes, this part of our anatomy was named after the man who first identified it, James Douglas. I prefer 'rectouterine pouch', but most doctors still use POD, so it is good to know what it means.

Figure 1.1: Pouch of Douglas

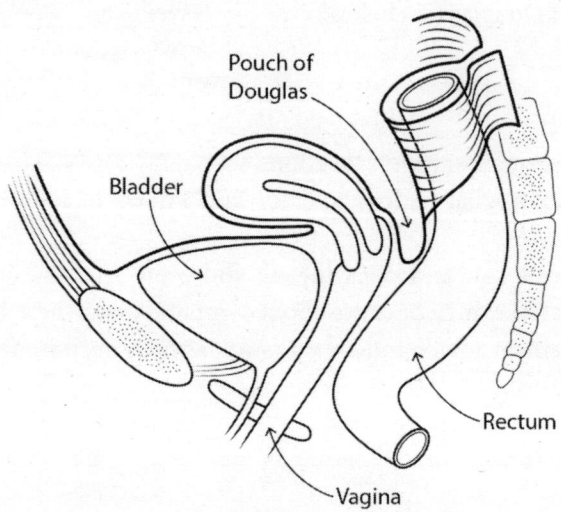

Extra-pelvic endometriosis

There is a common misunderstanding (yes, another one) that endometriosis is a pelvic disease. Disease beyond that particular area of the body (or 'extra-pelvic endometriosis') is still generally thought of as 'rare'. While the true numbers are not known, it is becoming clear that extra-pelvic endometriosis is not rare, it is just rarely looked for or diagnosed.

Pelvic endometriosis refers to disease in the reproductive organs and their surrounding tissue. This includes endometriosis of the ovaries, fallopian tubes, uterus, posterior cul-de-sac (aka POD; *see* page 21), ligaments (such as the uterosacral ligaments, which hold the uterus in place), the peritoneum and the pelvic sidewalls (*see* Figure 1.2). Extra-pelvic and extra abdominopelvic endometriosis refers to disease located anywhere else in the body, whether it is in your bladder, ureters, kidneys, bowels, diaphragm, lungs or nerves. The most common extra-pelvic locations are the gastrointestinal and urinary systems.

What is endometriosis?

Figure 1.2: Locations of pelvic endometriosis

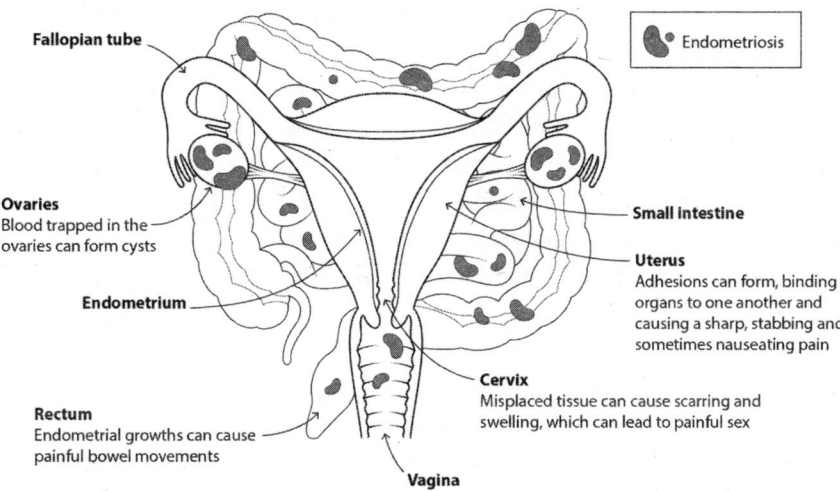

Dr Wendy Bingham, Executive Director of Extrapelvic Not Rare, an organisation devoted to increasing awareness and education of endometriosis as a full body disease, states that of the approximately 190 million people with endometriosis globally, '44 to 80 million of them have endometriosis among one or more body systems other than reproductive'. That would equate to an estimated 20–37 per cent of endometriosis patients having extra-pelvic disease.

Extra-pelvic disease can be very problematic. The involvement of vital organs can bring a whole new set of symptoms and worry about organ damage. Let's look at thoracic endometriosis as an example.

Thoracic endometriosis

Thoracic endometriosis involves endometriosis in the chest, including the lungs and diaphragm. The diaphragm is the most common form of extra-abdominopelvic disease, found in 1–12 per cent of patients. Symptoms include chest pain, shoulder and neck pain, and pain in the upper right quadrant (imagine the area below your ribs is divided into four quarters, with both the vertical and the horizontal lines passing through your belly button – your upper right quadrant is the top quarter on the right-hand side). Sometimes, thoracic endometriosis can even cause lung collapse (pneumothorax), which can be accompanied by bleeding in the chest (haemothorax).

These can be very serious medical issues, as Mr Francesco Di Chiara, a thoracic surgeon based in Oxford, UK, who specialises in endometriosis, explained when I spoke to him. In very rare cases, it can even be fatal. Thoracic endometriosis poses challenges to the multi-disciplinary model that endometriosis centres in the UK try to create. These centres often don't have access to thoracic specialists, which can make accessing appropriate care more difficult, especially in an emergency. Any hospital will have a gynaecology department, but for thoracics there are fewer than 30 centres spread over the UK. Within these thoracic centres, as far as Mr Di Chiara knows, there are 'around five thoracic surgeons with an interest in thoracic endometriosis'.

In terms of how endometriosis lesions end up in places like the lung, the diaphragm and the pleura, Mr Di Chiara believes we 'cannot rely on the old theory of retrograde menstruation'. For example, he told me about a case where endometriosis was found in the lung but not in the diaphragm. 'How did it get there? It just doesn't make sense that it would go from the abdomen, skip the diaphragm, and into the lung.' Instead, he believes there is likely to be a combination of factors at play, perhaps even 'different to the development of disease in the pelvis'. This belief is driven by the fact that 'thoracic endometriosis is often visually different to the disease we find in the pelvis' – yet another reason why it is so underdiagnosed.

Thoracic endometriosis is widely overlooked and underdiagnosed, which means its prevalence is hard to quantify. The literature varies, but the British Society for Gynaecological Endoscopy (BSGE) state that thoracic endometriosis may occur in up to 12 per cent of those with pelvic disease. However, we will see a common theme emerge throughout the book that the literature does not necessarily reflect what expert surgeons witness in their patients.

Mr Di Chiara feels that the reported numbers are staggeringly low. He told me that the medical gaslighting that patients with thoracic endometriosis face 'is the hardest part of the job for me', to the extent that it has 'made a dent in [his] trust in the medical profession'. Mr Di Chiara started his career as a cardiothoracic cancer surgeon, 'so every patient we saw, they were believed'. No one 'belittled their symptoms or overlooked their diagnosis'. When it comes to thoracic endometriosis, however, 'the most heart-breaking thing is that these patients have had to self-advocate for themselves, often for 10 years, before they even see me'. Mr Di Chiara firmly believes that the 'real numbers of those with thoracic endometriosis are massive, and we just don't know'. He elaborated that he 'only sees the tip of the iceberg, the patients who have managed to advocate

What is endometriosis?

for eight, 10, 15 years – the most determined ones, who also have the time for that self-advocacy and the financial means.' And it's not just the patients who have to fight for thoracic endometriosis to be taken seriously: 'I also have to fight to even take patients to theatre for biopsies'. In the select patients whom Mr Di Chiara is able to see and take biopsies from, the 'diagnostic rate is more like eight out of ten'. Obviously, these patients are already suspected of having thoracic endometriosis due to their symptoms, 'but even then I'm supposed to find five to ten per cent; instead, I'm finding 80 per cent.'

Mr Di Chiara fights to show his MDT, the medical community and the wider public that thoracic endometriosis is a very real problem, 'Because to me, it's obvious.' However, the lack of understanding means that 'even among endometriosis specialists, the very existence of thoracic endometriosis is debated', not to mention how best to treat it. Mr Di Chiara believes in patient choice, 'not in doctors imposing their ideas'. A trial of hormonal treatment, for example, may be a good option. 'But once you have that trial and it fails, I see the patient talked into trying again and again. So, you have years of hormonal treatments before the word surgery is even brought up.' This treatment pathway 'differs from that for pelvic endometriosis, where the established route is to try hormones for symptom management, then, if that doesn't work, surgery'. Instead, with thoracic endometriosis, the phase in which surgery is introduced is heavily delayed. 'Educating my colleagues about patient choice' is something about which Mr Di Chiara is clearly passionate: 'Patients shouldn't have to jump through a hundred hoops before seeing a thoracic surgeon with an interest in thoracic endometriosis.'

Surgery to remove thoracic endometriosis is often perceived as a 'nice-to-have' luxury, but Mr Di Chiara is trying to educate other clinicians that the disease 'is a highly debilitating condition that changes people's whole lives'. He hopes that his awareness and educational efforts will start to create a shift in understanding. 'I think doctors of a younger generation tend to focus on quality of life as justification for surgery,' he says, 'but older ones focus much more on raw mortality.' And that, he believes, drives a lot of the tension between surgeons, particularly within the National Health Service (NHS), where resources are spread increasingly thinly. He faces challenges among his clinical colleagues with misinformation about thoracic endometriosis, which, he argues, 'is not surprising considering it probably isn't even mentioned on most medical school curriculums'. During one thoracic endometriosis day he hosted for medical colleagues in his area, he revealed that many of his colleagues 'thought I performed the surgery just because the patient was complaining of chest pain' – a revelation that shocked me. Instead, he does the biopsy first, confirms the endometriosis and then carries out the radical surgery. 'It's a histological, pathological diagnosis, from tissue sent to a lab.'

Listening to Mr Di Chiara, I became very curious about how a clearly passionate, connected cardiothoracic cancer surgeon gets into thoracic endometriosis – a disease about which, by his own admission, he has to 'fight with colleagues to prove it even exists'. When he was studying for his final exam, thoracic specialists had two enormous books to study and learn the contents of. One of those tomes had 400 pages on benign conditions, with maybe 100 pages on pneumothorax (lung collapse). At the very bottom of this section were a couple of lines about catamenial pneumothorax, or lung collapse during menstruation: 'There are several reports of females suffering from catamenial pneumothorax whilst on their period.' Full stop. No images, no sources, no references. Nothing. But Mr Di Chiara found that sentence the most interesting thing in the entire book: 'How can hormonal changes cause lung collapse? I was so shocked that there wasn't more interest in that.' This interest and curiosity set him on his current path.

'Thoracic endometriosis is quite a scary disease. It has this label of being rare and benign. But honestly, it's hard for me to call it either of those things. I don't think it is rare, or benign. Once we have more acceptance that it is neither of those things, we will also receive more resources, more funding, and more research. Once we break this misconception, we will start to move forward.'

Mr Francesco Di Chiara's tips if you suspect thoracic endometriosis

- Social media is a great democratic source of health information. For all the misinformation, there is also great information. You should never take medical advice from a social media post, but you can find concepts, context and community. Use social media to find those surgeons who are truly specialised and interested in thoracic endometriosis and learn from them.

What is endometriosis?

> - Attend meetings online or in person with patient advocates and ask them questions about how they accessed care, what treatments they have tried and if they have any other tips or advice.
> - Don't let anyone, even an 'expert', dismiss your pain or tell you it isn't real.

We need to stop labelling thoracic endometriosis, and any type of extra-pelvic, or extra-abdominopelvic, endometriosis, as 'rare'. Despite the mounting data to support the prevalence of extra-pelvic endometriosis, the language used to refer to disease outside of the reproductive system makes it seem like an outlier. However, it is a very real prospect and reality for a large chunk of endometriosis patients, and it can often lead to life-changing surgeries and interventions. The persistence of the perception that extra-pelvic endometriosis is rare, unusual, atypical or any other synonym creates a bias in the minds of researchers and clinicians. It encourages the dismissal of symptoms and puts off those who allocate precious funds for research projects. It creates the notion, even if it is an unconscious one, that extra-pelvic endometriosis is a niche.

Doctors often end up misdiagnosing extra-pelvic endometriosis as other conditions – irritable bowel syndrome (IBS), urinary tract infections (UTIs) and even stress are diagnoses that often come before one of endometriosis of the bowel, bladder or chest. I cannot even remember the number of times that my chest pain, bladder issues or bowel issues have been put down to stress, despite my insistence that I believe them to be endometriosis related. Lo and behold, I've always, sadly, been proven right. One surgeon, instead of taking my symptoms of diaphragmatic endometriosis seriously, told me to put my hand in a bowl of ice and then notice how much longer I could keep my hand submerged if I thought happy thoughts. I kid you not: he thought I was thinking negative thoughts, which were causing my cyclical symptoms of thoracic endometriosis.

Recognising the prevalence and severity of extra-pelvic endometriosis is of paramount importance if we are to abolish the myth of endometriosis as a reproductive disease. We need to stop calling endometriosis a gynaecological disorder and start referring to it as the systemic inflammatory condition that it is. Until we do this, outdated beliefs will continue to hinder patients from receiving the expert, multi-disciplinary care they need.

What causes endometriosis?

Endometriosis is not a 'new disease'. It was officially first labelled in the 1800s, and it has even been suggested that diseases that could potentially be what we now know as endometriosis were included in Hippocratic medical texts going back thousands of years. Despite this, there is still no known cause of endometriosis.

Retrograde menstruation

One of the first theories to be established was the idea of retrograde menstruation, put forward by John Sampson (1873–1946), an eminent gynaecologist who also coined the term 'endometriosis' in the 1920s. Sampson's theory proposes that during your period, endometrial cells flow back into your body via the fallopian tubes. These cells then implant and attach themselves to different areas and organs, 'causing' endometriosis.

The problem is that Sampson's theory of retrograde menstruation has been debunked for numerous reasons. These include the following:

- Endometriosis cells are not the same as the cells lining the uterus, which are expelled during our periods. They are different in both structure and behaviour (*see* table on page 13).
- Approximately 90 per cent of people with periods experience retrograde menstruation, but the current endometriosis statistic is that it affects 10 per cent.
- Microscopic evidence of the process of retrograde menstruation leading to cell implantation leading, in turn, to endometriosis proliferation has not been found. All of the depictions of this process in published research and textbooks are illustrations; there are no photographs of this actually happening.
- Endometriosis has been found in girls who have not yet had their first period, post-menopausal women, foetuses, animals and even, rarely, men. Periods, or even a uterus, are not required for endometriosis to proliferate.

Even Sampson himself recognised that his theory did not account for all instances of endometriosis. However, this theory is still the most touted 'explanation' for endometriosis. It was the explanation that my first surgeon confidently gave me when I was diagnosed. It is still pushed and believed by medical schools, health organisations, media outlets, endometriosis charities, GPs and even many surgeons treating patients. This is a big problem. The theory of retrograde menstruation perpetuates the myth of endometriosis as a period issue. It excludes huge sections of patients who do not fit the 'menstruating' profile, and it raises huge barriers to accessing effective care and treatment.

So, if the cause is not retrograde menstruation, what is? Truthfully, and terrifyingly, we do not know. Endometriosis is often referred to as a disease of 'many theories' because theories are all we have, but none accurately accounts for all aspects of this incredibly complex condition.

Currently, a popular theory is Dr Redwine's idea of mülleriosis. The basis of this theory is that endometriosis forms during foetal development. That is, we are born with it. This could explain the presence of endometriosis in extra-pelvic locations, foetuses, animals and men. But it is still a theory.

Other theories include the following:

- Stem cells (which could help explain the cases in cis men)
- Immunological dysfunction
- Genetics
- Environmental toxins inducing cell changes
- Lymphatic spread

However, the evidence for each of these theories is limited and often conflicting, and no one theory can explain all incidences and locations of the disease. Mr Francesco Di Chiara, the thoracic surgeon we met earlier in the chapter, wonders whether a combination of processes might be at play: 'No one theory explains all the disease we see. I believe it's likely to be a mix of factors'. Mr Shaheen Kahzali, an endometriosis surgeon, agrees, even going so far as to wonder if we are actually dealing with separate disease mechanisms, each with its own origins and proliferation mechanisms. Speaking at an event, he explained, 'Endometriosis is a very strange condition. It is very unique. We have been putting everything under the umbrella of endometriosis, but we're possibly dealing with separate diseases' (superficial, deep and ovarian; *see* pages 15–16).

Why do we still not know what causes endometriosis, you might very reasonably ask? To put it simply, it is because of a lack of research. Endometriosis is severely underfunded, under-researched and misunderstood. When funds do become available, research has historically focused on profitable hormonal 'treatments' rather than gaining a deeper understanding of the disease, funding the training of experts or, we can hope, finding a cure.

Other theories that we can dismiss

Over the years, several more . . . unusual theories about the origin of endometriosis have raised their heads. Here are some of the more bizarre ones that the community has reported being told (genuinely!):

- Having sex while on your period
- Not having enough sex
- Delaying childbirth
- Being overly educated
- Being too ambitious
- Using tampons
- Not wearing socks and slippers enough
- Not fully getting over a previous breakup
- Straining too hard on the toilet

Is there a cure for endometriosis?

Oh, how I wish I could say there is. However, the bitter truth is that no, currently there is no cure for endometriosis.

Most 'cures' that are bandied about are based on the outdated and debunked notion that endometriosis is a menstrual condition. Under this (incorrect) theory, all we have to do is tinker with the sex hormones and reproductive organs and, easy-peasy, we can 'cure' the disease. The result of this thinking is that treatments designed to stop our periods or ovarian function, ranging from the contraceptive pill all the way to a full hysterectomy, are described as ways to cure, slow, stop or prevent endometriosis.

This is what happened to me when I was put on the contraceptive pill by a well-meaning GP when my periods started. I was 11 at the time, and my first period was the first sign that something most definitely was not

What is endometriosis?

'normal'. I remember crying, curled up on the floor of my parents' bedroom, unable to even straighten my body because of the pain. My mum took me to the GP, where I was put on oral contraceptives and told that I was just unlucky, that my periods were just heavy, just painful, and that they would settle down if I took the pill. And that was it. I ended up staying on hormonal contraception for two decades and all the while endometriosis was left to grow unchecked throughout my body. I cannot say this enough: stopping periods, through whatever means, may dampen the symptoms but it does not cure endometriosis. Treating pain is not the same as treating the disease. And the kicker is that endometriosis produces its own oestrogen anyway. So, stopping the hormone cycle, regardless of the method, will not stop the disease progressing.

I want to make it clear that I am not against hormonal treatments as part of your endometriosis care plan. If they help you manage your symptoms and give you some much-needed pain relief, that is excellent. I am genuinely so happy for you and hope it continues. However, what I am against is the promotion of the myth that these treatments will prevent, reduce or cure endometriosis. They can form a valuable part of a treatment plan, but their value and limitations must be explained to patients, and there must be monitoring in place to check for disease progression. Informed consent is always, always the key.

My mum underwent a radical hysterectomy in her 30s because it was believed then that this drastic and life-altering surgery was the cure for endometriosis. You would think we might have progressed in the last 30 years, but no – my friend was told in late 2024 that 'a hysterectomy is the gold standard treatment for endometriosis'.

A hysterectomy is not a cure for endometriosis. Hormonal contraceptives are not a cure for endometriosis. Menopause (natural, medical or surgical) is not a cure for endometriosis. Pregnancy is not a cure for endometriosis. Neither, come to mention it, are the cleanses, yoga, diets and all the other 'cures' thrown about online.

The closest thing we have to a cure, and the actual gold standard treatment for endometriosis, is complete excision surgery by a highly skilled endometriosis specialist, where the entire affected area is surgically removed. Done successfully by the right surgeon, long-term symptom relief can be achieved and recurrence rates can even be reduced. We will go into this in much more depth in the next chapter.

Skilled complete excision surgery is just the first step, however, and it should be part of a multi-disciplinary approach that may also include physical therapy, nutritional changes and other lifestyle approaches. It is not a cure, but it is the best we have for now. This is the treatment that we all deserve and should be able to access.

What are the symptoms of endometriosis?

Endometriosis is a complicated systemic disease that can be found in every system and organ of the body. This means that each individual case is unique, as will be the combination and severity of symptoms that are experienced.

To further complicate matters, the widespread and individualised nature of endometriosis symptoms, coupled with the severe lack of education around the disease, means that patients are commonly and repeatedly misdiagnosed with other conditions. IBS, stress, anxiety, costochondritis (inflammation of the cartilage connecting the ribs to the breastbone), even sexually transmitted infections (STIs) – all these were suggested before my doctor was even willing to consider endometriosis.

Your symptoms will depend on where the endometriosis is growing, but there are some common ones that likely indicate that the disease is present. How many of the symptoms listed below do you relate to?

Common symptoms of endometriosis (frequently misdiagnosed as 'just a bad period' or stress)

- Painful periods (dysmenorrhoea)
- Irregular periods
- Chronic pelvic pain
- Bloating (aka 'endo belly'; *see* page 38)
- Pain during ovulation ('mittelschmerz')
- Lower back pain
- Painful urination (dysuria)
- Constipation
- Diarrhoea
- Painful bowel movements (dyschezia)
- Pain during or after sex (dyspareunia)
- Pain after orgasm

What is endometriosis?

- Fatigue (*see* pages 35–36)
- Nausea
- Infertility or sub-fertility

Pelvic endometriosis symptoms (frequently misdiagnosed as 'just a bad period')

- Chronic pelvic pain
- Painful periods
- Pain during or after sex
- Bloating (aka 'endo belly'; *see* page 38)
- Irregular periods
- Lower back pain
- Hip pain
- Leg pain
- Infertility
- Miscarriage
- Ectopic pregnancy (where a fertilised egg implants outside the womb, usually in the fallopian tubes; unfortunately, it is not possible to save the pregnancy and, if left untreated, ectopic pregnancy can be dangerous for the woman)
- Painful urination
- Painful bowel movements
- Pain during ovulation
- Fatigue (*see* pages 35–36)
- Nausea

Thoracic endometriosis symptoms (frequently misdiagnosed as stress or anxiety)

- Chest pain (most commonly on the right side of the body, but not always)
- Shoulder pain
- Neck pain
- Coughing
- Shortness of breath
- Coughing up blood
- Lung collapse

Endometriosis

Bladder/urinary tract endometriosis symptoms (frequently misdiagnosed as urinary tract infections)

- Painful urination
- Frequent urinary tract infections (UTIs)
- Bladder retention (where you are unable to empty all the urine from your bladder)
- Flank pain (pain on the side of your back, just below your ribcage and above your waist)
- Lower back pain
- Hip pain
- Groin pain
- Increased urinary frequency (needing to urinate more often)
- Increased urinary urgency (a sudden, intense need to urinate)
- Blood in your urine

Bowel endometriosis symptoms (frequently misdiagnosed as IBS)

- Diarrhoea
- Constipation
- Nausea
- Vomiting
- Severe bloating
- Rectal bleeding
- Blood in stools
- Rectal pain
- Painful bowel movements
- Sharp gas pain
- Abdominal cramping
- Tailbone pain

These are just some of the symptoms that you may experience, grouped by the more common locations of endometriosis. You may find that you are experiencing others, so it is really important to get to know your body, track everything that is going on with it and start to connect the dots. One patient I spoke to realised that she was suffering with cyclical nose bleeds and it turned out she actually had endometriosis in her nose. Her nose!

What is fatigue?

Feeling tired and being fatigued are not the same thing. Very simply, tired is something you *feel*, while fatigued is something you *are*. All of us will relate to being tired at some point, even extremely tired, but not all of us will experience fatigue. Fatigue cannot be pushed through or ignored. When I am at peak fatigue, I describe it as going in to 'power-saving mode', and nothing can stop my body shutting down. This is not uncommon when it comes to living with endometriosis. In fact, a 2018 study showed that the second most frequently reported symptom was fatigue, with 77 per cent suffering from it. Table 1.2 breaks down some of the key differences between tiredness and fatigue.

Table 1.2: Tired versus fatigued

Tired	Fatigued
You generally recover after rest or sleep.	You generally do not recover after rest or sleep.
You can wake up, get out of bed and push through.	Waking up and getting out of bed can feel impossible – I describe it as feeling like my body is filled with concrete.
You can push through activities without burning out.	You are not able to push through; you enter 'power-saving mode'.
You can usually pinpoint why you are tired.	Individual events or activities may worsen it, but your quality of life is always impacted.
You can still function.	It feels like your body has been weighted down with concrete and you cannot function.

Fatigue is so much more than tiredness. It can also cause other symptoms such as headaches, vision problems, aching muscles, flu-like symptoms, impaired cognitive abilities, sleep disruption, mood changes and mental health decline – not an ideal bedfellow for endometriosis. Sarah is 38 and has been diagnosed with endometriosis in 2022. She says that 'the fatigue has just as much impact on my quality of life as the pain, to be honest. I permanently feel like I can't be the mum I wanted to be because of it.' Her two young children see her resting, and she's heard them say, 'Shhh! We can't play because Mummy needs to rest.' 'It breaks my heart. I have never told them that, and never would, but it's something they've picked up and absorbed.'

> Management strategies for fatigue can include pain management, lifestyle modifications, stress management and, importantly, support networks. Prioritising self-care and rest can be incredibly helpful, but sadly it is not always possible depending on your life situation. Whatever circumstances you are in, please use your support network. Whether that's a partner, a parent, a sibling or a friend, share with them what you are struggling with and ask for help. Our loved ones want to help us; we just have to let them in and let them know how.

Endometriosis is a spectrum disease, meaning that one patient's experience with symptoms can be wildly different from another's. Each symptom can range from mild to completely debilitating and can vary week to week, day to day, even hour to hour. Conversely, and this is really important to remember, not all endometriosis patients have symptoms. You could have 'silent endometriosis', which means you do not experience any symptoms at all. It is thought that up to 30 per cent of endometriosis patients are completely asymptomatic. Often, these patients are diagnosed 'accidentally', with endometriosis spotted during another procedure or when the individual is trying to conceive and experiencing difficulties.

I was writing off so many issues with my body as stress until I started properly tracking every single thing, however small or unrelated it seemed. Only then did I start to notice the patterns and connections and be able to advocate for myself more strongly.

'My symptoms aren't just around my period, so it can't be endometriosis, right?'

I have been told by so many doctors that unless a symptom is tied to my period, it is not endometriosis-related. Countless other endometriosis patients have heard the same.

Symptoms can often feel worse around your period. Indeed, your period may be the first and only sign that something is not quite right. However, this is not because endometriosis is a period disease. Instead, it is due to the endometriosis lesions responding to the variations in the hormone levels in your body at this point in your cycle. That is not to say that symptoms are

What is endometriosis?

restricted to the duration of your period. Sufferers often report symptoms throughout the entire month.

Unfortunately, the persistent narrative that endometriosis is a period- or uterine-related disease stops many clinicians from joining the dots and realising that endometriosis is the cause of suffering.

Lightning crotch

One symptom that many of us do not even realise is 'a thing' is something called 'lightning crotch', aka 'butt or fanny lightning'. This is a really common, but not widely spoken about, symptom of endometriosis – when I polled my Instagram followers, 99 per cent of those who responded said they had encountered it. It is an unpredictable, acute, stabbing or electric type of pain that can come on incredibly suddenly, taking your breath away and stopping you in your tracks. While it can be very painful, the intensity should pass relatively quickly (in seconds, not minutes). As the name (and nicknames) suggests, these lightning pains are usually felt in the vagina, cervix and/or rectum. This can make things pretty awkward if you are walking around and suddenly cry out and grab your vulva in public because it feels like someone has shot a lightning bolt up there.

Lightning crotch is thought to be caused by pressure, irritation or inflammation in the nerves and ligaments in the vaginal and/or rectal regions. Intense muscle contractions around the anus can also be a factor. Alternatively, it can be the result of endometriosis lesions around these areas. Basically, it is probably a mixture of things and doctors are not really too sure about it. However, it is a very common part of dealing with endometriosis, so please be vocal about it with your clinician if you are experiencing it and do not be embarrassed.

My Instagram followers also shared some of their own ways of describing lightning crotch before they realised it was a real thing – here are some of my favourites:

- Fanny daggers
- Butt javelin
- Like Zeus himself shot a thousand lightning bolts up my vagina
- Inner fanny zaps
- Shooty bum pain

Endo belly

Endo belly, or adeno belly, is the name for the extreme bloating and abdominal distention caused by endometriosis (or adenomyosis; *see* chapter 4). The abdomen becomes swollen and hard, often within minutes, and can cause a great deal of pain and stress, both physically and emotionally.

This isn't your typical food-baby bloating. Endo belly can last for hours, days or even weeks. It can cause severe pain and feelings of pressure, which can then radiate down to your spine, pelvis and legs, making it extremely difficult to move or get comfortable.

Endo belly is caused by inflammation, and there are lots of possible triggers for the inflammatory process. These triggers are likely to be different for each person, but they may include inflammation from endometriosis lesions, cysts and endometriomas, fibroids, adenomyosis, trigger foods, constipation, other bowel issues and the point you are at in your menstrual cycle.

It can come on incredibly quickly and change your appearance in a matter of minutes. This, along with its unpredictable nature, is bound to have an effect on your body image. Adding salt to the wound, the size and shape of endo belly can often mimic the look of a pregnancy – a cruel irony from a disease that can impact fertility in a number of ways. I've been stopped multiple times and asked how far along I am . . .

If you suffer from endo belly, try the following:

- Make a note of your triggers and try to avoid them where possible.
- Soak in a warm bath.
- Use a body pillow to help you get comfortable and allow you to rest.
- Drink peppermint tea.
- Have outfits ready that still make you feel confident but are also endo-belly friendly.

How does endometriosis cause pain?

Endometriosis can be exceptionally painful. Although not everyone reports pain symptoms, where pain is present it can often be debilitating. In 2018,

What is endometriosis?

the NHS listed endometriosis as one of the top 20 most painful conditions a human can suffer with. But why is it so painful?

As we have seen, it used to be thought that endometriosis cells behaved like the lining of the womb each month, shedding and bleeding during a period. This blood would then, the theory went, become trapped, with no way to escape the body, which would cause pain. However, we now know far more about how endometriosis lesions are structured and behave and that this 'shed and bleed' narrative does not reflect reality. Mr Mikey Adamczyk, consultant gynaecologist and endometriosis surgeon, explained to me how endometriosis generates pain in a number of interacting ways: 'Endometriosis causes severe pain due to a combination of inflammation, adhesions, nerve involvement and hormonal sensitivity.' Endometriosis thrives in an inflammatory environment, but it also 'triggers inflammation that then irritates surrounding nerves'. Adhesions add another layer to the pain picture: 'Scar tissue, or adhesions, form as the disease progresses, binding organs together and causing pain.' This pain can then be intensified by the involvement of nerves: 'Endometriotic lesions often develop their own nerve supply' in a process called angiogenesis, and can also invade nerve-rich areas, increasing pain even further. Since the tissue responds to hormones, it becomes increasingly inflamed during certain points in the cycle, 'leading to heightened pain during menstruation'. Finally, we need to add in the complexity of organ involvement: 'When endometriosis affects organs like the bowel or bladder, it causes additional pain specific to these functions'. You can see how all these different mechanisms make endometriosis pain exceptionally complex and often debilitating. Mr Adamczyk adds, 'Living with ongoing pain can also lead to increased pain sensitivity and psychological distress, further worsening the pain experience.'

What does this mean in practice? Living with pain for a prolonged period can lead to something called 'central sensitisation' (*see* page 141). This is a controversial term as doctors who do not fully understand the mechanisms underpinning endometriosis can often use it to dismiss patients, but it is a very real phenomenon where the body comes to expect pain after being in a heightened state for a long period of time. *It does not mean the pain is in your head*; it means *your central nervous system has adapted the way it processes pain*. Mr Adamczyk, who has a special interest in neuropelveology (the diagnosis and treatment of problems with the pelvic nerves), believes that understanding nerves and our entire nervous system is 'absolutely crucial to managing endometriosis effectively'. It is obviously important to understand pelvic nerve anatomy to be able to deal with endometriosis on or near nerves; but understanding the entire neuroanatomy is 'really about grasping the entire pain pathway'. A crucial point here is that pain itself 'isn't actually the pathology – it's information that is being sent to the brain. This means that the real problem doesn't necessarily have to be where the pain is felt; it could lie anywhere along the nerve's pathway'. This is known as referred pain and, for example, can often account for the leg pain described by many endometriosis patients. 'This understanding is vital for anyone treating endometriosis, especially in those complex cases where pain is severe or seems to radiate throughout multiple areas,' concludes Mr Adamczyk.

Endometriosis and periods

As I mentioned earlier, my first period was the first time I noticed my endometriosis. Endometriosis announced itself with a bang during that first period, and I have not felt 'well' since. Each month when my period came, I thought I was dying: the pain, the blood loss, the clots, missing school and work, the passing out, the vomiting . . . and did I mention the pain? This is a common theme among endometriosis patients; it is often reported that endometriosis symptoms start with the onset of puberty and, hence, periods. Despite knowing that endometriosis is not itself a period condition, it would also be wrong to say that endometriosis has nothing to do with our periods. Let's investigate the relationship a little further.

Endometriosis symptoms can truly reflect the fact that this is a full-body disease. However, some of the most common symptoms are related to periods: painful periods, heavy periods, irregular periods and passing clots. Many endometriosis patients also report symptom changes during their periods. Some only feel symptoms during menstruation. Others feel certain symptoms throughout the month, with additional symptoms kicking in during their period. Others still have symptoms every day but report that their symptoms intensify during their period.

Common treatment options for endometriosis often revolve around stopping periods, ovulation or your entire cycle. These include hormonal pills, intrauterine devices (IUDs), injections for chemical menopause or, infuriatingly, suggestions such as getting pregnant or having a hysterectomy. To be clear, none of these cure endometriosis. They may, however, result

What is endometriosis?

in symptomatic relief, allowing us to live more of our lives and giving the appearance of reduced disease.

After reading this far, and maybe reflecting on your own endometriosis and its relationship to your period, you might find yourself thinking, 'To be honest, Jen, it's starting to sound like endometriosis might be a period condition after all!' And I would totally understand that, especially if your symptoms started with your first period, are heavily linked in type and timing to your period, worsen during your period and you start to feel a little better after taking treatments designed to stop your cycle. However, the relationship between periods and endometriosis is a very complex one. Endometriosis is not the endometrium (womb lining), but changes and fluctuations in our body during our menstrual cycle can trigger endometriosis lesions and their inflammatory response (*see* page 10). This means your symptoms may flare in response to your hormonal cycle, and you may feel relief from these symptoms if your cycle is controlled or stopped altogether.

Why, then, is shutting down this cycle not a cure for endometriosis? The answer is that endometriosis also produces its own oestrogen, which means it does not rely on the hormonal cycle to grow.

For decades, I thought my period was 'normal'. I thought it was probably a bit heavier than other people's, and I knew it was painful, but I thought – and was repeatedly told by doctors – that this was okay. That it was expected. That 'half the world has periods', to 'stop being dramatic' and to 'get on with life'. But normalised does not mean normal. In a society where menstrual health education has a very long way to go, most of us don't actually know what a 'normal' period is. We go to the doctor's because we have a concern, but we are told, 'That's perfectly normal'. We end up with a warped sense of normality that helps no one, with symptoms being normalised that really should not be. Let's flip the script and not worry about what is 'normal'. Instead, let's look at period red flags. What makes a period abnormal? What signs and symptoms should we be looking out for that we know need investigation and support?

Painful periods

Painful periods are *not* normal. Periods may cause some discomfort, but you should be able to ease this with over-the-counter pain medication. Any pain that interferes with your life, stops you going to school or work, causes you to miss social engagements or is not relieved by paracetamol or ibuprofen needs to be investigated. Your period should absolutely not be causing you so much pain that you vomit, pass out, are bedbound, burn yourself with hot-water bottles or are in floods of tears. Never allow a doctor or anyone else to gaslight you into thinking this is normal. Your pain is real, and you deserve an explanation for it.

Heavy periods

The medical definition of a heavy period is 80ml of blood loss across a cycle. However, most of us are not collecting and measuring blood in little jugs, so how can we know if we are passing too much blood? Look out for the following symptoms:

- Needing to double up on period products
- Flooding through period products, clothes or bedsheets
- Needing to change period products every hour
- Fatigue, shortness of breath or feeling faint

If you are experiencing heavy periods, please visit your doctor and have them investigate the cause. There are also medications available, such as tranexamic acid, a non-hormonal medication, usually in the form of a tablet, to help blood to clot and reduce heavy bleeding (*see* page 84).

Passing large blood clots

Passing clots is a perfectly natural part of a period, so do not panic if you notice this happening. However, if the clots are larger than a 10p piece (UK), you should see your doctor.

Decidual casts

These are most easily described as a 'super-clot', where the entirety of the lining of your womb comes out in one piece, often retaining a vague uterus-like shape. They are extremely painful and are often accompanied by intense cramping. We know very little about them, but they are thought to be caused

What is endometriosis?

by hormonal changes such as those brought on by ectopic pregnancy (*see page 33*), miscarriage or being on hormonal medication, which many of us with conditions such as endometriosis are. Decidual casts can be extremely alarming if you do not know what they are. I have passed three in my life and they were three of the worst periods I have ever experienced, which is saying something. If you think you have passed a decidual cast, take a photo and go to your doctor.

Length of bleed

The average length of a period is five days. If you are regularly bleeding for longer than seven days, this should be investigated.

Length of cycle

Anything between 23 and 35 days is considered 'normal'. Anything outside of this should be investigated.

Regularity

The average length of a menstrual cycle varies from person to person, but regularity is important. If you are the type of person who can never plan when your period will appear – maybe your cycle is sometimes 21 days, sometimes 40, sometimes 90 – this irregularity should be investigated.

Changes to your norm

A 'normal' period is exceptionally hard to quantify because they vary so much from person to person. It is always helpful to chat with your friends and family about periods – this helps destigmatise them and can provide a good sense check about your own – but the most important comparison you should be making is with yourself. Have your periods changed in any way? Have they become longer, heavier, more irregular or more painful? If there are any changes to your norm, get to the doctor and ask for investigations.

If you can relate to any of these red flags, even just one, please do visit a doctor and insist on an investigation. For too long, these red flags have been trivialised and normalised, but I repeat: normalised does not mean normal. And remember, painful periods, heavy periods or irregular periods are symptoms, not diagnoses. The root cause should always be investigated. If your doctor dismisses your concerns, see another one. See as many as it takes for them to take you seriously.

It is important to note here that you can have textbook periods and still have endometriosis. You might have a light, relatively pain-free regular period and have endometriosis. Conversely, you can have all the above red flags and not have endometriosis. However, there are many conditions that can interfere with periods, some of which are covered in chapter 4, and you deserve an answer for your suffering.

Finally, do not forget that while periods often exacerbate symptoms for many endometriosis sufferers, you can experience symptom flares at any point during your cycle.

What is a flare-up?

When you are diagnosed with endometriosis, or any chronic illness, a word you will likely hear a lot is 'flare' or 'flare-up'. This is when your symptoms suddenly intensify. A flare can last from a couple of hours to days or even weeks.

Flares can be set off by a huge variety of triggers, including your period, certain foods, stress, physical activity, illness, inflammation in the body – the list goes on, and will be unique for each of us. Flares can build up or they can come on extremely quickly, which can cause a great deal of anxiety and distress, especially if they happen in public.

Flare-ups are physically debilitating, but they also cause a significant strain on our mental health. Their unpredictable nature means that we do not know when they will arise, how long they will last or which symptoms will join the party. As a result, it is easy to start avoiding activities and hiding away out of fear of triggering a flare. This, obviously, hugely impacts our quality of life and adds to the sense of isolation we often already feel when battling endometriosis.

So, what can you do to help? Start keeping a flare diary to try to spot any patterns in your flare-ups. Do they happen when you eat particular foods? When you overexert yourself? After sex? Doing this helped me realise that my top triggers were stress, overexertion, caffeine, alcohol, my period and ovulation. Knowing what is likely to bring on a flare can help you either avoid those triggers or come up with a plan to lessen the symptoms or make yourself more comfortable. I barely touch alcohol now, for example. I also take a 'flare-up' kit with me everywhere I go. It contains things like my pain medication, fans, drinks, nausea bands, a transcutaneous electrical nerve stimulation (TENS) machine, water, a heat pad, spare underwear, period products and a fold-up walking stick.

Taking out even some of the unpredictability of flare-ups can help you feel a tiny bit more in control and can be a massive help for you and those supporting you. You will find more on flare-ups in chapter 5.

Who can suffer from endometriosis?

Endometriosis does not discriminate; however, once again our old friend – the period-related-disease myth – rears its ugly head. Because endometriosis was historically considered a uterine condition, it was assumed that only women of reproductive age could suffer from it. Unfortunately, this leaves a significant number of sufferers out of the equation, such as younger girls, those who are pregnant, those who are post-hysterectomy, those who are post-menopausal or going through chemical menopause (where the use of certain medications, for example hormone blockers or some chemotherapy treatments, puts you into menopause temporarily) – the list goes on. We will explore the factors that lead to some populations being particularly overlooked when it comes to endometriosis diagnosis and treatment in chapter 7.

Allowing this 'endometriosis is a period disease' narrative to continue is seriously harmful. It stops sufferers in any of the categories mentioned above from accessing help. I experienced this first-hand nearly 11 months after my endometriosis excision surgery and hysterectomy (the latter was for adenomyosis; *see* chapter 4). I ended up in A&E due to severe pain that was all too familiar. I insisted to the first gynaecologist I saw that it was endometriosis-related and I needed to be seen by the endo clinic at the hospital. Their response was, 'But it can't be gynaecological because you don't have gynaecological organs'. We are so close to grasping the point that endometriosis is not a gynaecological condition, but the lack of education and the low level of awareness instead meant I was not given the treatment and support that I desperately needed. Twenty-four hours of sitting in severe pain in an A&E waiting room later and I was discharged with emergency referrals to three separate departments.

You do not need to have periods, or a uterus, to have endometriosis. You could not have started your periods yet or be post-hysterectomy, in chemical menopause, in surgical menopause, in peri-menopause, post-menopausal, pregnant, on hormonal medication, a trans man or even a guinea pig (yes, really!).

Karla Robbins is an endometriosis patient who has also been diagnosed with a condition called Mayer–Rokitansky–Küster–Hauser syndrome (MRKH), a reproductive disorder characterised by an absent or undeveloped uterus and cervix. It can also lead to the shortening of the vaginal canal. I first came across Karla's story after I posted on Instagram about how endometriosis can persist without a uterus, for the reasons listed above, and Karla messaged me saying that MRKH is another example that is nearly always overlooked. In all honesty, I had never heard of the condition, so I wanted to give Karla the chance to share her experience here.

'My periods just never started,' she says. 'We went to the doctor when I was 15, but they said it's normal and to just wait . . . We went back when I was 16 and said that this isn't really normal for our family – even my younger sister had started her period by then.' Karla was in increasing pain. She was sent for an ultrasound, and she can still clearly remember the sonographer's face. 'She said to my mum, "I can't see anything; I can't see a uterus".' What followed was a bit of a blur, but Karla was sent for an MRI. 'My kidneys and ovaries were there, my vaginal cavity was there, but my body had never produced a uterus.' A laparoscopy was the next step, where Karla was formally diagnosed with MRKH and endometriosis, after nodules of disease were also identified. 'The endometriosis was a shock. I didn't even know what it was, but it did make a lot of sense of things.'

From the age of 15 to 18, Karla doesn't really feel like she processed everything: 'I was more aware of how everyone around was affected, so I put them first.' At 18, she had surgery to remove the endometriosis lesions and any underdeveloped tissues caused by the MRKH. She struggled with depressive episodes, viewing herself as 'a mutant' during this time. I asked Karla if she feels accepted by the endometriosis community, where we still see images of uteruses used as a type of mascot for the disease (you will notice there is no uterus on the cover of this book), and she responded, 'I don't feel like I'm not accepted; I just think people don't know. It's just not recognised.' Karla acknowledges that MRKH is a rare disease, thought to impact one in 5000 of those born with gynaecological anatomy, but, 'as someone born without a uterus, but who still suffers from severe endometriosis and chronic pain, it would be nice if there was some acknowledgement'. Demonstrating a level of humility that I could only wish I'd had at 22, Karla knows that 'it's not malicious . . . it's not a deliberate exclusion', but the incorrect focus on endometriosis as a uterine condition is difficult for her. 'It makes me feel really isolated and excluded . . . It takes me back to those thoughts of, "I'm not a woman without a period" – someone actually said that to me once.'

This idea that you have to have a uterus to have endometriosis is problematic for so many reasons. It is also just incorrect, as my own hysterectomy and Karla's MRKH prove. And cis men have also been found to have endometriosis. The cases are *exceptionally* few – currently around 20 – but if we have never known to look for it before, how many more men throughout history have had endometriosis and slipped through the cracks? No one knows.

Whoever you are, and whatever life stage you are in, your pain is valid and you deserve treatment and relief from your symptoms.

Is endometriosis hereditary?

For lots of people, the first time they hear the word endometriosis is when they are diagnosed. That wasn't the case for me as my mum was diagnosed in her 30s, when I was a toddler. The inheritability of endometriosis is another area (shock horror) lacking in research, but the studies that have been undertaken show that there is an increased frequency of endometriosis in first-degree relatives. This 'familial clustering' means that if your mother has endometriosis, like mine, then you are around seven times more likely to also suffer from the disease.

If you have a close relative who has endometriosis and you are suffering with endometriosis symptoms, please see a doctor. The reverse is likewise true: if you have endometriosis and a close relative also has symptoms, then encourage them to seek medical help.

You can also have endometriosis even if no one else in your family has the disease. Please do not dismiss your symptoms because there is no endometriosis in your family.

How is endometriosis diagnosed?

We have already seen that the process of obtaining an endometriosis diagnosis is complicated, and we will talk more in chapters 2 and 3 about how to advocate for yourself and navigate this particular minefield (hopefully a lot more quickly than the statistics indicate). For now, let's focus on how endometriosis is actually diagnosed.

The gold standard for endometriosis diagnosis is laparoscopic surgery, also known as 'keyhole surgery'. This is a type of surgery, performed under general anaesthetic, which is classed as 'minimally invasive' due to the small incisions. The surgeon makes small cuts in your abdomen through which a laparoscope, a thin tube with a light and camera, and other surgical instruments are inserted to review your internal organs. The number of incisions will depend on your individual circumstances and where endometriosis is suspected and found. During this surgery, the goal is to identify all areas of disease and remove them at the same time. The procedure should be undertaken by an endometriosis specialist. Samples should then be sent away for testing and confirmation.

Now, you might be thinking that surgery is a pretty invasive way to achieve a diagnosis. Surely there is a better method than that? You would be right, but the diagnosis of endometriosis is not simple and is not the same for each person.

On your journey to an endometriosis diagnosis, you will likely encounter at least one of the following diagnostic methods, none of which are perfect or foolproof:

- Medical history: A detailed and accurate medical history can tell a clinician a lot. However, as we saw earlier, endometriosis symptoms are so wide-ranging, individualised and dynamic that it often does not occur to us, nor to the clinician, that they can be connected. Education of clinicians is paramount to changing this, but, until then, medical history is not a reliable method and is very rarely how a diagnosis is given.
- Physical examination: In expert hands, a physical examination, both internal and external, can provide a good clinical indication of endometriosis. It is very rarely used to diagnose endometriosis on its own, but in combination with other methods it can create a compelling argument for the presence of the disease.

What is endometriosis?

- Ultrasound – abdominal (external) and/or transvaginal (where a wand-like instrument is inserted into the vagina)): An external and/or internal ultrasound scan is often one of the first steps in trying to ascertain whether or not you may have endometriosis. The trouble is that endometriosis does not always show up on ultrasound scans. Sometimes, an ultrasound scan is completely clear but a patient has surgery and endometriosis is found. Sometimes, a scan shows some signs of endometriosis, then surgery shows the disease is more extensive than the ultrasound picked up. Sometimes, and sadly this is all too common, an ultrasound scan is clear so the patient is dismissed, but they have extensive endometriosis with organ involvement. The latter is exactly what happened to me.
- MRI: An MRI (*see* pages 78–82) is another diagnostic method that you are likely to be referred for, and one should always be undertaken prior to a laparoscopy to aid surgical planning. An MRI is more likely to show endometriosis, particularly DIE (*see* page 15) and OMAs (*see* page 16), and may also show other conditions such as adenomyosis or fibroids (*see* chapter 4). It is still not a guaranteed method for diagnosis, however, and, as with ultrasound, endometriosis can be missed. My MRI showed endometriosis, endometriomas and adenomyosis but did not reveal the extent or full organ involvement. That only became apparent during surgery.
- Laparoscopy: As mentioned earlier, laparoscopy is currently the gold standard for diagnosis and is when most of us will receive a confirmed, definitive diagnosis of endometriosis. However, to reiterate, it absolutely must be performed by someone who truly understands endometriosis, knows all the different ways it can present (it can be blue, grey, white, brown, red, yellow or even translucent!) and can identify and excise all disease. The surgeon who performed my first surgery missed significant disease, which went on to choke my ureters and put me at risk of double kidney failure. Choose your surgeon carefully! Remember, you do have a choice (*see* chapter 3, where we go into more detail on this).

As you can see, and you may have experienced yourself, we do not have an easy time with getting a diagnosis. Each stage can come with its own hoops to jump through, delays, anxiety and pain. And it's absolutely terrible that surgery, with all the consequences and risks it carries, is currently our best hope for an accurate diagnosis.

There are those who believe that, as technology improves, we can shift the gold standard away from surgery and towards medical imaging (i.e. scans). But for now, the thing to remember is that a clear scan does not rule out endometriosis. Again, the education of clinicians, at all stages, is incredibly important. If they do not know what to look for, they simply will not see it.

Diagnostic tests

There is a lot of talk at the moment about various research projects claiming to diagnose endometriosis via a 'simple' test. Whether it's using urine, blood, menstrual blood, saliva, even faeces, there are lots of promises being made about the future of endometriosis diagnosis. And yes, it would be wonderful to be able to receive a diagnosis without waiting an average of a decade or having to undergo surgery. But these tests are still in very early stages of testing and development. Until robust studies (known as randomised controlled trials) have been undertaken, the findings replicated, and the information made fully available, the information surrounding these tests is simply marketing.

One test that does seem to be on the right track is called Endotest, a saliva-based test, developed by a French company. But even this, at the time of writing this book, still needs much more evidence, and accessibility is a major issue, with a single test costing nearly £1,000.

It's great to see research into fast, non-invasive tests for endometriosis. It would certainly help reduce the woeful diagnosis times. But it is much too early to be celebrating just yet. And we need to remember that diagnosis is only one piece of the puzzle. Do doctors have the appropriate education and training to connect our symptoms and order the test in the first place? What happens after the test? Are there enough experts with enough experience? What is the overall strategy for managing endometriosis care?

And as Mr Shaheen Khazali, endometriosis surgeon, explains, 'If we don't fully know what this disease is, and what causes it, how can we accurately and reliably test for it?'

How is endometriosis managed?

We know that endometriosis has no cure, but that does not mean there are no ways to manage our symptoms and try to improve our quality of life. Treatments can broadly be split into the following categories:

- Lifestyle changes: Dietary changes, movement, stress reduction, trigger identification and avoidance
- Non-hormonal medical intervention: Painkillers, drugs to reduce bleeding (e.g. tranexamic acid)
- Hormonal medical intervention: The pill, a coil or IUD, injections to stop your cycle (i.e. chemical menopause)
- Surgery

Endometriosis has a wide range of symptoms that will vary among patients. The treatment options that are recommended to you will also vary according to what you are struggling with, the impact on your quality of life and your goals.

Your clinician should discuss all options in detail with you. This discussion should include all the pros and cons of each option and explore your personal preferences. A plan should then be devised between you and your doctor, with the emphasis on your choice. Clinicians usually advise giving a treatment a set period of time (usually between three and six months) to see if it is working, but if you have any concerns during that period, please seek medical advice.

We will be going into the various treatments in much more detail throughout the book, but for now it is important to remember that they are very much about symptom management, not cures. The closest thing we have to a cure is surgical excision, where the disease is cut out by an experienced, skilled endometriosis excision surgeon, but sadly, even this is not a magic wand and access to these experts is frighteningly difficult.

Endometriosis and fertility

Fertility is an incredibly personal and intimate topic, so before we get stuck in, I just want you to know that whatever stage you are at, and whatever your fertility goals are, you are not alone. Endometriosis is an area riddled with misinformation, as is fertility. Combine the two and the result can be overwhelming and confusing. It is one of the areas that has also fallen victim to oversimplification when the reality is anything but. I will do my best to share the latest that we know about the relationship between endometriosis and fertility, but there is no one-size-fits-all approach and, sadly, we still do not fully understand the connection.

Issues with fertility do not just encompass the initial conception but may also include miscarriage, ectopic pregnancy (*see* page 33) and the inability to carry a baby to full term. This section is referring to all of these scenarios.

Fertility is, understandably, an area of huge concern for many who are diagnosed with endometriosis. I want to clarify that an endometriosis diagnosis is not also an instant infertility diagnosis. Sadly, it is a part of the picture for many, but that does not necessarily mean it will be for you. Even with severe endometriosis, natural conception is possible. That said, it is thought that infertility can affect 30–50 per cent of endometriosis patients.

'There is no question that endometriosis affects fertility, but it is very nuanced,' says endometriosis surgeon, Mr Shaheen Khazali, during our conversation. 'We don't understand which type of endometriosis affects fertility most, but a combination of changes in anatomy, quality of eggs and egg reserve, and also other associated conditions such as adenomyosis, can all affect fertility.'

This is another area where the available data and research can be confusing. 'The evidence suggests that surgery excising endometriosis probably improves the chances of spontaneous conception,' Mr Khazali explains. 'Studies have also shown that patients with failed in vitro fertilisation (IVF) who then go on to have excision can improve their chances of getting pregnant.' His extensive experience in the operating room seems to back up this early data: 'There are also lots of case series that show that good surgery and complete excision of endometriosis can lead to good fertility outcomes – with up to 60 per cent getting pregnant and carrying a pregnancy successfully to term.' However, and this is where things get a little more complicated, when operating on endometriomas (blood-filled cysts, typically found in the ovaries; *see* page 16), 'we are going to reduce the ovarian reserve, almost certainly'. This then raises the question of whether it is the right thing to do. Should endometriomas be excised, and what is the price of that in patients where fertility is a priority? This is where egg freezing may enter the chat, and you might be looking to harvest eggs before any ovarian surgery.

What is endometriosis?

Often, people will find out they have endometriosis while already undergoing fertility treatment such as IVF, after suffering from no other symptoms or having them dismissed as normal. Endometriosis, in its usual complex fashion, can affect fertility in multiple ways, as follows:

- Sex can be painful – an initial stumbling block that can provide significant hurdles to natural conception.
- OMAs (*see* page 16) can damage ovarian tissue and impact egg reserve.
- Adhesions can distort the woman's anatomy, making implantation and subsequent development of the embryo problematic.
- The long-term effects of endometriosis symptom management options are unknown, but research is emerging to say their prolonged use may have sustained negativity that we do not yet fully understand.

However, early intervention can improve outcomes, even in cases of advanced disease. The Center for Endometriosis Care advises that 'for those with stage I–II, the chance of conceiving after excision is between 80–85%, almost the same rate as if you did not have endometriosis. Those with stage III will have a 70–75% chance of conceiving and those with stage IV is between 50–60%'. Remember, the traditional endometriosis stages were developed in relation to fertility so these figures are not particularly suprising. Mr Khazali stresses that, just as surgery is not a cure for the disease, it also does not reverse fertility issues in all patients. 'We know that endometriosis and infertility have very close ties, we understand some things about the reasons for the fertility issues,' but surgery is not a magic fix for everyone, even in the most capable hands.

Despite endometriosis up to doubling the risk of infertility, in a recent report published in the UK, 58 per cent of endometriosis patients would have liked fertility support but were not offered any. Only 44 per cent of patients were even asked by a medical practitioner if their fertility was important to them. If you are currently struggling with fertility, please know that support exists, including in the National Institute for Health and Care Excellence (NICE) guidelines for endometriosis management (*see* pages 77–78). Who is performing the surgery – and how – is the key to increasing the chances of a positive outcome. Make sure you are seeing a skilled, experienced endometriosis specialist, and come up with a plan together. Fertility is a hugely personal and emotional topic but remember that an endometriosis diagnosis is not an instant infertility diagnosis too.

A note on fertility: pregnancy, despite what has been taught for many years, *is not a cure for endometriosis*. Some women may experience a temporary reduction in symptoms due to the interruption of their cycle, but this is not a cure. Many women note that their symptoms return almost immediately after giving birth, with some saying those symptoms are worse than ever. A baby is not a prescription. It is also absolutely wild to suggest to someone with a disease that can double the risk of infertility to just casually conceive anyway.

Endometriosis in children and adolescents

Endometriosis also affects children and adolescents. While most of the information and advice provided in this chapter applies to these younger patients, we also need to look at the unique challenges in this age group.

Many experts believe that endometriosis is 'present from birth', but when a girl's periods start, the 'oestrogens stimulate the endometriosis cells to start flourishing'. Despite not being a period disease, endometriosis patients commonly recall their symptoms starting with their periods during adolescence. Research seems to support this anecdotal evidence, with 'at least 60% of teens diagnosed with endometriosis presenting with symptoms within 6 months of menarche; 80% within 3 years'. Despite this, it takes years to achieve an endometriosis diagnosis. What's going on? Why are so many young people not finding answers to their pain?

When I went to see doctors during my teenage years, I was invariably told variations on the theme of 'painful periods are normal', 'they will settle down', 'you're just one of the unlucky ones' and 'teenage girls are prone to being a bit dramatic'. And I'm not alone. Although the true prevalence of endometriosis among this age group is unknown, an American College of Obstetricians and Gynecologists report in 2018 revealed that 70 per cent of teens suffering from pelvic pain are later diagnosed with the disease. Meanwhile, 82 per cent of participants in a 2014 study on the topic had never even heard of endometriosis, simply accepting the pain as normal and carrying on the best they could. However, the symptoms unavoidably spill over into other areas of life, leading to missed school or reduced performance, loss of social opportunities, increased isolation and the mental distress caused by living with these symptoms and medical gaslighting. Twenty to 40 per cent of adolescents report having to

What is endometriosis?

miss school or experiencing a decline in academic performance. Not listening to these teens and denying them diagnosis and early intervention is creating issues that will influence their lives for decades to come.

Endometriosis was once thought to occur only very rarely in teenagers – it was seen as a disease of middle-aged women. Sadly, although this myth has softened over the years to include slightly broader demographic criteria, there is a stubbornness that persists around age. Many doctors, particularly GPs, who are our first line in medical treatment, believe that endometriosis is not possible in younger patients. Even when a GP does consider endometriosis a possibility, the next step is usually an ultrasound scan. As we will learn (*see* pages 79–81), this comes with its own set of difficulties, with the scan often coming back 'clear' so the investigations stop. The preferred type of ultrasound for the best chance of spotting endometriosis is a transvaginal, or internal, scan (*see* page 79). This may not be desired by the patient or their parents, so sometimes only an abdominal scan is performed. While in expert hands, and in the right circumstances, this can still provide an excellent picture of the situation, 'as always, it comes down to who is performing and interpreting the scan and how,' explains Dr Wendaline VanBuren, expert sonographer. When I tell her of one patient who, at 14 years old, was told she 'couldn't possibly have an internal ultrasound because she would no longer be a virgin', Dr VanBuren sighs. 'These procedures are entirely medical and should never be sexualised . . . but it is always the patient's choice.' She stresses that appropriate counselling and expert intervention is even more important in situations with adolescents with suspected endometriosis. 'We need it to be one good scan,' she says. We also need to make sure we are providing education to sonographers on early disease presentation in adolescents, such as thickening of the uterosacral ligaments. If a transvaginal ultrasound is decided against, or even denied, Dr VanBuren suggests pushing for an MRI instead to give the best chance of disease identification.

I was not one of the 82 per cent of teens who had never heard of endometriosis. My mum was diagnosed with the disease when I was a toddler. When I first experienced symptoms, she was able to spot the early warning signs that reminded her of her own experiences and we went to the doctor's early on. She mentioned her medical history and her concerns but was made to feel like she was 'pushing her own experience on to her child', like she was 'paranoid' or 'neurotic'. Despite my mum advocating for me, despite me being so convinced throughout my 20s that I had endometriosis that I nicknamed it

'Edna' when talking to friends, it took me over two decades to even be seen by a gynaecologist – let alone an endometriosis specialist surgeon.

Currently, very few surgeons in the UK operate on adolescent endometriosis patients. Even fewer would be classed as experienced, expert endometriosis specialists. Many adolescents end up under private care, with their parents often paying out from savings or even entering debt. One such parent, Mike, explained that seeing his daughter in crippling pain 'destroyed me'. 'I felt like a failure. I promised the day she was born that I would do everything I could to protect her. But this disease beat me. I couldn't take her pain away no matter what I did.' He and his wife took their daughter to the GP. At first, the doctor suggested that they were paranoid, perhaps even exaggerating their daughter's symptoms and making her feel like they were worse than they actually were. Eventually, as her symptoms worsened, they found a GP who would listen. Their daughter was referred to a gynaecologist, who told them that 'yes, it was likely to be endometriosis, but she was too young to be operated on. They suggested chemical menopause drugs until she turned 17, which would have been four years away'. These drugs are intended for short-term use only. Long-term use can be associated with any number of issues for the patient, and we still do not know the full risks associated. Appalled at the suggestion, Mike and his wife found a specialist who ran a private clinic and who operated on the 14-year-old girl, discovering and excising severe endometriosis. It cost Mike and his wife around £15,000. 'The whole lot went on a credit card . . . We couldn't afford it, but I would have done anything to help my girl at that point.' A year after his daughter's surgery, Mike tells me that she is doing amazingly well. 'She's my little girl again. She can attend school, she has friends that she goes out with, she's funny and bright . . . I thought we had lost that version of her forever.'

Despite numerous patients saying that early intervention with expert excision surgery can increase positive patient outcomes in both the short and the long term, this position is not without its controversies. Some surgeons argue that putting a teen through invasive surgery, with all its associated risks, is perhaps not the best way forward. Endometriosis surgeon Mr Shaheen Khazali takes a balanced view: 'You shouldn't treat this group of patients categorically differently than any other patient,' he firmly states when we speak. In other words, they should not be denied treatment because of their age; instead, nuance and individual circumstances and goals should always be the key factors. Without early intervention, he explains, 'you have to consider that you are letting that pain settle, becoming chronic' and moulding that young person's identity and future. 'You are allowing a lot of problems further down the line.' He also stresses that if the teen's 'quality of life is very severely impacted', they would be a good candidate for surgery. However, he adds that, as with any aspect of endometriosis care, things are not as black and white as we would like them to be. 'Some surgeons believe that endometriosis should always be immediately surgically removed.' Others refuse to operate at all, even dismissing and ignoring patients. 'Those are the two extremes and the "right" answer is somewhere in between. Finding that balance is the art', because there is always the 'worry about causing more problems, such as adhesions and scar tissue'.

Other global endometriosis experts, such as surgeon Dr Shanti Mohling, slightly disagree; remember how in the Introduction I said that even global experts differ on certain aspects? Dr Mohling believes that 'endometriosis causes scarring and complications much more than the surgery with proper excision'. But where she agrees is that 'we need to listen to our teenagers in pain and not be afraid to operate when it's indicated'.

Sadly, what often happens is that teens presenting to their doctors with endometriosis symptoms are immediately put on hormonal interventions, often with very little explanation as to what they are, how they work, what the risks are or what other options are available. These interventions can mask symptoms, allowing disease severity to worsen unchecked. They can be lifelines for many, including adolescents. In my case, they certainly meant that my symptoms were confined to the duration of the 'withdrawal bleed' – and no, no one told me that I could run the packs back to back and avoid that week of excruciating pain each month. I only learned that a few years ago. However, they are not curative, and as soon as we come off the drugs, for whatever reason, we often find that our symptoms come back with full force or even worse than ever.

Endometriosis patient Natalie had her first surgery at 12 years of age to investigate her symptoms and, despite being told that the surgeons saw endometriosis lesions, she was still told that she was 'too young' to have endometriosis. The doctors refused to add the disease to her medical records until she was in her 20s. 'I'm still dealing with the consequences of not being believed for so long when I was younger,' she says. After multiple failed IVF rounds, Natalie started therapy, which she describes as 'illuminating'. She realised that 'not being listened to, in any context, is hugely triggering' for her, and it 'took me a long time to realise that comes from not being believed as a child about my pain. It has had a huge, lifelong impact on me.'

Making sure you are seen by a true endometriosis specialist team (*see* pages 109–14) is always of utmost importance when considering your options, and this is especially true with young patients. When it comes to surgical imaging, healthcare professionals need to know the optimal protocols, what to look for in terms of the disease and its impacts and how to accurately interpret the findings. Then, if surgery is pursued, the surgeon needs to understand all disease presentations, to look everywhere and to remove what is found without leaving remnants behind. It seems that the visual appearance of endometriosis may even be different in adolescents compared with adults. In younger patients, endometriosis lesions are 'typically clear or red', making them difficult to identify for surgeons unfamiliar with the complexities of the disease. Nobody wants to see adolescents undergoing repeat surgeries because of incomplete removal that leads to disease persistence, or subpar technique leading to further issues. It should not be a case of teens being wheeled into operating theatres up and down the country to have surgery performed on them by general gynaecologists just to say they've had the surgery. No one is advocating for that. But expert intervention, at an early stage, could change lives.

I am often asked, when giving talks and presentations, 'How would your life be different if you had been believed when you were 11 years old?' When I was first asked this question, I became emotional, and I actually cried about it when I got back home – because I had never even considered it. I had never considered that a world where my pain and symptoms were believed at that young an age was a possibility. To wonder what my life could have potentially been if I had not had to live for over 20 years in excruciating pain, and to now live the rest of my life with the permanent consequences of those decades, was overwhelming. It felt like grief. I never want a future generation to have that moment. We have to do better for adolescents when they speak up about pain.

Why does endometriosis sit under gynaecology?

We know that endometriosis is not simply a gynaecological disorder. It is a full-body disease occurring, by its nature, outside of the uterine cavity. Despite this knowledge, endometriosis patients are seen by gynaecology departments all over the world. We are often treated by general gynaecologists who frankly do not have the experience or education to fully understand the disease and to optimally treat patients. Endometriosis is also still seen as an obscure period issue.

So, what are the options? Some of us believe that endometriosis should be removed from the gynaecology department – that its association with gynaecology perpetuates this myth and can hinder access to appropriate care. As long as endometriosis is linked to the uterus, the 'logical' thinking will be that removing the womb will solve the problem. According to the Center for Endometriosis Care, hundreds of thousands of unnecessary hysterectomies are performed in the United States each year due to the lack of education on endometriosis. Research also shows that endometriosis expert centres worldwide (more on these on pages 111–113) have a lower rate of life-changing surgeries such as stomas and bowel resections, despite handling far higher volumes of these complex cases.

It seems clear that not only would endometriosis being its own specialism improve patient outcomes, it would also raise the profile of the disease, attracting more specialists and funding. It could also help tackle the abysmal UK gynaecology waiting lists, revealed to be (at the time of writing) a staggering 763,694 women. We would fill Wembley Stadium eight and a half times. And the situation is worsening.

Removing endometriosis from the confines of gynaecology could also greatly improve patient comfort. Only those of us who have had to sit in a packed waiting room filled with expectant mothers, waiting to be seen for our infertility or hysterectomy consultation, will understand the heartbreak.

However, it is not as simple as creating a whole new department for a single condition. The resourcing alone would be an astronomically high barrier. Instead, argues Mr Mikey Adamczyk, gynaecologist and endometriosis specialist, 'endometriosis needs to become a completely separate subspecialty' (subspecialties are specific areas of a particular area of medicine, with their own curricula, training programmes and examinations). This subspecialty, he believes, should still sit under the broader heading of gynaecology, similar to gynaecological oncology (gynae cancers). 'As gynaecologists and endometriosis surgeons, we know the anatomy of the pelvis better than anyone else, and we're trained in complex surgery. But we need to be trained properly, with specialised, high-level skills *specifically for endometriosis*, and we need the resources to support these complex procedures.'

He goes on to say, 'a gynaecological endometriosis surgeon should be like the captain of the ship, leading a team of specialists from other fields to give patients the absolute best care. With a cohesive team and the right support, we can manage these complex cases with the depth and precision they deserve.' This multi-disciplinary approach to endometriosis care is the key to long-term positive patient outcomes, something we will explore in much more detail over the coming chapters.

Support for endometriosis as a subspecialty is gaining traction. Katie Boyce, Board Certified Patient Advocate, aka @endogirlsblog, says, 'We have to get doctors to stop operating when they are in over their head. And the way to do that is by creating a subspecialty for endometriosis. Until then, they will carry on, because that is what their training told them they can do.' We have a clear subspecialty for urogynaecology. We have one for gynaecological oncology. Now we need to have one for endo-gynaecology.

Loss of endometriosis knowledge

Something that genuinely shocked me when researching this book was how much we do actually know about this disease and how to improve patient outcomes. And that isn't new information. By the end of the 1930s, endometriosis had been reported on the lungs, bowel, bladder, lymph nodes, cervix and ligaments. Nearly 100 years ago, we had proof that this is a full body disease, not something confined to the uterus, or even the pelvic organs. Endometriosis was also reported among teens, something which some ill-informed modern-day doctors still insist is not a possibility. We even knew, in 1957, that endometriosis symptoms can occur at any point in the cycle, not simply confined to our periods, something that I know I was certainly told impossible numerous times by countless doctors over the years of trying to find answers.

In 1957, a new drug was launched that would change the face of endometriosis care until this day. The hormonal contraceptive pill was introduced initially to treat menstrual disorders and some of the first to be given this novel treatment were endometriosis patients, marking

What is endometriosis?

a move away from surgical treatment for the disease. This is despite, as Katie Boyce, BCPA, @endogirlsblog tells me, excision surgery being 'known to be the most effective method for decades'. These excerpts from publications in 1935, 1947 and 1950 illustrate: 'the most efficient treatment is radical excision', 'we have excised localised endometrial implants with satisfactory relief and have been gratified to see our patients bear children', 'based on excision…in four fifths of cases…the symptoms entirely disappeared.' But the introduction of the cheaper, more readily accessible ablation surgeries, combined with the advent of hormonal symptom management masquerading as treatment, meant that much of this knowledge was lost, held only by a small number of specialists. And so, relatively recently, the myths that we will have heard time and time again became entrenched as accurate knowledge.

Endometriosis myth busting

- **Endometriosis is not just a bad period:** Endometriosis is a full-body condition with symptoms to match. It is not a period condition, but periods are relevant to the conversation and often a warning sign that endometriosis might be present. Conversely, you can have a 'textbook' period and have endometriosis.
- **Endometriosis is not rare:** Endometriosis is thought to affect one in 10 women. More recent studies show that this is closer to one in seven. It has the same occurrence rate as asthma or type 2 diabetes.
- **Endometriosis is not cured by the pill:** No medication cures endometriosis, but there are some that can provide symptomatic relief.
- **Endometriosis is not a disease of reproductive age women:** Endometriosis has been found in patients as young as six and in patients many years post-menopause.
- **Endometriosis is not rogue endometrium:** There are numerous significant differences between endometriosis and endometrium. They are not structurally, behaviourally or visually the same. Endometriosis does not act like a mini period each month, shedding and getting trapped.

Endometriosis

- **Endometriosis does <u>not</u> mean you won't be able to have children:** Infertility is a big part of the discussion about endometriosis, and many patients do struggle. However, an endometriosis diagnosis is not an infertility diagnosis. Many endometriosis patients are able to conceive and carry a full-term pregnancy naturally.
- **Endometriosis does <u>not</u> equal severe pain:** Endometriosis is a spectrum disease and is highly individual to each patient, including the symptoms present and the effect they have on quality of life. Some patients are in daily debilitating pain, but others are completely asymptomatic, suffering no pain at all.
- **Endometriosis is <u>not</u> a pelvic disease:** Endometriosis is a full-body disease, having been found in every organ and system of the human body. The spleen was the last organ to join the party, having been documented in 2022.

Chapter 2

Dealing with the system – how to get help

'Are you sure you're not just wanting attention?' – GP

Hopefully, you now have a pretty solid understanding of what endometriosis is. So, how do you translate that knowledge into accessing medical support? That is what this chapter is going to focus on, taking you through getting a diagnosis, medical interventions, symptom management and the importance of choosing your surgeon wisely. Let's start at the beginning with diagnosis.

Diagnosing endometriosis

It is notoriously difficult to receive an endometriosis diagnosis. Worldwide, the average diagnosis time is eight to 10 years. In the UK, the average is eight years and 10 months, with Northern Ireland and Wales facing the longest waits of nine years and five months and nine years and 11 months, respectively. Black and Hispanic endometriosis sufferers could be waiting double this time, but to be honest, we have no idea how bad this disparity truly is due to an alarming lack of data about demographic differences (*see* chapter 7 for more on this topic). The team that published the above diagnosis times are now working with a grass-roots charity, Cysters, to understand diagnosis times in people of colour.

Even more worrying is that the length of time for which we are waiting for a diagnosis is actually *increasing*. Things are not improving; they are getting worse, despite Dr Ken Sinervo of the Center for Endometriosis Care telling us that 'the earlier endometriosis is diagnosed and treated properly, the better the outcomes are for those struggling'. 'Delays in the diagnosis of endometriosis are common and are associated with worsened quality of life and greater medical costs.'

Endometriosis

Why is a diagnosis helpful? Sounds a ridiculous question, I know. Believe it or not, there are still doctors asking why we even want a diagnosis, believing it is 'just to feel better now [we] have a label', as one charming medical professional told me. Some doctors take that idea even further, believing that a diagnosis is as good as treatment. A diagnosis can be many things, but treatment it is not. Instead, a timely diagnosis could mean the following:

- Relief and validation, especially after medical and societal gaslighting for years
- The ability to track and manage symptoms more effectively
- The ability to access appropriate and effective treatment options
- The ability to make better healthcare and lifestyle choices for ourselves
- Access to support schemes such as a Blue Badge or financial assistance (*see* pages 197–199)
- The ability to communicate our struggles and needs more effectively to loved ones, employers and others (*see* pages 72–73)
- Earlier intervention, which could save organs and fertility
- More accurate data for research and resource allocation
- Increased awareness and dialogue around historically taboo issues
- Decades of life back for sufferers
- A reduced cost and resource burden for the NHS
- A boost to the economy

Given the clear benefits of an earlier diagnosis of endometriosis, why is it taking so long? It is a murky, toxic soup made up of internalised misogyny, societal taboos, a lack of research and prioritisation and the diabolical state of endometriosis education for clinicians.

Take four common problem areas for endometriosis sufferers: menstruation, bowel issues, infertility and painful sex. Each one on its own is still, infuriatingly, considered taboo – something we don't talk about, that we just get on and deal with ourselves. Layer them together and you end up with a super-taboo. And these stigmas run deep. Even I, who talk openly every day about my story and journey with this disease, have only just begun to talk to my husband frankly about the bowel issues I am suffering with thanks to endometriosis on my bowel. We have been together for 14 years, but I still feel awkward talking to him about constipation, bowel movements and rectal bleeding. It is not my fault or something to beat myself up about; it

Dealing with the system – how to get help

has been drilled into me since childhood by a society that does not talk about these health issues. I grew up in an era where the advice in magazines was 'if you're staying over at your boyfriend's house and need to use the toilet, lay tissue paper in the bowl and run the tap so he won't know what you're doing in there' and T-shirts were literally emblazoned with slogans like 'girls fart rainbows and glitter' (I'm eternally grateful to my parents for never dressing me in those!). Then there are periods, which are seen as something only women should know about. Boys don't need to learn about them. Periods are inherently 'dirty'. Period products are referred to as 'feminine hygiene' or 'sanitary' products. Even in 2025, my local supermarket was still signposting tampons and pads this way.

All that said, it is definitely true that more of us are speaking up. However, we are not being listened to, taken seriously or believed. Research by the charity Endometriosis UK in 2024 revealed the following:

- Seventy-four per cent of respondents had attended five or more GP appointments with symptoms before receiving a diagnosis.
- Forty-seven per cent had visited a GP 10 or more times with symptoms prior to their diagnosis.
- Fifty-two per cent had visited A&E at least once due to the severity of their endometriosis symptoms prior to diagnosis.
- Twenty per cent reported seeing a gynaecologist (the specialty within which endometriosis currently sits) 10 or more times before being diagnosed.
- Seventy-eight per cent of those who later received a diagnosis of endometriosis reported an experience of medical dismissal and/or had the severity of their symptoms questioned by healthcare practitioners. This was an increase from 69 per cent just four years earlier.

Medical gaslighting is increasing in line with diagnosis times. It is always important to remember that correlation does not equal causation, so in this instance we cannot say that one is causing the other, but I would put money on it being a factor.

I have never heard a doctor speak so honestly about medical gaslighting as I did when talking with Dr José Eugenio-Colón, a surgeon specialising in endometriosis excision at the Center for Endometriosis Care in Atlanta, Georgia. 'Doctors learn how to gaslight patients,' he admits. 'I had an attending doctor tell an endometriosis patient who was experiencing painful sex, "Sex can't hurt that bad and, if it does, get yourself a man with a smaller penis"... it's medical abuse.'

> ### Medical gaslighting
>
> Medical gaslighting occurs when a healthcare professional ignores, downplays or dismisses a patient's concerns, normalises them or questions their validity and severity. Alongside leading to diagnostic delays and the consequences of missed and misdiagnoses, medical gaslighting can lead to mental health impacts for the patient, making them question themselves or put off seeking (even emergency) medical help, and, in severe cases, causing post-traumatic stress disorder (PTSD).

Doctors themselves usually cite that the disease is complex, often presenting as other conditions and differently in each patient, making a diagnosis difficult. However, the issues run much deeper. The reality is, many doctors do not know what to look for because they do not understand endometriosis. This is particularly true when it comes to extra-pelvic, and extra-abdominopelvic, endometriosis (*see* pages 22–23). If you believe that endometriosis is a period condition, then of course you will put symptoms occurring outside of menstruation down to something else. Diaphragmatic endometriosis becomes costochondritis; bowel endo becomes IBS (*see* page 27). Endometriosis is, shockingly, not taught as a mandatory component of many medical school curricula. Those that do include it usually reduce it to a few slides in the gynaecology section. It is not nearly comprehensive enough for a disease that impacts as many people as it does. At the start of 2024, the University of Cambridge, regarded as one of the top medical schools in the world, had no formal endometriosis education as part of their medical curriculum. When I found out, I contacted them, and we set out to change that. I am proud to say that endometriosis is soon to be officially part of the curriculum for future doctors there – not just for gynaecologists, but for all specialisms. The next step is to encourage other medical schools to follow suit, because we need a fundamental change in education at every single touchpoint of the endometriosis pathway. Until that happens, diagnosis times will remain unacceptably high and doctors will continue to operate based on the outdated, handed-down information that keeps us in the dark.

So, how can we harness all this context about why there are diagnostic delays to our advantage? How can we use it to help us navigate the first hurdle of endometriosis care?

Educating yourself

The first step, in my opinion, is understanding that doctors generally are not misogynists, out to make our lives more difficult. There are so many cheaper, faster and easier ways to achieve this than putting themselves through medical school and all that entails. Doctors are operating with the information they have, within the guidelines of a system that works against patients and doctors alike. Of course, there are exceptions. Doctors are humans and have internalised (and sometimes not so internalised) biases, just like we all do (more on this in chapter 7). It sounds so basic, but understanding this perspective truly helped me navigate medical appointments and deal with medical gaslighting in a gentler way. I no longer question myself like I did for so many years; instead, I remind myself that the doctor probably doesn't have the level of knowledge and understanding required on this topic. I then either go back armed with guidelines and research or I find a new doctor.

The knock-on effect of realising that many doctors simply do not appreciate the complexities of endometriosis was understanding that I then had to. Luckily for me, my brain processes things by understanding them and educating myself. Even if you are not like that, if you have or think you have endometriosis, you are going to have to learn about the disease. A lot. It should not necessarily have to be that way, but sadly it is the best way to advocate for yourself and make sure you receive the best treatment. The great news is that you are reading this book, so you are already arming yourself with a level of information that will outstrip that of many in the medical profession.

Accessing information about endometriosis might seem easy. Over the last few years there has been a welcome increase in awareness about the disease. There are articles, celebrities talking about their own experiences in magazines, radio segments and mentions on TV, and as you scroll through social media you will more than likely encounter videos and posts explaining aspects of endometriosis. It is a favourite topic among doctors on social media, who know that it will garner high rates of engagement from a population starved of answers. The problem, and it is a big problem, is that not all of the content being produced is accurate. Endometriosis advocates spend hours each week emailing organisations, media outlets and social media accounts trying to correct misinformation. Sometimes, we will get a response from a receptive source who is willing to learn and update the piece. More often than not, however, we are ignored and the content enters the perpetuity of the internet, ready to be discovered by those starting out on their journey and looking to understand their symptoms and options.

Doctors are often quick to say, 'Be careful on the internet'. One surgeon even warned me that 'there's a lot of angry women on there, with a lot to say'. When doctors talk about the misinformation that persists when it comes to endometriosis, most of the time the first thing that they raise is social media. It's true that there is a lot of misinformation on platforms such as TikTok and Instagram, but there are also advocates and endometriosis experts reaching millions of people who have been let down by traditional sources. My challenge to any doctor who cites social media as the first problem is to ask why patients feel the need to turn to social media for their health literacy in the first place. Usually, it is due to a combination of medical gaslighting (*see* page 66) and misinformation coming from the medical institutions themselves.

It is infuriating to know how much misinformation exists, particularly from seemingly reputable sources such as the NHS, national charities and doctor-influencers, some with hundreds of thousands or even millions of followers. It makes it exceptionally difficult to say 'educate yourself' when the information out there is a minefield. The whole purpose of this book is to carefully bring everything that we currently know together.

But social media, used wisely, remains a fantastic resource. Mr Francesco Di Chiara, thoracic surgeon, even says it is the first place he would go if he was trying to understand the disease. 'It is the perfect way to understand context . . . and it can be updated instantly,' he tells me. A lot of the information currently presented by more traditional sources is outdated and has to go through a whole process to be updated and republished. On the other hand, social media can provide up-to-date information in a few minutes. I sometimes, only half-jokingly, say that 'social media saved my organs'. Because, while surgeons were telling me that my continuing pain was in my head, endometriosis advocates online pushed for me to seek a second, expert opinion. I might have lost both my kidneys had I listened to the original doctors.

How do you know if the content you are looking at is reliable and accurate?

Sadly, the answer is not as simple as looking for the doctor or account with the biggest number of followers. Here are some tips to keep in mind when educating yourself about endometriosis:

- Are there any red flags in their information? For example, do they state that endometriosis is the lining of the womb or that it acts like a mini period?
- Do they give sources for their statements?
- If so, are those sources trustworthy? Is it always the same people being cited? Is the research conducted rigorously?
- If they talk about 'new treatments' or 'new drugs', were double-blind randomised controlled studies undertaken? Were they human trials or mouse models (*see* page 257)? You can find this out in the methodology section of the research itself, or you can ask in the comments.
- Are they stating unknowns as 'facts'? For instance, are they saying that endometriosis is definitely caused by one process or another?
- Are they providing a balanced, nuanced view?
- Are they able to give further information when asked?
- Are they willing to discuss the topic and be open to learning and updating information?

Remember never to take medical advice from social media.

When it comes to looking at sources outside of social media, research papers can be interesting, but they may seem daunting and inaccessible if you are not used to reading and interpreting them. And let's be honest here, you shouldn't have to wade through scientific journals to the point where you should probably have an honorary PHD just to understand your diagnosis. I can't think of a single other condition where that would be expected. Thankfully, there are incredible sources of information out there, many of which I have listed at the back of this book. Endometriosis is so complex and nuanced, and we know nowhere near enough about it. And what we do know is not being filtered through to medical education and practice. The more we can understand, the better we can advocate for ourselves in medical settings and in our broader lives.

Symptom tracking

Part of educating ourselves is understanding what is going on with our own individual bodies. Knowledge of the disease mechanics is great, but knowing how they interact with your unique physiology is vital.

Symptom tracking helped me to finally get a GP to understand just how much endometriosis was ruining my life and kick-started my diagnosis process. The first thing I did was keep a diary and track everything. It wasn't anything fancy – I literally used my paper diary and a pen because none of the fancy apps that were on the market would 'recognise' my long cycle as valid (eye roll). When I tried to input a cycle length as 74 days into one app, there was a pop-up saying it was 'incorrect'.

There are other things to consider when it comes to your choice of tracking method too. Your data is valuable, and that includes your reproductive and health data. Imagine how much a company that sells products would love that data to target the right adverts to you at exactly the right time. About to start your period? Here are adverts for period products, chocolate, comfy clothing and pain relief methods. Trying to conceive? Here are products or supplements designed to help you with that. There is even a research paper that goes into how consumer behaviour is influenced by our hormonal cycle. It declares that during ovulation, the peak fertility time, 'women nonconsciously choose products that enhance appearance (e.g. choosing sexy rather than more conservative clothing) . . . driven by a desire to outdo attractive rival women.' So, knowing that you are ovulating, marketers could start sending you adverts for red lipstick, high heels, tight clothing and anything else that apparently makes us 'sexy'. If it sounds ridiculous, that's because it is. However, it goes to show just how many companies could be interested in your reproductive data – and, terrifyingly, it goes far beyond shopping choices.

In a world that seeks to heavily control the reproductive rights of women, the security of that data is paramount. In 2022, users in the USA deleted

Dealing with the system – how to get help

period tracking apps in droves after Roe *v* Wade (which guaranteed women the right to an abortion up until the point of foetal viability, approximately 24 weeks) was overturned by the Supreme Court. This removal of choice gave rise to concerns that the menstrual cycle data held by those apps could be used to prosecute women. In 2023, the Information Commissioner's Office (ICO) in the UK announced that it was conducting a review of period tracking apps to understand how they process and protect users' data. In 2024, the ICO released a statement saying, 'We haven't found any evidence these apps are using . . . data in a way that could cause . . . harm. However, our review has highlighted there are improvements app developers could make to ensure they are meeting all their obligations to be transparent with their users and keep their data safe.' As a result, many of us remain nervous about data security, which goes beyond an app sharing your information with companies or the state. It also refers to who could physically access the app and the information within it, something that could be incredibly dangerous in a relationship involving domestic violence or in cultures where there are very strict ideas about female autonomy and reproductive freedoms. A 2024 study by researchers at University College London and King's College London backs these concerns. Dr Ruba Abu-Salma, one of the study's authors, explains that, 'while female health apps are vital to the management of women's health worldwide, their benefits are currently being undermined by privacy and safety issues. Mismanaging or leaking reproductive health data can lead to dire consequences, with blackmail, discrimination, and violence being among the worst.'

It is entirely up to you whether you choose to track your symptoms using a specialist app, a wearable device, your phone calendar or pen and paper. However, it is important that you are confident in the security of any app or source to which you add this data. Make sure you read those terms and conditions that we all, let's be honest, so casually agree to. Important factors to look out for are as follows:

- Your data is stored safely and securely – encrypted, stored locally and password protected. Just saying that your data is kept safe and not sold is not enough. These agreements can be changed. The data must be encrypted to be truly safe as this means the company itself cannot access your data to share it with others.
- Data is not shareable with third parties or law enforcement.

- It is easy and quick to delete your information.
- No unnecessary data is tracked without your knowledge; this could include your location or your camera and microphone.

What to track

Once you have chosen your method of symptom tracking, it is time to actually track. When I was tracking my symptoms, I wrote down every single one that I was experiencing, whether or not I thought it was related (I had no idea back then just how much of what I was going through was connected to endometriosis). Provide your doctor with as much data as you possibly can. Note down things like the following:

- Type of symptom
- Location
- Intensity
- Sensation – what does it feel like?
- Duration
- Triggers – what makes it worse?
- What eases it?
- Timing – is it cyclical? Constant? At certain times of the day?
- What impact does it have on you and your life?

To give you an example, this is lifted from my symptom diary, written on 9 November, 2021:

Severe pain in my pelvis. It feels like someone has put electric cake beaters inside me, turned them up to max and they're scraping the insides of my pelvis with them. On top of that it feels like someone is ramming a blade into my hip socket and twisting it. It's pretty constant now, always there but the intensity can suddenly increase. Pain level 9. No pain meds are helping. Completely debilitates me. I can't do anything.

Be as descriptive as possible. Try not to say generic things like 'my stomach hurts'. Really paint a picture of the type of pain you are feeling. I used to really struggle with this, so I came up with a glossary of terms I could refer to. Providing myself with the language to communicate really helped me articulate what I was going through, not just with my doctors but with my husband too. He understood 'I feel like I am being repeatedly stabbed and clawed in the uterus' much more than 'My period is so painful'. If you are struggling to describe your pain, here are some common ways to describe endometriosis pain:

- Stabbing
- Burning
- Electrocuting
- Ripping
- Pulling
- Radiating
- Twisting
- Cutting
- Exploding
- Drilling
- Bruised
- Barbed wire
- Battery acid
- Gunshot
- Heavy
- Scraping
- Clawing monster

Rating your level of pain

A lot of us struggle when it comes to rating the severity of our pain. I know that I certainly used to have no idea what to say when asked to rate my pain on a scale of 0–10, so I used to just pull any number out, usually between 5 and 7, without any understanding of what that number meant. There are so many issues with asking people to rank their pain in this way. First, I'm pretty confident in saying that most patients aren't actually sat down and told what each number represents. Second, pain is so subjective, and if we are not educated on what the numbers mean, their helpfulness is called into question somewhat. Finally, the usefulness to the endometriosis community is even more questionable. Endometriosis pain (type and intensity) can vary dramatically hour to hour, let alone day to day, and we are also far more likely to downplay and normalise our pain thanks to being expected to put up with it and having our experiences questioned for decades. There have been numerous attempts to simplify the scales or adapt them for chronic illness patients who do not quite 'fit' into the traditional scales. That said, the majority of the medical profession still uses the 0–10 scale (*see* Table 2.1), and you will likely be asked along your endometriosis journey to give your pain a number.

Table 2.1: The Mankoski Pain Scale

Number	Description
0	No pain.
1	Very minor annoyance – occasional minor twinges. No medication needed.
2	Minor annoyance – occasional strong twinges. No medication needed.
3	Annoying enough to be distracting. Mild painkillers are effective (ibuprofen/paracetamol).
4	Can be ignored if really involved in work but still distracting. Mild painkillers relieve pain for three to four hours.
5	Cannot be ignored for more than 30 minutes. Mild painkillers reduce pain for three to four hours.
6	Cannot be ignored for any length of time, but you can still go to work and/or participate in social activities. Stronger painkillers (codeine) reduce pain for three to four hours.
7	Difficult to concentrate, interferes with sleep. Can still function with effort. Stronger painkillers only partially effective. Strongest painkillers (morphine) relieve pain.
8	Physical activity severely limited. Can read and converse with effort. Nausea and dizziness set in as factors of pain. Stronger painkillers have minimal effect. Strongest painkillers reduce pain for three to four hours.
9	Unable to speak. Crying out or moaning uncontrollably – near delirium. Strongest painkillers only partially effective.
10	Unconscious. Pain makes you pass out. Strongest painkillers only partially effective.

This scale is not a perfect system. Those of us suffering from conditions that cause long-term pain, like endometriosis, are able to operate differently from someone without chronic illness at the same pain rating. Why? Because we have had to. But understanding the pain scale has allowed me to realise that currently:

- My best days are a level 6.
- My average days are level 7–8.
- My bad days are level 9.

- And during my flares I experience level 10.
- I cannot remember a time when my pain was less than a 6.

Having this knowledge allows me to 'speak the same language' as my medical team and to far more accurately articulate what I experience. I'll be honest, I still get looked at and asked, 'Really?! Are you sure?! You don't look like you're in that much pain.' Before I understood the pain scale, I might have said, 'Oh, maybe not; maybe it's a 4 then.' At least now I am absolutely confident in my answers when asked for a number. It can also be hugely helpful to use the pain scale to explain to your loved ones how you are feeling at any given point.

If you are more of a visual person, it can be helpful to create pain maps. This is where you illustrate exactly where you are feeling pain, using colour or shading to signify different types and intensities. You end up with a heat map of your body that can be really useful to explain your pain. I found this particular way of tracking really helpful for noticing cyclical patterns, especially ones that I did not realise were connected. For example, I knew I suffered with chest pain. I have for years. Ambulances have been called, electrocardiograms (ECGs) undertaken, scans performed. The result is usually 'nothing to worry about; probably just stress' or 'costochondritis' (*see* page 32). When I started doing these pain maps, I noticed that the chest pain was always in the same spot and always occurred in the run-up to my period. I brought it up with my endometriosis specialist, and investigations for thoracic endometriosis began. You can find templates for the outlines of the human body, front and back, for free online.

Advocating for yourself during appointments

In an ideal world, you would experience a symptom and visit your GP, who would listen, believe you, assess you and refer you on to the appropriate specialist for treatment. Unfortunately, as we have seen, this does not happen very often when it comes to endometriosis. Many of us stumble at this first hurdle and are sent away with a prescription for the contraceptive pill, a misdiagnosis or even nothing at all. Learning how to advocate for yourself in these appointments is a huge part of making sure you are receiving the right treatment and are being heard. So, you have educated yourself on endometriosis, you have tracked your symptoms and have lots of data and patterns to show your doctor, but what do you do in the appointment itself?

Endometriosis

For years I would attend GP appointments and say, 'I have exceptionally painful and heavy periods'. That immediately put into the mind of the doctor that I was there to discuss periods. Now, I advise people not to do that. Instead, say, 'I would like to discuss the endometriosis symptoms that I've been experiencing'. Reframe the conversation away from 'just a bad period' right from the start.

Take your data. Make sure you bring any information you have tracked with you and show it to your doctor. I used to feel so embarrassed doing this, worried the doctor would roll their eyes and think I was being 'too dramatic'. However, Dr Nighat Arif, women's health GP and advocate, empathically tells me otherwise: 'I love it when patients bring their data in! We only get a certain amount of time together, so it is incredibly helpful to have all of that background knowledge and get a real snapshot of the issue.'

Have someone accompany you to your appointments if possible. This can be helpful in so many different ways. They can simply be a silent supporter, they can remind you of things you want to bring up, they can take notes for you and they can speak up and advocate for you if you feel you are not being listened to. Whoever the person is, make sure that you communicate clearly with them before the appointment which role you would like them to play. It is sad to say, but sometimes it can be very helpful if the person accompanying you is a man. I have noticed an enormous difference when my husband is in the room rather than just me, and this is an experience echoed around the world.

Keep as detailed records as possible. You can take notes or record appointments. Sign up to the NHS app, MyChart, so that you can access your medical records and results, and always ask for copies of scans, reports, photos and so on. I know that medical admin is a nightmare and can feel like a full-time job in itself, but keeping on top of your records is an important part of advocating for yourself and your body. If a doctor declines to refer you or offer a particular treatment, ask them to put a note on your record saying that they are refusing. Sometimes this in itself is enough for them to change their mind, but either way it should be noted.

Before you leave your appointment, make sure you ask what the plan is now. If there is nothing more the GP (for example) can do, then to whom and where will they be referring you? When should you book a follow-up appointment to chat about progress and how you are getting on? Pin the

Dealing with the system – how to get help

doctor down for next steps to keep the conversation going and make sure you are not just sent off with no support.

What then happens if you have educated yourself about endometriosis, tracked your symptoms and advocated for yourself during the appointment, and the doctor still tries to tell you your symptoms are normal? First, remind yourself that your pain is valid and deserves to be investigated. Do not internalise the dismissal and start questioning your own experience. Next, find another doctor. Ask for second, third, fourth opinions – however many it takes to find out what is causing your pain. Dr Aziza Sesay, GP and women's health campaigner, explains to me that a good tip is to ask your practice which doctor has a special interest in endometriosis or women's health and then ask to see them. 'It doesn't mean that they're an expert, but it does mean that they at least have an interest in these areas and issues such as endometriosis are more likely to be on their radar.'

Living with endometriosis is exhausting in so many ways. Fighting to be heard and believed is an experience that so many patients share, but it is important to keep going.

NICE guidelines

It is impossible for a single doctor to know everything about every condition, especially a GP or primary care provider who may see any number of conditions within a single day. In the UK, there is a body called NICE whose responsibility is to establish care pathways for individual conditions and presentations, which are then used by clinicians to support patients in getting diagnoses and treatment. They are also used by medical schools to set curricula for future doctors, by policy makers and by research bodies.

They can also be used by patients to advocate for themselves during medical appointments. The NICE guidelines for endometriosis were updated in November 2024 and, while they are far from perfect, they can be used as a tool when you come up against any resistance from healthcare providers. For example, the guidelines are very clear that doctors are not to 'exclude the possibility of endometriosis if the abdominal or pelvic examination and ultrasound scan are normal and recognise that referral may still be necessary even with a normal scan' – something that has long been a stumbling block for receiving an endometriosis diagnosis. If your doctor is telling you that your scan is clear and therefore you cannot have endometriosis, as mine did, you can bring up the NICE guidelines and request further investigation and referral.

Again, these guidelines are not perfect, and a lot of changes need to be incorporated to bring them in line with the latest disease knowledge, but they are the framework that our medical system uses. It is therefore important that we understand them and use them to our advantage where we can. I highly recommend reading through the guidelines and using them if you need a little extra power in your corner. You can even print them out and take them with you if needed. There is a link to them in the Resources section of this book.

Medical imaging for endometriosis

I will never forget the day in November 2021 when a GP finally said to me, 'Hmm, yes, it does sound like endometriosis could be present – let's investigate'. It was the first time in 22 years that I moved past the hurdle of even being taken seriously, and it kick-started a succession of scans, tests and, ultimately, surgery. Hopefully, this section will help you navigate this part of your own endometriosis journey and understand how to overcome any barriers that may come up along the way.

The first step was the GP asking about my symptoms and the effects they had on my life. I had begun tracking my symptoms by this point, so this was simple and I was able to provide detailed information. The GP also asked if there was a family history, which I was able to confirm. As my appointment happened over the phone during the pandemic, I did not have a physical exam at this point, but you may find that your doctor performs one at this stage.

I was then sent for imaging. At some point in your endo journey, you will encounter at least one type of medical imaging. The most common are the following:

- Abdominal ultrasound (external), where a handheld scanner is used on your skin

Dealing with the system – how to get help

- Transvaginal ultrasound (internal), where a handheld scanner is inserted vaginally
- MRI, where you lie down and move into a tube-like scanner that uses strong magnetic fields and radio waves to produce a detailed picture. They are painless, but noisy! You will be given ear protection and will always be able to communicate with the person performing the scan. Your consultant may also ask you to have a contrast dye or muscle relaxant added through a cannula to increase the chances of spotting endometriosis.

Ultrasound

The first step is usually ultrasound. This is a scan that uses high-frequency sound waves to create an image of the inside of the body. An abdominal ultrasound is done non-invasively, with the scanner outside your body on the surface of your skin, but it may not show as much detail and should not be the only imaging offered to you. A transvaginal ultrasound, where a narrow gel-covered probe is inserted into the vagina, is able to provide a better view of the pelvic anatomy.

Transvaginal ultrasounds

There is a stubborn myth that sadly persists that having a transvaginal ultrasound is akin to sexual penetration. Heartbreakingly, this results in some women being denied access to this imaging, particularly if they are young or in cultures where virginity is equated with an individual's value.

For the avoidance of any doubt, a transvaginal ultrasound is a medical procedure that has nothing to do with virginity. If your doctor is refusing you a transvaginal ultrasound, you can ask for a second opinion or for a referral for an MRI. Likewise, if you find transvaginal ultrasounds too painful, or if it is not a procedure you are comfortable undertaking, then push for an MRI scan instead.

If you are having a transvaginal scan and find it uncomfortable or painful, please let the sonographer know.

There is a lot of discussion about ultrasounds and their usefulness in detecting endometriosis. As with most things to do with this disease, the relationship is complicated. We hear from patients time and time again that their ultrasounds came back as 'clear' or 'normal', but then they go on to have surgery where extensive endometriosis is discovered. This was certainly the experience I faced. I was told, 'There is no sign of endometriosis on your ultrasound, so no further action is needed'. Fast forward five months and I was in surgery having superficial, deep and ovarian endometriosis removed (*see* page 15). This is far from an unusual experience. So, what is going on? Is endometriosis undetectable by imaging? Or is it not being detected by those operating and reading the scans? The truth is a mixture of both.

Specialised skills are required when it comes to medical imaging. Specialist endometriosis sonographers are needed to both perform the scan and read the images, which will give a much higher likelihood of detecting any existing disease and its effects. Some endometriosis clinics do have specialist endometriosis imaging staff, but not all. We desperately need to train more sonographers in how to spot the signs of endometriosis and how to sensitively perform the scans to maximise the chance of disease detection. Someone who is passionate about driving this is Dr Wendaline VanBuren, a radiologist who is a specialist in endometriosis imaging. 'Endometriosis can be detected by imaging, but it is complex,' she explains when we talk. 'Endometriosis has several different manifestations and understanding these different presentations and how they can be perceived on imaging is critical. Provided that we have:

- Dedicated protocols for endometriosis detection by both ultrasound and MRI
- Individuals trained in the expert interpretation of the images

then we are able to see endometriomas and deep disease with very high levels of confidence.'

When it comes to SPE (*see* page 15), also known as peritoneal disease, the story gets trickier. These deposits are often not visible on medical imaging, despite being the most prevalent form of the disease. The result, as Dr VanBuren tells me, is that 'the vast majority of endometriosis patients are not being diagnosed by imaging'. Dr VanBuren believes that, when it comes to the difficulties with detecting superficial disease, this is due to the technical limitations of current technologies; however, she confirms that, with the right operator, 'we are able to diagnose the most severe and most complex types of endometriosis'.

Dealing with the system – how to get help

But, why are so many patients, even those with deep or ovarian endometriosis, still being told that their scans are 'normal'? 'It comes down to the lack of uniformity in imaging protocols and appropriate education for disease detection,' Dr VanBuren explains. The lack of consistency means that sometimes the procedure itself, the interpretation of the findings or even both may not be up to the standards required for such a complex disease. This can result in even deep disease, endometriomas or other key indicators, such as kissing ovaries, being missed. During endometriosis awareness month in 2024, I was asked to be part of a webinar for the British Society for Gynaecological Endoscopy (BSGE). A fellow panellist, consultant gynaecologist and ultrasound specialist, Dr Susanne Johnson, aka Gynaecology Ultrasound on YouTube, summed it up perfectly, 'If you don't know what you're looking for, you're not going to find it.'

Kissing ovaries

'Kissing ovaries' are a distortion of normal anatomy, where the ovaries are pulled behind your uterus, thanks to endometriosis and/or adhesions. The ovaries can then either partly or completely touch, or 'kiss' each other. It can be spotted on scans and is strongly associated with moderate to severe endometriosis. They are usually an indicator that deep pelvic endometriosis is present although not everyone who has deep endometriosis will develop them. Studies suggest that in cases of 'kissing ovaries', the chances of having stage IV endometriosis are eight times higher than in cases where the ovaries are in their 'usual' position.

Kissing ovaries are not only linked to disease severity, but also to fertility issues and increased pain. Not as romantic as the name would suggest, hey?

However, even in a perfect environment, Dr VanBuren stresses throughout our entire conversation that if a scan is read as 'normal', this should never mean the investigations stop there. 'A "normal" scan would never rule out the disease; you may still have superficial disease which cannot be detected even with expert interpretation. It can infer a statement about disease complexity but can never rule out disease.' Even MRIs, which 'can detect additional disease sites that an ultrasound did not pick up', may not highlight all disease, particularly if there is not 'blood vessel involvement' in those particular areas.

If your ultrasound comes back clear, *do not let your doctors tell you that you therefore do not have endometriosis*. The absence of evidence is not evidence of absence. Push for referral to an endometriosis specialist centre (*see* pages 111–113) for further investigation.

The different types of endometriosis (*see* pages 15–18), the limitations in current technology and the gaps in education mean that expert surgery remains the only definitive way to diagnose endometriosis and assess its full extent. However, imaging remains a key part of the endometriosis pathway and improving its application should be a priority. If we could achieve Dr VanBuren's ideal scenario of dedicated imaging protocols and expert interpretation, these techniques could achieve the following:

- Identify the involvement of and risks to organs
- Monitor disease progression or persistence
- Aid fertility planning
- Map disease for surgical planning (MRI scans)
- In some cases, diagnose endometriosis without the need for a diagnostic-only surgery
- Reduce the diagnostic delay, allowing earlier detection and intervention

Symptom management

Once endometriosis is suspected and you have been placed on a waiting list for imaging and/or a referral to an endometriosis centre (more on these on pages 111–113), your doctor will look at managing your symptoms. There are a few ways to do this, but remember that all of these methods are for symptom management only. There is no cure, but there are ways to deal with the effects of endometriosis. If a doctor is telling you that any of the below is a cure, this is a red flag and you should seek another opinion because they do not understand the disease.

That does not mean you should not try any of the below methods if you would like to. We all know how much we desperately need relief, but we should absolutely know the pros, the cons and the limitations of all the options. Informed consent is key. All options should be discussed in detail with you by your clinician, and they should then ask you what your preferences are based on your goals and quality of life. A plan should then be devised based on all of this, with emphasis on your choice. Usually, clinicians advise giving treatment a set amount of time to assess how it is working, but if you have any concerns within that time frame, please seek medical advice.

As we've seen, endometriosis has a wide range of symptoms that vary in type, location and intensity for each patient. This means treatment options need to be equally tailored and individualised. This section will look at some of the major symptoms, but please remember that if you are struggling with any other symptoms, seek advice from your doctor.

Medical options

Broadly speaking, medical interventions for endometriosis fall into two camps: non-hormonal and hormonal.

Non-hormonal options

Pain is the most common endometriosis symptom, so one of the first options offered to patients is pain relief. This typically includes the following:

- Over-the-counter medication, such as paracetamol or ibuprofen
- Prescription non-steroidal anti-inflammatory drugs (NSAIDs), such as diclofenac, naproxen or mefenamic acid
- Prescription opiates – stronger analgesics such as codeine, morphine or tramadol

NSAIDs can be extremely helpful in reducing inflammation – an environment in which we know endometriosis thrives. However, sometimes they are not enough and opiate-based pain relief is also required. You could also be one of the unfortunate ones who cannot take NSAIDs, maybe due to pregnancy, allergies or other conditions, (welcome to the club!) and therefore have to rely on other methods of pain relief. Opiates come with their own issues, particularly with long-term use. Side effects such as constipation, nausea, vomiting, fatigue and dizziness can exacerbate the already-present issues associated with endometriosis. On top of that, opiates also carry the potential for your body to develop a tolerance to the medication, where you start needing higher doses to offer the same level of pain relief, and are known to be highly addictive.

If you are suffering from heavy and/or prolonged periods, your doctor may offer you a medication to help reduce bleeding, such as tranexamic acid. Tranexamic acid is an anti-fibrinolytic drug, which means it works by inhibiting the process that dissolves clots, reducing blood loss. It is usually taken three to four times per day while on your period, but your doctor may advise you to take it for longer depending on your situation. It is not unusual to experience iron deficiency if you suffer with heavy bleeding. Your doctor should run tests to check your levels. If appropriate, options include iron tablets or even infusions to help manage your symptoms.

Many of us struggle with nausea. Whether that is caused by the endometriosis, another condition such as adenomyosis (*see* chapter 4), a side effect of medication or the by-product of living in pain, there are things that can help with nausea. Drugs such as cyclizine hydrochloride, a type of antihistamine, might be suggested. I've personally had great results for what had become debilitating nausea with this medication, but, as with any treatment, it is not suitable for everyone so make sure you chat with your doctor about the best option for you.

Hormonal options
Before we dive into the hormonal options that might be offered to you, we need to clear up some misconceptions. Hormones and their role in endometriosis management are the source of most of the conflicting information swirling around this disease and can lead to a lot of confusion and distress among patients.

No hormonal intervention can reduce, reverse, slow the development of or cure endometriosis lesions. There is some evidence coming through that hormonal medication may be able to reduce endometriomas (haemorrhagic cysts in the ovaries), but this is not true of superficial or deep disease. Where did this confusion come from? It goes back to our old friend, the myth of endometriosis as a period and uterine condition. If we misguidedly accept that endometriosis is a menstrual condition, then of course it follows that tweaking or stopping the menstrual cycle will also stop the disease. This then leads to the notion that menopause (natural or chemical) will cure the disease, or even that the complete removal of the womb, a hysterectomy, is a cure. Sadly, this is still promoted in clinics today.

Alongside the belief that endometriosis is structurally the same as the endometrium comes the belief that tinkering with the sex hormones and reproductive organs can cure the disease. However, as we have learned, endometriosis creates its own oestrogen anyway, so stopping the hormonal cycle, through whatever method, *will not stop disease progression*. On top of that, we all have slightly different hormone receptors, so there is no guarantee that how one patient reacts will be the same for another. Some of us experience symptom relief with hormonal treatment and can regain our quality of life. For others, it has no effect. Others still suffer greatly with side effects, which can range from weight gain and migraines to depression, mood changes and even suicidal thoughts. The key thing to remember is that none of these hormonal treatments is a cure, none will stop superficial or deep disease progression and we are all completely unique.

There are numerous hormonal options available that may help your symptoms. Each has pros and cons. Let's look at three different types: combined hormonal treatments, progestin-only treatments and gonadotrophin-releasing hormone (GnRH) treatments.

Combined hormonal treatments

Combined hormonal treatments contain synthetic forms of two hormones: oestrogen and progestin (the synthetic form of progesterone). They work by inhibiting follicular-stimulating hormone (FSH) and luteinising hormone (LH) and, therefore, ovulation. The most common types are the combined contraceptive pill or the contraceptive patch. These methods usually have a 'withdrawal bleed' (simulating a period), but they can also be taken continuously. The aim is to reduce the pain associated with menstruation. They can be successful for many patients, but can also come with significant side effects, including headaches, nausea, mood changes, weight gain, bloating and skin changes.

Progestin-only treatments

Progestin-only treatments are another option and include the mini pill, Provera, Depo injections, the contraceptive implant and, as many of us will encounter on our endo journeys, the Mirena coil, an IUD. An IUD is inserted into the uterus and provides progestin locally, working to inhibit ovulation. This local application means that it is usually considered to provoke fewer, and less severe, side effects than other hormonal interventions, but again, this depends on the person. As with combined hormonal treatments, for some people this method of symptom management has worked incredibly well and given them back their life. For others, it can be ineffective or come with mild, moderate or severe side effects.

Inserting and removing IUDs – managing pain

It is important to include a note here on the insertion and removal of IUDs, which can sometimes be extremely painful, particularly if you have a condition such as endometriosis or adenomyosis. I am not saying this to try to scare anyone out of having an IUD for symptom management but to make sure you know that those who perform these procedures are often not aware of just how painful they can be if you have endometriosis.

The Faculty of Sexual and Reproductive Healthcare provides guidelines and recommendations for pain relief for IUD fittings. Key points to be aware of are as follows:

- Experiences are different for everyone. Pain can range from none to severe and clinicians may underestimate a patient's pain and anxiety.
- Clinicians should support patients and let them know they can pause or stop if the pain is too much.
- There should be an assistant in the room to monitor the patient for signs of pain and distress and to keep them comfortable and distracted.
- Pain relief options should be discussed and offered to all patients.
- Pain relief should be proportionate. Options could be local anaesthetic injections, spray or gel containing lidocaine or even general anaesthetic.
- If the clinic performing the insertion or removal cannot provide sufficient pain relief, the patient should be referred elsewhere.

For some reason, despite this guidance, patients often undergo IUD insertion or removal without any anaesthesia or even an offer of pain relief. Recently, a friend who nearly passed out during the insertion was told to 'just go home and have a cup of tea; you'll be fine'. You do not have to persevere through pain. You might be interested to know that a male counterpart to the IUD, ADAM, is currently undergoing human trials as a male contraceptive. Despite being inserted during a 'quick, minimally invasive procedure', it has already been approved for local anaesthesia. And you'll be pleased to hear that ADAM works 'without affecting sensation or ejaculation'. Couldn't have that male pleasure impacted now, could we?!

Just know that if you are one of the people who find IUD procedures painful, you are not weak and it is not in your head. You are fully entitled to adequate pain relief – if it is not offered, ask for it. If your clinic does not have the facilities to provide the level of pain relief you request, you can ask to be referred elsewhere. Remember that each person's experience will be different, so do what is right for you and try not to compare yourself with others. And, as always, remember that an IUD cannot reduce or cure endometriosis, but it may provide symptom relief and allow you to reclaim some quality of life.

GnRH analogues

GnRH analogues induce a chemical menopause in the patient by effectively switching off the ovaries and preventing oestrogen production. They include drugs such as Zoladex, Lupron and Prostap and are primarily given as (one-off or monthly) injections or tablets. Again, these drugs are not cures. When they were first introduced, the manufacturers used to state that they reduced disease. But they have retracted this, now stating clearly that they only 'treat the symptoms associated with endometriosis' or aid 'management of endometriosis'. It is infuriating that two of the largest producers of these medications still boldly and confidently have the basic facts about endometriosis wrong on their websites. There are references to endometriosis as 'lining tissue' (i.e. endometrium), and stating that 'the tissue that has grown outside of the uterus responds the same as the tissue inside.' That is a fight for another day. The important thing to note here is that even they do not claim to cure, reduce or prevent the growth of the disease.

In the UK, the NICE guidelines (*see* pages 77–78) mention GnRH analogues and they are widely used. That said, experts such as Mr Shaheen Khazali are strongly against their use. Mr Khazali tells me when we speak that he 'very rarely, almost never' uses them. Why? In his opinion, they 'should never have been included in the guidelines' as there is no robust evidence that 'they do anything positive for the patient'. The use of GnRH analogues 'may even be harmful' for the patient, he continues, although he stresses that this is also yet to be definitively proven. However, he says, there are some early indications that may 'suggest that levels of ovarian function may not come back to normal following the use of GnRH analogues'. This lack of conclusive evidence either way, coupled with the suggestion of potential longer-term fertility effects, is enough 'to put a question mark in my mind and it's enough for my patients to be worried about it'. There is always a grey area, and in some rare cases Mr Khazali will still use these drugs in limited circumstances, but 'as a blanket policy, I do not agree that we should be using GnRH analogues.'

Mr Khazali acknowledges that this is an area where his clinical practice deviates from the guidelines, but he believes there is a drawback in how the guidelines are established. Guidelines are often based on data from randomised controlled trials. This is the gold standard in clinical trials, designed to give the most accurate findings on which to base recommendations. However, which trials get funding and by whom is a highly political process. Creating guidelines based on these limited studies neglects the wealth of knowledge, particularly regarding long-term positive patient outcomes, that exists within endometriosis specialist centres (*see* pages 111–113).

These medications are absolutely not a long-term solution due to the side effects and other risks associated with the prolonged use of GnRH analogues, such as the well documented risk to bone density and potential for osteoporosis. As these drugs place the patient in a chemically induced menopause, hormone replacement therapy (HRT) should be provided to help mitigate some of the associated risks, which include menopausal symptoms but also longer-term issues such as reduced bone mass, osteoporosis and fertility impacts. As Mr Khazali explains, the balance between the potential benefits of these drugs and the risks that come with them 'does not lean towards the benefit'.

Your doctor may suggest a course of GnRH analogues while you wait for surgery to help with your symptoms. It is entirely your choice but there are some things to bear in mind:

- These are very strong medications that come with some serious potential side effects. Make sure you are fully informed and know what these are and what to expect.
- They should only ever be taken in the short term.
- Why is your surgeon suggesting them? If it is to improve your quality of life while you wait for surgery, that is one thing. If they are saying you *must* take them before they will operate, this is a red flag.
- Short-term GnRH analogue use is part of the process if you are undergoing egg retrieval prior to surgery, for example if you are undergoing IVF or having an oophorectomy (surgery to remove one or both ovaries) as part of your procedure owing to severe ovarian disease.

Dealing with the system – how to get help

There is some controversy surrounding the use of GnRH analogues before surgery, with many of the global experts I spoke to for this book saying they can lead to missed disease and an increased chance of repeat surgeries. We know that any hormonal intervention, including GnRH analogues, cannot shrink, remove or 'clean up' (as is often heard) endometriosis lesions, but they can reduce the inflammation caused by hormonal fluctuations in the cycle, which is why they provide symptomatic relief for some patients. However, removing this driver of inflammation can, frustratingly, make the disease more difficult to identify during surgery. This makes the surgeon's job harder, leading to missed disease if the surgeon is not fully trained in what to look for. Unless your surgeon is a highly specialised endometriosis expert, they are unlikely to have the level of skill required to ensure complete excision of all disease.

Some surgeons are known to recommend hormonal medication after surgery to 'clear up' anything left over. This is another major red flag for multiple reasons – it means the surgeon is not confident that all the disease was removed, and it shows that they do not understand the mechanics of endometriosis. No drug will 'mop up' any lesions that are left behind. They can, however, help to reduce period pain and related symptoms. That is an entirely different discussion, and it is up to you whether you would like to pursue it.

For some patients, hormonal medications are a lifeline when it comes to dealing with endometriosis-associated symptoms, but, as we've explored, others suffer with terrible side effects and cannot tolerate these options. Decisions need to be made on a case-by-case basis – we patients are all unique, and our treatment plans should be individualised too. The most important thing is informed consent and shared decision-making. Your doctor should take the time to explain all the options to you, including all risks and limitations. Only then can you make the best decision for you and your body. If you do decide to try hormonal options, then there should also be a follow-up plan in place, to see how you are getting on, discuss any side effects and adjust course if necessary. Ask your doctor as many questions as you need to. You are not being difficult; you are advocating for your health and your future.

Hormonal interventions and their relationship with endometriosis are a contentious area. Many patients are very happy with the symptom management that they provide, while others suffer with side effects that they either cannot tolerate or that they just put up with in order to gain some reduction in their pain or other symptoms. The biggest concern is patients not being given full and accurate information about the risks and limitations of hormonal options when it comes to endometriosis management. Many of us are still being told that these drugs will halt, reduce or even eliminate disease because that is what doctors are still being taught, either at medical school or when training in gynaecology departments. Others, myself included, are put on hormonal medication and told nothing. The result is that disease progression is allowed to happen unchecked, hidden by the suppression of the most severe symptoms. We are still being put on these drugs, sometimes at incredibly young ages, and left to get on with things. The long-term effects of this approach are not fully understood yet, but recent research indicates that there could be lasting impacts on androgen (sex hormone) receptors, bone density and brain structure, function and connectivity, and that these effects may not reverse once the pill is stopped, as was once thought. More research is urgently needed to confirm the type and longevity of these changes, but research looking at this aspect of hormonal medication, or the development of alternatives, is sadly rare. Instead, hormonal medication is very big business, projected to grow to US $37.22 billion by 2032, and research often looks at the more profitable aspects of healthcare.

Education about the interaction between these drugs and endometriosis needs updating urgently, otherwise this cycle (pardon the pun) will never be broken.

Rebound endometriosis

This is a very new term, introduced by Dr Andea Vidali, MD, an endometriosis specialist surgeon in New York. According to Dr Vidali, Rebound endometriosis is a 'dramatic worsening of endometriosis symptoms or the appearance of new lesions following the cessation of oral contraceptives, other hormonal suppression treatments or pregnancy.' As the body's natural hormonal cycle and ovulation resumes, the hormonal surges are thought to intensify the symptoms felt by the patient. Dr Vidali also believes rebound endometriosis can be seen in endometriosis patients who have miscarried or suffered pregnancy loss, and who then report significantly higher pain levels.

Its existence as a pattern 'highlights the need for greater awareness and research into the complex interplay between hormonal regulation and endometriosis, and the importance of ensuring patients are better prepared and supported when transitioning off hormonal therapies, post-partum or following miscarriage'.

When I heard the term 'rebound endometriosis' for the first time, something clicked inside my brain. I finally had the terminology to describe what happened when I came off the pill after 22 years. I normally describe it as feeling like I'd been hit like a truck. Within three cycles I was unrecognisable, bedbound from pain almost every day, burning my skin with hot-water bottles, being sick and passing out. And it's a pattern I see in so many of us when I listen to others' stories. While rebound endometriosis is still very much just a concept, it is one that I hope sparks research and provides evidence-based validation to the experiences that we have been suffering with for decades.

Exacerbated Endometriosis is a similar but different concept, also suggested by Dr Vidali. This is where pre-existing endometriosis becomes more aggressive, symptomatic or expansive in response to external factors like the hormonal stimulation during IVF. This is likely linked to the elevated oestrogen levels and inflammatory responses during IVF, which can fuel the activity of endometriosis lesions. Natalie, an endometriosis patient whose story I shared on pages 57–58, can definitely relate to this concept, describing her 'endo going bonkers' after five rounds of IVF treatment. Dr Vidali says that this does not mean we should not be providing IVF for those who need it, but it is again something to be aware of and provide support for.

Lifestyle and home-based methods

Medical interventions are not the only ways in which we can manage endometriosis symptoms; there are methods we can try ourselves at home. Now, I know from my own experience that when I first heard the words 'holistic methods' or 'lifestyle methods', I rolled my eyes – hard. After decades of being told 'try yoga', 'eat this food', 'avoid this food', 'have more sex', 'have less sex' and even 'try drinking celery juice' (yes, really), I was cynical about anything that wasn't 'medical' in nature. However, these symptom management options are not to be dismissed. If you think about it, endometriosis is a full-body disease, so it makes sense that symptom management should also be holistic, looking at the whole picture.

These methods are not cures. They will not shrink the disease, reverse it or prevent it from progressing. However, for many of us endometriosis sufferers, they are what help us get through the day, living with this disease as best we can. They can help us better manage flares, daily life and the wait until diagnosis or surgery. But there is no silver bullet when it comes to symptom management. I wish that I could wave a magic wand and write out a list of things that will work for everyone, but the reality is that not all of these options will be appropriate or accessible to everyone. Lifestyle options are just as nuanced and individualised as medical options. As the saying goes, we may all be in the same storm, but we are not all in the same boat.

This section by no means provides an exhaustive list, and you may find that you are using some of these methods already. As usual, what works fantastically for one person might have no effect whatsoever for someone else.

Heat

Hot-water bottles, electric heat mats, hot baths – I don't think I have spoken to a single person suffering with endometriosis who has not turned to heat at one point or another to soothe their pain, whether it is chronic or an acute flare-up. It is a very effective method, and I now boast a rather impressive collection of hot-water bottles in various shapes and sizes, microwaveable bags, plug-in electric pads and even a heated bed sheet that covers the entire mattress (bliss for back pain!).

While heat is the go-to method for many of us, it comes with its own 'side effects' and risks, namely, erythema ab igne (err/i/thee/muh ab ig/nay). Also known as 'toasted skin syndrome', erythema ab igne is the development of a 'lacy' pattern of redness after prolonged exposure to a strong heat source such as a hot-water bottle or heat mat. The reason the skin forms this toasted appearance rather than a traditional burn is that the heat source, while extremely hot, is not scalding. Lengthy exposure to this heat causes changes to the elastic fibres that make up your skin, as well as to the microscopic blood vessels at the skin's surface. This means that over time, more and more heat is required to feel relief, and the toasted skin worsens.

The only way to lessen toasted skin syndrome is to completely remove the heat source; that is, stop using hot-water bottles or heat pads. The affected

Dealing with the system – how to get help

skin should return to normal with time, but chronic sufferers may find that it takes months or years to fully heal. However, if the toasted skin is severe and the skin is darkly pigmented, the damage may be irreversible.

I suffer from erythema ab igne and have had permanent marks on my lower abdomen and upper thighs for years now. I find it impossible to give up heat as it forms one of my primary methods of pain management and provides me with so much relief. I have therefore had to make my peace with these marks, but I do still have to be very careful to avoid burning the top layers of skin and causing blistering. I do this by alternating heat with other methods, avoiding the maximum heat settings and keeping an eye on my hot-water bottles for signs of deterioration.

My experience with toasted skin syndrome and doctors has not been great. When the marks are spotted, I am often looked at as if I am deliberately committing self-harm, rather than it being seen as a sign of desperation for pain relief and an indication of just how severe my symptoms had become. One surgeon called me a 'silly girl'; I was a 33-year-old woman who had been fighting for 22 years for someone to believe me and was relying upon the only methods I could access to relieve my pain. I would love to see erythema ab igne included in medical training as a warning sign and a prompt to ask the patient about their pain and why they need to use so much heat. It might just save someone years of suffering.

Hot-water bottles

Did you know hot-water bottles have an expiry date? If your hot-water bottle has occasional use, you should replace it every two years to avoid the risk of the rubber perishing and causing you nasty burns.

The important part there is 'occasional use'. Chances are, if you have endometriosis or any chronic illness, you are probably using your hot-water bottle a lot more frequently than might be expected. This means you need to check it regularly and replace it even more often than advised.

Every hot-water bottle should be stamped with a production date. The number is the year of manufacture, and each 'petal' shows the month. Each dot within a petal is a week. The hot-water bottle in

Figure 2.1 was manufactured towards the end of April 2021. With regular use, I should have disposed of it at the end of April 2023.

Figure 2.1: Example of a hot-water bottle production date

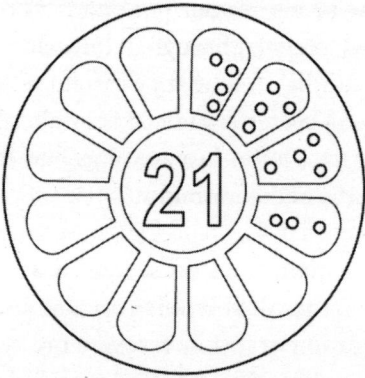

However, at the end of 2021, while sitting in bed, scalding hot water suddenly leaked over my lower abdomen and upper thighs. When we took the hot-water bottle cover off, we were shocked to see that the rubber had burned and perished only six months after the manufacturing date. It wasn't faulty; I was just using it far more than the manufacturer would expect, which massively shortened its life (by 75 per cent in this case). Please, if you use your hot-water bottle a lot, especially daily or multiple times a day, check it before using it. Take it out of the cover and look for cracks, discolouration, bulging or any other changes. It might just save you a lot of extra pain and scarring.

Baths

When my symptoms were at their worst, between my two surgeries, I practically lived in our bath. The hotter the better, it was sometimes the only thing that soothed the pain – particularly the pain that I felt deep in my hips and pelvis. The heat helped, but there was also something about the relaxation element that helped my muscles, tight from pain, gently release. Please be careful with hot water and do not burn yourself. Also, be careful getting in and out of the bath; if you can, have someone to assist you and take particular care if you are unsteady.

Dealing with the system – how to get help

TENS machines

TENS machines have long been used in maternity settings, but they can be brilliant for easing endometriosis pain too. They have saved me on numerous occasions, particularly when I am out of the house with no access to heat. You stick pads where you are feeling pain and then adjust the settings to send out electrical currents to block your perception of pain. They are a short-term fix, but they have seen me through many a flare-up. There are so many brands available, including some that target endometriosis patients. Some have wires, others are wireless; some include a heat setting; and others are skin-toned (in a range of shades) so are more discreet. You don't need the priciest one – just find one in your budget that suits your needs.

Diet

Talking about diet in relation to endometriosis is such a personal topic and can bring up a lot of strong feelings. The truth is, despite what you will see across social media, there is no magic diet for endometriosis. Endometriosis is a disease of nuance and diet triggers are no exception. As soon as I set up my Instagram account to talk about endometriosis, the algorithm immediately set to work and served me post after post of various diets that promised to heal my endometriosis 'naturally'.

I was told all of the following:

- Don't eat gluten
- Eat gluten, but don't eat dairy
- Go vegan
- Go carnivore

The advice was so conflicting, and one plan practically eliminated every food group going.

It is a difficult one because diet can potentially help symptom management. Endometriosis is a condition that thrives in an inflammatory environment. So, it follows that a broadly anti-inflammatory diet will reduce bodily inflammation and may help symptom management. However, this does not have to be extreme. What is most important is to eat a balanced, healthy diet and to find out what your own personal triggers are. For me, caffeine and alcohol are two major ones. Consuming them will guarantee a flare-up, so I now avoid them as much as possible. Someone else could be fine with alcohol but flare up after having chilli, for example. Finding out what your individual triggers are and tweaking your diet accordingly is far more helpful than eliminating huge swathes of foods indiscriminately.

There are elimination diets that are designed to help you identify these triggers, but these can be extreme. If you would like to undergo an elimination plan, please consult with your doctor, who should be able to refer you to an appropriate nutritional specialist to guide you. I did not undertake an elimination diet. Instead, I found that as a by-product of tracking my symptoms and flare-ups carefully, I was able to identify which food and drink triggers were the culprits for me.

Diet is an extremely personal and subjective topic. On days when you are bedbound from pain, exhaustion and other symptoms, you are probably not thinking about heading to the kitchen and whipping up a nutrient-dense, colourful plateful of balanced anti-inflammatory foods. You just need to get some calories in you to give you enough energy to survive the day. You are far more likely to be grabbing anything you can before curling back up with your heat pad. And that is fine. Do what you need to do. Other times, when you feel terrible and are in constant pain, you just want your favourite comfort food. That is okay too. Mine is macaroni cheese and will never not hit the spot. Sadly, patients can feel like they are judged for this – that they are not taking their disease seriously enough or are even 'causing endometriosis'.

Endometriosis patient Blessing says, 'I joined a group for living with endometriosis and the subject of food came up. It was like a competition for who could cut out the most and who could survive off the most extreme diet. I made some small steps, which definitely helped me day to day, but I was always made to feel like it wasn't enough. I left the group when the "expert on nutrition" who was brought to speak to us basically told me that the food from my culture was "bad" and "causing my endometriosis". They said that if I wanted to heal, I needed to "stop eating all that and have a proper diet".'

This insensitivity to our individuality is a common theme in discussions around diet. Clare, who was diagnosed in her late 20s, lost her job due to the impact endometriosis has had on her. She does some freelance work when she can, but money is tight and she struggles financially. The last time she was seen at her endometriosis clinic, one of the members of staff told her that unless she is willing to put the effort into overhauling her diet, why should they perform expensive surgery on her? The diet plan they then gave her consisted of organic produce, grass-fed steak, fermented drinks, wild salmon, an abundance of fresh fruit and vegetables and whole grains. Sounds wonderful, but Clare, like many others, simply cannot afford it. 'I broke down as soon as I got home,' she says. 'I have no money because endometriosis means I can't work. Without money, I can't afford what they're telling me to buy. And if I don't buy that food to prove I am "serious", then they didn't want to offer me surgery. I feel trapped.'

There are so many reasons why someone might not be able to follow a 'perfect' diet, even if one did exist that was universally successful for endometriosis. We are all just doing the best we can, within the context in which we live, with the resources that we have, in any particular moment. That is more than good enough.

Movement
Hands up if you have ever told someone you have endometriosis and they asked if you have tried yoga to fix it? It has become a bit of a running joke in the endometriosis world: 'Yes, I have endometriosis. And yes, I've tried yoga.' Movement, or exercise, is another area that can elicit eye rolls and controversy. I get it. We all know the health benefits of exercise, but when you are curled up in agonising pain, the last thing you want to do is go for a run – and woe betide anyone who suggests it. However, movement does not have to mean punishing gym workouts or running marathons – although if that is what works for you, go for it! You do not need me to tell you that exercise, both cardio and strength training, is vital for your long-term health. But, as with diet, this is an area that can lead to a lot of anxiety among patients, a lot of comparison and, sadly, a lot of judgement. Remember that movement does not have to always be a workout. It can be as simple as a gentle stretch, a small walk, or some mild exercises performed while lying on your bed.

When we are in pain, particularly when that pain persists for a long time, our bodies tense up. Over time, this can cause increased pain and even issues with tissues such as those in the pelvic floor, bladder or bowel. Stretching can be fantastic to help ease these muscles and soothe this aspect of your pain over time. We'll delve more into how and why when we discuss pelvic floor physiotherapy (*see* pages 142–145), but for now, just know that micromovements also count when we are talking about lifestyle changes. You can search YouTube for routines designed specifically for when you are menstruating, for pelvic pain or for whatever it is you are struggling with. Do whatever feels right for your body each day, but a small amount of movement daily really can make a difference. And when you are really in the trenches of a flare, Child's pose (*see* Figure 2.2) is my ultimate go-to.

Figure 2.2: Child's pose

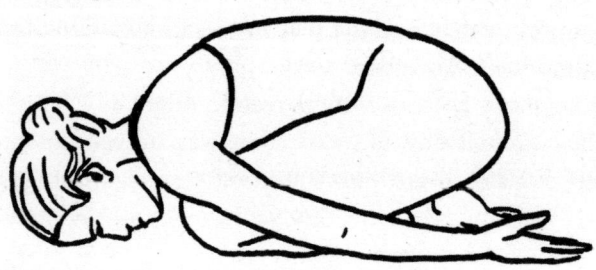

Stress reduction

I know how infuriating it is to be told that stress is the problem, especially as someone who was dismissed medically for two decades and told 'it's just stress' more times than I care to remember. To be clear, stress should never be used to dismiss you when you have concerns about your health, but the truth is that reducing stress as much as possible can help with symptom management. It is a bit of a cruel joke because living with endometriosis is inherently stressful. Maybe I wouldn't be so stressed if I wasn't living in constant pain, worried about fertility, on the brink of losing my job from health-related absences, constantly fighting to be believed by doctors, dealing with a mountain of medical admin, worrying that the intimacy in my relationship is being harmed – you get the picture. Stress and pain are a vicious cycle and form the most toxic co-dependent relationship you can imagine.

So, how do you break the cycle? Try to find ways to reduce your stress: being in nature, going for a walk, reading, playing videogames, crafting, watching the latest series to drop, painting, soaking in the bath, getting a massage, gardening or whatever it is that relaxes you, try to do more of it. On the flip side, think about the situations that stress you out. They could be related to work, social situations or family, and again they will be unique to you. Once you have identified them, try to avoid them. If you cannot avoid them, try to think of ways to lessen your exposure to them or come up with strategies to cope.

Dealing with the system – how to get help

One strategy to help reduce stress levels is breathing. I know that sounds a bit patronising – you are reading this book, you are alive, you know how to breathe. However, most of us do not breathe optimally. With lives packed with stress and, as is often the case with endometriosis, pain, we tend to breathe too quickly and not deeply enough. It's understandable. But taking deep, regulated breaths can help not only to reduce stress but also to get through a flare-up. Try this simple diaphragmatic breathing technique and practise it consistently. Once you have mastered it, you can use it during times of stress (physical or emotional):

- Take a deep breath in through your nose, allowing your chest to expand and your belly to soften. Place your hand on your belly to feel it rising as you inhale.
- As you breathe in, visualise your muscles and body relaxing.
- Breathe out normally and relax.
- Repeat five times or as many times as needed.

You know the score by now. Stress reduction is not going to cure your endometriosis, but reducing stress-induced inflammation in your body may help day-to-day symptom management.

Sleep is also linked to stress reduction. Again, I really do understand how difficult it can be to prioritise quality sleep, especially when you are flaring, in pain that your strongest painkillers do not touch, are unable to find a comfortable position, are dashing to and from the bathroom and are paranoid you might leak blood on to the sheets. However, doing what you can to improve your sleep as much as is possible is another way to reduce inflammation and potentially manage your symptoms. I now have a very detailed, precise bedtime ritual and sleep set-up that involves an early dinner, a warm bath, an audiobook, a specific room temperature, my heated sheet but a cool pillow, a very particular sleep position, a body pillow and numerous other requirements that, even so, don't always work. 'Painsomnia' (insomnia brought on by pain) is still a semi-regular occurrence for me, but I do what I can to minimise it. Sometimes, that means turning down social events because I know they will keep me up too late; this is always disappointing, but I am learning to protect the boundaries that help me mitigate the disruption caused by my exhaustion and symptom flares.

Pacing

We have all been there. We have been feeling awful for a while, unable to do half of the things that we needed to (if that), let alone anything fun. So, when that magical moment comes when we feel like we have a bit more energy, and maybe are in less pain too, we feel like we want to achieve as much as possible. We push ourselves, perhaps because we feel like we missed out when we were flaring or because we simply do not have a choice and must catch up. The problem is, this ends up becoming a perpetual cycle of boom and bust. In order to break out of this cycle of flare-up and overexertion, we need to practise pacing. This is the process of balancing activities with rest, allowing for more consistent and sustainable levels of activity without causing our symptoms to flare up. There is a lot of information about pacing available online. If it's something you would like to explore, you can ask your GP to provide you with some resources to get you started. We will also explore it in more detail in chapter 5 (*see* pages 196–197). Again, though, it is always worth bearing in mind that some people's life circumstances will not allow or accommodate pacing.

Massage

This does not have to be a full-on spa day with candles and plinky music – although, to be honest, that would be very lovely. Massage can help with adhesions, muscle tension, relaxation and even constipation. Constipation is a very common symptom among those with endometriosis. It can be caused by endometriosis on or near the bowel (remember how tightly packed in everything is), or it can also be the result of medication side effects, particularly if you are taking codeine-based pain relief.

A method called the 'I Love yoU' (ILU) massage (*see* Figure 2.3) can be used to help alleviate constipation and even some pain. Always work from left to right and use some cream or oil on your skin:

- Start by forming the letter 'I', stroking with moderate pressure from your left ribcage down in a straight line to your left hip bone. Repeat 10 times.
- Next, form the letter 'L' by stroking, again with moderate pressure, from your right ribcage, across to your left ribcage and then down to your left hip bone. Repeat 10 times.

Dealing with the system – how to get help

- Lastly, form the letter 'U' by moving up from your right hip bone to the bottom of your right ribcage, across to your left ribcage and down to your left hip bone. Repeat 10 times.
- Finish with one to two minutes of clockwise circular movements around your belly button to stimulate the small intestine.

Do this routine once daily and you should begin to notice some improvements. You can even get your partner to help you with this, although they might have something else in mind if you suggest a couple's massage!

Figure 2.3: The 'ILove yoU' massage technique

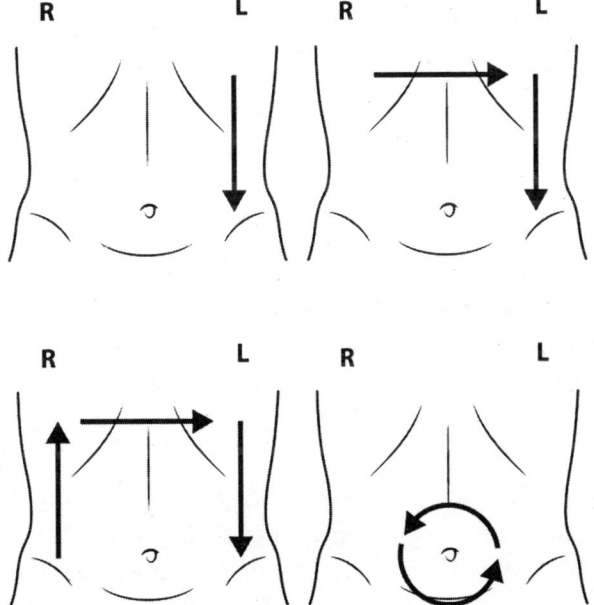

Nausea relief
Nausea is a symptom that a lot of endometriosis patients suffer with. Whether it's from the condition itself, a side effect of medication or just a by-product of living in pain, nausea comes up time and again in patient stories. We covered medical options earlier in this chapter (*see* pages 83–91), but I've found a few non-medical ways of helping to manage my nausea too. Hopefully, something here might work for you:

- Iced water: Sipping cold water really helps when nausea strikes. I like to put ice and water in an insulated cup to keep it extra crispy. Ice lollies can also help.
- Mints: These are especially handy when you are out and about. I always have at least one packet of strong mints on me at all times. A peppermint tea can also help soothe symptoms.
- Keep hydrated: This sounds basic, but it really can help.
- Cool packs: I have ice blocks in various shapes, including one like a curved sausage that wraps around my neck. When nausea really hits, I use the ice blocks on my pulse points (back of the neck, wrists, etc.) to great effect. Be careful when using items straight from the freezer so as not to harm your skin.
- Eating: Try not to avoid eating, even though it is likely the last thing you feel like doing when you are nauseated. If you skip food but still take your medication, you are more than likely going to end up in a vicious, nauseous cycle. Have something small, light and plain if needed.

Combined approaches

Since there is no cure, treatment is not straightforward, and it is likely that a combination of approaches will make up your symptom management plan. For example, you may find that an IUD, anti-inflammatory pain relief, tranexamic acid, pelvic floor relaxation, heat and a TENS machine could be a winning combination for your symptoms. Maybe you do not want any hormones and prefer to manage your symptoms with dietary changes, movement, heat and some pain relief only during flares. It does not matter what your combination looks like as long as you understand the options and have chosen what works best for you at that time.

Endometriosis and the 'wellness industry'

After years of dismissal and gaslighting, endometriosis patients are often desperate for validation and relief. This opens wide gaps that businesses and entrepreneurs try to fill with cynical products, programmes and protocols promising to heal us. Whether it is an extreme diet, expensive supplements or 'womb-healing protocols' promising to 'reconnect you to your divine feminine and banish endometriosis for good' (yep, that was a real sales pitch!), the holes in the healthcare system leave us vulnerable to those looking to make money from our physical and emotional suffering. Most of the accounts and websites making these blanket promises have something to sell. From monthly pills with very little, if any, robust evidence supporting their claims to online courses that can cost thousands (yes, really!), endometriosis can be a profitable business.

When I was first diagnosed, all of these options and products constantly telling me what I was 'supposed to be doing' left me confused, overwhelmed and, to be honest, with a sense of guilt. It made me feel like I wasn't doing enough to help myself. Every time I had one of the supposed 'bad' foods, for example, I felt like I wasn't taking this seriously enough and that my pain was my fault. Let's just clear this one up right now. Nothing that you do, don't do, take, don't take, eat or don't eat has caused your endometriosis.

If you would like to try any of these options to see if they make any difference for you, then please, feel free. It is entirely your choice. But do so fully informed, with a critical eye and from a place of curiosity rather than one of vulnerability or desperation for relief.

Endometriosis and A&E

Eleven months after my second surgery, I was at home. I was in my usual amount of pain and then, out of nowhere, it felt like someone was playing Kerplunk with my pelvis but using knives instead of straws. I cried out and fell to the floor. My husband is pretty well-versed in my pain flares by now, but this was something we hadn't dealt with for over a year. After trying all our usual methods to calm the flare, nothing was working and I could barely speak or see straight through the pain. We rang 111, the non-emergency helpline, and told them my medical history, and they advised we go straight to A&E and request immediate gynaecological assessment. They offered to send an ambulance, but we assured them that my husband would take me straight away.

At A&E, I spent 24 hours on a hard plastic chair, by far the person with the longest wait in the department. It took five hours for me to be given any pain relief, and my husband had to go up and ask for more each time I became due. At one point, I was left for 10 hours without being spoken to or seen at all. I begged for a bed, a trolley, anything to be more comfortable, but nothing was available, so I was left curled up in the corner, crying and vomiting from pain.

Eventually, a consultant gynaecologist came along and admitted that nobody knew what to do with me. They told me they could not put me on a gynaecology ward because I had 'had a hysterectomy and don't have gynaecological organs any more'.

After 24 hours, I was exhausted. I was not being given any treatment beyond what I had at home and, to be honest, I just wanted my bed. So, I was discharged with emergency referrals for an MRI and for colorectal, urogynaecology and endometriosis clinic appointments. Eight months later, I'm still waiting for half of those 'emergency' appointments.

The sad reality is that many endometriosis patients end up seeking emergency care at some point in their journeys and have stories that are very similar to mine. According to a report by the All Party Parliamentary Group on Endometriosis, 53 per cent of patients have had to visit A&E due to the severity of their symptoms, while 27 per cent went three or more times. Despite that, only 2 per cent were investigated for endometriosis during their time there. After my experience, I conducted my own informal poll on Instagram, answered by over 1,100 endometriosis patients. Fifty-six per cent answered that they had been to A&E, but a shocking 88.8 per cent of those individuals felt like their symptoms were not taken seriously. Official reports often cite figures on A&E attendance but often miss those of us who need to go, who need to access treatment or pain relief, but do not, for fear of dismissal or lack of understanding. It is frightening that we have been gaslit so much that we now gaslight ourselves and don't get the help we need.

In my very quick Instagram survey, which had respondents from all over the world, 32.2 per cent had considered going to A&E but cited reasons such as 'previously dismissed', 'they don't understand endometriosis' or 'they won't believe me' as reasons for not seeking emergency care. Others have been accused of 'drug seeking' or told to 'go home; it can't possibly be that bad'.

Our collective experiences in emergency departments highlight the lack of understanding and education around conditions such as endometriosis. It is an issue that has long term-ramifications, putting endometriosis patients off seeking emergency care for other aspects of their health too. As Julia, one of the respondents to my Instagram poll, describes, 'Unless I have something visibly wrong with me, like a broken bone, I won't go to A&E. It scares me when I think about it. I could be having a heart attack without knowing it, but I wouldn't go to A&E because of how many times they've just sent me away and told me to get on with it. Living with such extreme pain for so long has become so normalised. It's hard for me to understand what's okay to deal with and what isn't.'

Our medical and education systems are currently failing endometriosis patients and need to do better. Please know that your pain is valid. If you are unable to manage your pain at home, seek medical support.

Evidence-based medicine

Evidence-based medicine is a term bandied about a lot in the Western medical world and is what influences the care and treatment you receive as a patient. It is 'the conscientious, explicit, and judicious use of current best evidence in making decisions about the care of individual patients', integrating 'clinical experience and patient values with the best available research information'. Sounds great, yes? Surely, we should be able to let the experts decide how to treat us. However, what does being an 'expert' mean? What happens when clinical education about the disease is practically non-existent? What happens when the 'current best evidence' is outdated at best and incorrect at worst? And what happens when the research is so scant and was funded by organisations with explicit agendas? How can this environment, the very one we find ourselves in as endometriosis patients, result in positive patient outcomes?

There are three distinct parts to the definition of evidence-based medicine:

1. Current best evidence
2. Clinical experience (findings and knowledge from expert surgeons)
3. Patient values (your goals, your desires and your priorities)

Currently, however, there is an overwhelming emphasis on point 1 only, to the detriment of clinical and patient experiences. This leads to the precise situation in which endometriosis patients find ourselves, with gaps in knowledge, average diagnosis times of nine years, patients being operated on by surgeons who do not understand the disease, the loss of organs, ineffective and potentially damaging treatment options and a 50 per cent infertility rate. We cannot continue to view endometriosis care purely through the narrow scope of 'current best evidence'. All three lenses of evidence-based medicine need to be given due consideration and balanced appropriately. That balance is an artform, as the three may conflict.

As we've already seen from endometriosis expert Mr Shaheen Khazali, his clinical practice sometimes deviates from the guidelines created by bodies such as NICE or the European Society of Human Reproduction and Embryology (ESHRE). These bodies seek to aggregate all of the current research findings about endometriosis to create a roadmap of sorts for clinicians to follow. However, as we have seen, research is limited in its reliability and impartiality. The result is a disconnect between the guidelines and patient outcomes. The experiences of both the clinician and the patient are being neglected. Professor Trish Greenhalgh, a doctor and healthcare academic, describes a 'dissonance . . . when trying to apply research findings to the clinical encounter often occurs when we abandon the narrative-interpretive paradigm and try to get by on "evidence" alone.' That is, when doctors stop listening to patients and disregard their symptoms, relying instead on outdated research, disagreements and poor outcomes are inevitable.

Doctors are under more pressure than ever. They are trying to operate in a system that is stretched beyond capacity, with ever-increasing demands on their knowledge, their time and their skills. Can you imagine being a GP, given 10 minutes to take a history, perform examinations and decide on a treatment for what could be any condition, illness or symptom? There is no way they can know all of the care pathways for every single issue. Guidelines exist to help doctors streamline the process and identify appropriate care pathways, but medicine, particularly in a situation as complex as endometriosis, is not 'an algorithm,' says Mr Khazali. An exceptional doctor, in any specialty, will not simply read the guidelines and check off the steps like a tick-box exercise. They will use critical thinking, exercise the judgement and discernment they have established through experience, consider what the patient desires and focus on empowering that patient to make the best choice for themselves. David Sackett, widely referenced as 'the father of evidence-based medicine', describes 'integrating individual clinical expertise with the best available external clinical evidence from systemic research' and the 'thoughtful identification and compassionate use of individual patients' predicaments, rights and preferences'.

If your doctor, whether it's your GP or the doctors you see in hospital or a specialist clinic, is not considering your concerns, goals and preferences when discussing a treatment plan, it is time to see a different one.

Tips for navigating endometriosis with your GP

Unless you are diagnosed 'accidentally', after an emergency or when seeking fertility or other treatment, your first experience with navigating the healthcare system with suspected endometriosis is likely to be your GP. When we spoke, Dr Nighat Arif, women's health GP and campaigner and author of *The Knowledge*, was kind enough to share her top tips for advocating for yourself in that setting:

- Keep a symptom diary and tracker. This really helps me as a doctor – I need that data. Even if your pain is 0, log it. Having no pain does not mean you don't have endometriosis, just as a clear scan doesn't rule it out.
- Go in saying what works for you and what doesn't. What treatments have you tried? What helps your symptoms? What makes them worse? You can identify these through your tracker too.
- Ask to see the GP specialising in women's health. You should be able to see who this is on the practice website, but you can ask if you are not sure.
- Be prepared to be armed with more information than your healthcare provider has. Diagnoses like endometriosis or adenomyosis are not on the radar of as many GPs and clinicians as we would like to think. And even if they are aware of them, they might not know what the latest NICE guidelines are. Familiarise yourself with them, and even take them in with you.
- Ask for a second opinion. Even with 17 years of experience, I don't mind if a patient would like a second opinion and I will always facilitate one.

- If, after all of that, you feel like you are still not being listened to, escalate it to the practice manager or the Patient Advice and Liaison Service (PALS), the NHS patient complaint service. Don't be nervous or uncomfortable making a complaint. When you lodge a grievance, the situation doesn't change just for you but for all the others who come after you.

Chapter 3

Understanding endometriosis care and surgery

'I'm a gynaecologist. If it's good enough for the NHS, it should be good enough for you too.' – gynaecological surgeon

Hopefully, while all this investigation and symptom management is going on, whether you are suspected of having endometriosis or the disease has been confirmed through scans already, you will also be referred to an endometriosis specialist centre or clinic. Ideally, this should all happen concurrently, especially given the exceptionally long average wait times for both diagnosis and specialist appointments. It should be a multi-pronged approach rather than a simple linear pathway.

As we have explored in earlier chapters, endometriosis is a complicated disease that we know nowhere near enough about. It is currently barely taught at medical school level and the level of knowledge among the general clinical population is not where it needs to be. Mr Mohamed Mabrouk, endometriosis surgeon and president of the European Endometriosis League, sums up the situation during a phone call: 'We currently have a mess in endometriosis practice'. He explains that 'the majority of GPs have no idea what endometriosis is', and even most gynaecologists 'just don't get it'. Even within gynaecology, the medical specialty under which endometriosis sits, knowledge about the disease is scarily outdated and rarely taught. It therefore follows that endometriosis patients need to be seen by clinicians who truly understand the disease and how it presents, operates and manifests. We need to be seen in specialist endometriosis clinics that work in a multi-disciplinary environment.

Multi-disciplinary care

As we know, endometriosis is a full-body disease, found in every organ and bodily system (*see* pages 20–21). It needs a treatment approach that matches its multi-disciplinary nature. The exact makeup of your multidisciplinary team (MDT) will vary depending on where the disease is growing, your symptoms and your longer-term goals. Your MDT may include the following:

- GP
- Specialist endometriosis surgeon
- Specialist endometriosis nurse
- Specialist sonographer or radiologist
- Urology surgeon
- Colorectal surgeon
- Any other supporting surgeons required, such as thoracic
- Pelvic floor physiotherapist
- Mental health support
- Fertility specialist
- Dietitian
- Pain management specialist

This kind of collaborative approach is the 'key for success' and 'makes all the difference' for both surgeons and patients, Mr Mikey Adamczyk, consultant gynaecologist and endometriosis surgeon, tells me. 'Sure, as skilled endometriosis surgeons, many of us can technically perform a segmental bowel resection (where part of the small intestine is removed) or a ureteric reimplantation (surgery to reposition the tubes connecting the kidneys to the bladder). But that's not really the point. The real question is whether we're fully equipped to handle the complications that can come up from something like a segmental resection. And honestly, the answer for most would be no.' That's where a solid MDT comes in – 'one where we know each other and are comfortable bouncing ideas around even mid surgery'. The benefits are not just for the surgical team. 'These surgeries are incredibly complex,' he continues; often, 'we're dealing with anatomy distorted beyond recognition, which means we have to bring our best to each case'. It's vital 'not just for managing the technical challenges, but for giving the best possible care'.

A key part of your broader MDT should also include support at home. This is just as important as your medical team and could be a partner, parent, sibling, friend or pet. It does not matter who it is, but never underestimate their importance. Living with endometriosis can be a lot to deal with and having this support can make the world of difference to your quality of life.

Think about what your current MDT looks like. Do you have any gaps where you could use some additional support? If so, speak to your GP or your endometriosis clinic about referrals.

Specialist endometriosis centres

In the UK, an organisation called the British Society for Gynaecological Endoscopy (BSGE) has established a network of centres and clinics designed to support patients with endometriosis to access specialised care in a multi-disciplinary environment. These centres must meet a set of criteria in order to become accredited by the BSGE and they are widely regarded as 'centres of excellence' for endometriosis care in the UK. There is a very severe demand and supply issue when it comes to specialised endometriosis care. This is not a phenomenon unique to the UK; everywhere in the world, demand for these services far outstrips the supply of highly experienced, skilled endometriosis specialists. At the time of writing, the BSGE lists 79 centres across the UK. That's 79 centres to serve the estimated 2 million endometriosis patients currently in the UK, meaning that each centre is, on average, expected to cater for over 25,000 of us. As ever, though, it's not that simple as these centres are not equitably spread across the four countries of the UK. Seventy of the centres are in England, four are in Scotland, four are in Wales and a solitary one is in Northern Ireland. Twenty-three per cent of all centres are located in London or Greater London.

These centres are not miracle fixes. Remember, there is no cure for endometriosis, and that includes surgery. However, the rationale behind the BSGE accreditation is that these clinics are staffed and operated by clinicians who understand the nuanced nature of endometriosis and are equipped to manage even the most complex cases. Let's look at these criteria, shall we? To become accredited by the BSGE, a centre must demonstrate the following:

- A dedicated consultant-led endometriosis service devoted to endometriosis patients
- Sufficient workload to maintain surgical skills for complex cases
- A named supporting colorectal surgeon to attend cases involving the bowel
- A network of other supporting clinicians, such as urologists, pain management specialists and pelvic floor physiotherapists

Endometriosis

- Data collection to drive a database of cases and outcomes
- An endometriosis specialist nurse
- Annual submission of a sample surgical video of 'laparoscopic excision of severe recto-vaginal endometriosis that required dissection of the pararectal space'. In other words the centre must submit a video showing removal of endometriosis around the vagina, rectum or areas between them.

You can certainly see that the aim is to create a standardised high level of care for endometriosis patients, particularly where cases are more complex and involve organs. Unfortunately, that aim, worthwhile as it is, does not seem to be currently reflected in patient care. Patient reported experiences and outcomes vary widely among centres and sometimes even within them.

Patients, advocates and endometriosis experts are calling for the BSGE to strengthen their accreditation criteria, in particular when it comes to workload. The current requirement is that 'at least 12 cases of rectovaginal endometriosis which require dissection of the pararectal space are treated by surgery each year' per surgeon at the clinic. This is in comparison to the hundreds of endometriosis surgeries, including complex cases, that are performed annually by specialists worldwide. This, of course, does not mean there should be a conveyor belt of patients undergoing rapid, slapdash surgery, but the evidence is clear that high-volume expert surgery following a structured, standardised approach improves patient outcomes. Discussing low complication rates in endometriosis surgery despite the increasing complexity of cases, a 2024 paper cited 'the surgeon's learning curve, high surgical volume and adherence to a structured approach'. The lead surgeon referenced in this research, Mr Shaheen Khazali, averaged nearly 140 surgeries per year for eight years: a bit different from the minimum of 12 required by the BSGE.

This is just one example of where the BSGE could really raise the bar for endometriosis care standards. Another would be to stipulate the sole use of excision surgery as opposed to ablation, a superficial treatment that leaves the underlying disease intact (*see* page 115). Many surgeons at BSGE centres exclusively use excision instead of ablation, but others do not. Again, this lack of standardisation is harming patient outcomes and resulting in repeated surgeries. Endo patient Lucy tells me that, under the care of a BSGE clinic in the North of England, she underwent 24 ablation surgeries. 'They just

Understanding endometriosis care and surgery

told me that I would need surgery at least once a year because it would keep coming back. I didn't know any better.' Eventually, she travelled to another centre, hundreds of miles away, and underwent excision surgery. 'That was nine years ago. I still have some symptoms, but that's probably due to the damage of so many operations. I have my life back. I didn't need 25 surgeries. I needed one, done right.'

BSGE centres are not perfect, but they are currently the best option we have in the UK for accessing specialist endometriosis treatment on the NHS. They are staffed by many incredible clinicians working hard to try to improve patient outcomes and lives. However, they are not immune to the stubborn myths about endometriosis and the legacy of a lack of education and updated training. So, it falls to us, again, to make sure we have done our research, understand our options and are confident in both the treatment and the person performing it. This is especially important when the topic of surgical intervention comes up.

Finding an endometriosis expert

Normally, with any other condition, we would go to the GP and get referred to a specialist doctor, whom we would trust and rely on to treat us. As we've seen, as endometriosis patients we have to do our homework to make sure we are seen by someone who actually understands the disease, the treatment options and the long-term outcomes. But what does that homework look like, and how do we actually find an expert?

The first step is to educate yourself, which, by reading this book, you are already doing. You need to understand the disease and what the current evidence says in order to spot any red flags from doctors.

There are groups online that provide shortlists of surgeons, based on patient experiences, such as Nancy's Nook on Facebook. Bear in mind that Nook is a self-education tool and does not recommend individual surgeons. Instead, see it as a starting point for you to then do your own research. There are also websites that claim to rate and check surgeons and certify them as experts. Here, you need to be aware that surgeons can pay for spots on these sites and the vetting process is controversial among patients and surgeons alike. Surgeons submitting their work for review are, of course, going to highlight their best work, which may not be representative of their overall approach. Social media accounts and support groups can be great places to chat with other patients about their experiences with doctors, which may also help inform your decision.

Ultimately, however, it will come down the conversations you have with a surgeon. Think of it as interviewing them. There are questions later in this chapter to help you with that. I know one patient who had consultations with six different surgeons before choosing who she wanted to perform her operation. You need to choose someone who aligns with your preferences, needs and goals.

Endometriosis surgery

As we've explored, alongside medical options and lifestyle changes, surgery plays a large role in endometriosis management. Surgery is still classed as the 'definitive' way to diagnose endometriosis, largely due to the limitations in performing and interpreting medical imaging that we have already covered (*see* pages 78–82). This means that, even now, you may still have to undergo invasive surgery to find out if you have endometriosis and to what extent.

Diagnostic surgery

Sometimes, patients undergo surgery purely for diagnostic purposes before then being referred on to an endometriosis specialist for surgery for disease management. This is less than ideal for several reasons:

- These surgeries are often performed by general gynaecologists with little experience of complex endometriosis.
- Undergoing invasive surgery purely to diagnose endometriosis leads to multiple surgeries, increased scar tissue and adhesions, missed disease, organ damage, increased waiting times, lengthy recovery periods and so much more.

Understanding endometriosis care and surgery

Instead, diagnosis and disease removal should be undertaken at the same time by a skilled surgeon who is an expert in and solely dedicated to endometriosis.

The surgical procedure for endometriosis is usually referred to as a 'laparoscopy', but this simply describes the method of access. A laparoscopy is a surgical procedure in which an instrument (a laparoscope) is inserted through the abdominal wall to permit surgery. It is also known as keyhole, as opposed to open, surgery.

Once the surgeons are 'inside', there are two types of endometriosis surgery that are far from equal. It is important to know the difference and to make sure your surgeon uses the correct method. I did not know this before my first surgery, otherwise I would never have had it. It was only after that surgery, still in debilitating pain, that I started the process of finding out as much as I could about endometriosis and discovered the critical importance of the type of surgery and who performs it. This information did not come from any surgeon, any medical professional I saw in a patient–doctor capacity or any organisation (NHS or charity). It came from taking it upon myself to learn and talking to countless patients, advocates and experts. Please take your time to really absorb and understand the information in this section, as it may just change how you decide to proceed with your treatment.

The two methods are ablation and excision. To explain them simply, let's use the analogy of a weed.

Ablation surgery

Ablation surgery is a superficial treatment where the surgeon burns, or 'destroys', visible endometriosis lesions. However, this only destroys disease on the surface, leaving the deeper 'roots' intact. Recurrence of symptoms after ablation is very common and can be rapid. Burning can in fact make things worse as it creates a 'sticky' surface, allowing more adhesions to occur, and can also damage surrounding tissues. Ablation is also connected to poor fertility outcomes as a result of damage to tissue and egg reserves. Destroying the disease on-site also removes the chance of sending a sample of the tissue to the lab for diagnostic confirmation. Despite this, ablation is still shockingly the most commonly performed surgical technique for endometriosis as it is cheaper, simpler and quicker than the alternative.

Excision surgery

Excision surgery, by contrast, is where the surgeon cuts out the disease, including the 'roots'. This is especially important in patients with deeply infiltrating disease where endometriosis is deeply embedded (*see* page 15). Heat energy is often used to excise the lesions, acting as a knife that cuts through tissue rather than destroying the cells on site. Cutting the disease out at the root is the established 'gold standard' in endometriosis care and allows the cells to be sent away for laboratory testing and diagnosis. A 2018 study reinforced the importance of taking biopsies: 'meticulous histological confirmation should still be the first step in the laparoscopic diagnosis and treatment of suspected endometriosis'. This is particularly important to avoid 'unnecessary, prolonged medical treatment and operations' and 'delaying the proper treatment measures from being applied'. I should note here, though, that false negatives can occur even at this stage. If you have had surgery, had tissue removed and sent to the lab, and the result came back negative for endometriosis, even this does not necessarily rule out endometriosis. Any number of things can happen to tissue samples and testing conditions are not always uniform.

As ever with endometriosis, the absence of evidence is not necessarily evidence of absence, but only by excising tissue is it possible to analyse the tissue and obtain a definitive, pathological diagnosis. Speaking to Dr José Eugenio-Colón, endometriosis specialist, he agrees wholeheartedly. 'Absolutely we should be sending tissues away to the lab. What are we even doing if we're not confirming what disease is present?! And the only way to achieve that is excision.' Even endometriomas (aka ovarian endometriosis, chocolate cysts or haemorrhagic cysts; *see* page 16) should be excised. Simply draining the cyst may cause short-term symptom relief, but to protect against recurrence and avoid negative fertility impacts, the entire cyst, including its contents and wall, must be carefully removed.

Sclerotherapy

An alternative method for endometriomas is a procedure called sclerotherapy, but this is not yet widely used. Sclerotherapy is where the endometrioma is flushed with a solution, a mix of water, sodium chloride, sodium lactate, potassium chloride and calcium chloride, filled with a 96 per cent ethanol (alcohol) solution and left while the surgeon continues operating. The alcohol breaks up the cyst wall, which is then extracted. A small section, not exposed to the alcohol, is sent away for testing. The aim of endometrioma sclerotherapy is to protect the ovarian tissue and preserve as much as possible while also effectively removing the disease. This is a particularly attractive option for those for whom fertility is a concern, and it shows great promise. In a 2020 study, recurrence of endometriomas was observed in 9 per cent of patients who received sclerotherapy and pregnancy occurred in 57 per cent of those desiring to conceive. This was supported in a 2023 study, where 40 per cent of those with pregnancy intent conceived post sclerotherapy and 11.8 per cent had disease recurrence. More traditional methods of endometrioma management see recurrence rates ranging widely, with one 2023 study suggesting rates from 29–56 per cent after two years. We can only hope that further training happens to make this option more widely available.

Comparing surgical methods: ablation versus excision

A study published in 2023 followed endometriosis patients who underwent either ablation or excision surgery. In the group receiving excision surgery, there was improvement in most symptom areas and quality of life measures, while the participants who underwent ablation indicated either no improvement or worsened symptoms and quality of life.

You might think that excision must be a new treatment, something that very few surgeons have had access to training for or even an experimental option. But no. As far back as the 1850s, doctors were known to 'dig out the endometriosis nodules with blunt scissors, or even their own fingernails'. In the 1930s, the first reports of laparoscopic surgeries for non-diagnostic purposes were published, including for the treatment of adhesions and abdominal biopsies. As early as in 1952, it was reported that 'one should excise . . . all evident endometriosis'. In 1985, the first video laparoscopy excision treatment of advanced endometriosis was reported by Camran Nezhat, MD. So, we can see that excision of endometriosis has a long history, although it was muddied by the introduction of hormonal medication in the 1960s.

Even excision is not a cure. However, it is the closest thing we have and, when performed by expert endometriosis specialists, has the lowest chance of disease recurrence or persistence and offers long-term symptomatic relief for many patients. Figures vary, but global experts report that recurrence rates after expert excision surgery can be as low as seven to 15 per cent depending on disease type and location. Without this skilled approach, recurrence rates are estimated at up to 50 per cent within five years.

I asked Dr Rebecca Mallick, consultant gynaecologist and endometriosis surgeon, and BSGE Vice President, for her opinion on ablation versus excision: 'Ablation surgery is easier to perform and more widely available within the UK. However, ablation surgery can leave disease behind and may also be associated with increased scarring and potential for increased pain.' On the other hand, 'laparoscopic excision surgery is associated with significantly greater reductions in pain symptoms compared to ablation surgery'. It is Dr Mallick's opinion that excision surgery should be the way forward for endometriosis surgical management. 'We need to train more surgeons in excision surgery to make it more widely available to all.'

Dr José Eugenio-Colón, endometriosis specialist at the Center for Endometriosis Care, sums it up clearly when I asked him what he thought about ablation surgery: 'Ablation does not work for endometriosis.'

Had I known all of this in 2022 I would never have undergone ablation surgery.

A note on recurrence

Recurrence is always a risk; otherwise, expert excision would be a cure for endometriosis. However, it is important to differentiate between genuine disease recurrence and persistence. If not all lesions are identified and excised completely during surgery, they are likely to continue to cause symptoms and to proliferate. Lesions are also known to grow and change appearance over time. It could also be that disease that was not active at the time of the surgery becomes symptomatic at a later time.

No one wants multiple surgeries for the rest of their lives, but, heartbreakingly, this is what many patients are told when they are advised they have endometriosis. These repeat surgeries are actually harming us and costing the NHS time, resource and money.

Understanding endometriosis care and surgery

Mr Shaheen Khazali, lead endometriosis surgeon at the Centre for Endometriosis and Minimally Invasive Gynaecology (CEMIG) in England, agrees. During our conversation he explains an NHS mantra, "GIRFT" – Getting It Right First Time. 'This is particularly relevant with a disease such as endometriosis and yet it is completely forgotten.' When talking about patients having multiple, repeat surgeries, he is particularly passionate. 'Sixty per cent of my patients have already had two or more surgeries by the time they come to me. But the first surgery is the best surgery. It is the best chance we have to help this patient.' He sums it up pretty much perfectly: 'We need to be getting these individuals diagnosed earlier, referred to the right people, in the right place, the first time. It would save so much time, resource and, most importantly, suffering.'

In a webinar, Dr Ken Sinervo, Medical Director of the Center for Endometriosis Care and an expert excision surgeon, hammered the point home: 'Any doc that says you will likely need repeat surgeries every six to 12 months is a quack and you should leave immediately. Eighty-two per cent of our patients only need one surgery; 2 to 4 per cent need a third.'

Personal stories

At this point, I want to share two stories that really highlight how important accessing expert care truly is. Both of them were shared with me while writing this book and have stayed with me ever since. One is from a patient, Heather, and one is from a surgeon, Dr José Eugenio-Colón.

Heather was diagnosed with endometriosis in the mid-1980s when she was 19. She jokes that it 'only' took her five years to receive the diagnosis and says that she believes her doctor 'did the best with what he knew'. Heather entered a pattern of approximately 'two surgeries a year, for 10 years, with multiple rounds of Lupron (a GnRH) in between'. As she started learning more about the disease, she became increasingly angry about the care she had received so far. 'I remember thinking that if I could just see the celebrity OBGYNs of the day, the ones featured on Oprah, then I could buy better health.' Heather took out loans and credit cards and borrowed money from family to achieve her goal. 'The first doctor told me I had endo because I didn't get along with my mother. The second told me, aged 25, that I should have a hysterectomy and would never be able to have children.'

Endometriosis

Heather was introduced to Dr David Redwine in 1995 by Nancy Peterson, a nurse, creator of Nancy's Nook (the endometriosis education platform), and an endometriosis patient herself. Dr Redwine introduced Heather to the concept of expert excision and referred her to someone who could help. Before that surgery, Heather was in excruciating pain and her 'gallbladder exploded' due to endometriosis. She made it to her planned surgery, where they removed all of the endometriosis, treated the adhesions caused by the emergency gallbladder surgery and told Heather that she could in fact have children after all. Three weeks later, Heather fell pregnant. After having her son, she was still in pain and suffering from heavy bleeding, contributed to by a diagnosis of adenomyosis and fibroids that was mentioned for the first time during this expert surgery. 'No one ever mentioned it to me before.' She decided to undergo a hysterectomy. That was in 1998 and, after 22 surgeries in total, was the last time Heather was operated on for endometriosis.

When I spoke with Dr José Eugenio-Colón, he generously shared his experience and reasons for becoming an endometriosis specialist. Although it is a sad tale, it highlights just how important this expert knowledge is. 'I was a general obstetrician gynaecologist (OBGYN) on an amazing programme, and I loved it. I was doing a lot of surgeries there, and for two days a week I also worked in a clinic in a medically underserved area with a high volume of Hispanic patients. So, I was exposed to patients of all different cultures and socioeconomic statuses.' One of the patients at this clinic had endometriosis. 'I treated her with the little knowledge I had as a board-certified OBGYN here in the US, which was pain medication, birth control, Lupron (a GnRH), "it's in your head", "it can't be that bad" and more gaslighting . . . then I took her to surgery.' When Dr Eugenio-Colón looked inside this woman's pelvis, he 'saw a mess'. He 'took some biopsies, burned some stuff' and told her that I couldn't do anything else. ...General OBGYNs are not trained to deal with all that drama,' he says, so 'I sent her to oncology, who told her that the only option was a hysterectomy. She was in her mid-20s and wanted children in the future.'

'I told her I couldn't do anything else except more Lupron, but she had bad side effects with that . . . She disappeared for a month or so, then came back and her pain was horrible. Her mum told her to tell me what she had done. She had tried to commit suicide. She told me, "You didn't want to help me." I cried . . . I felt like I sucked as a surgeon and as a person.'

This experience triggered Dr Eugenio-Colón into wanting to train further to avoid another case like this one. 'I went back for more training at a fellowship, despite colleagues telling me it was pointless.' But he felt like, despite the high surgical volumes he was undertaking, he was not doing enough. 'Part of my fellowship was with Dr Sinervo at the Center for Endometriosis Care. When I saw what Dr Sinervo was doing, it blew my mind. I knew then I'd dedicate myself solely to endo and I told Dr Sinervo I would stay for as long as he'd have me.'

Our level of knowledge around endometriosis has increased since Dr Eugenio-Colón was working in that clinic a decade ago, but many of us will still relate to his description of the treatment plan he provided for his young patient. So, why are we in the position where suboptimal surgeries are being performed on patients, despite what we now know about this disease? 'In the end, it all comes down to education, awareness and quality control,' explains Mr Mikey Adamczyk, consultant gynaecologist and endometriosis surgeon. 'If we're not equipping clinicians with up-to-date, evidence-based knowledge, they simply won't have the tools to give patients the care they deserve. Endometriosis has long been underfunded and neglected in both research and education. Because of this, a lot of clinicians are simply repeating what they were told by their mentors years ago', continuing the cycle of misinformation and outdated practices. 'We need broader awareness of endometriosis across the medical community and, importantly, quality control to ensure that the most current information is used in practice' and to improve patient outcomes. 'The only way to get better at endometriosis surgery is to solely dedicate yourself to endometriosis as a specialism,' says Dr Eugenio-Colón. 'You can't be a general gynaecologist. You can't be delivering babies. You can't be distracted'.

Sadly, patients from the UK and many other countries around the world are having to travel overseas to access the levels of expert care they need. Endometriosis campaigner Rey, @reythewarrior, travelled from Scotland to Bucharest in Romania for their second surgery, and shares their story with us here. 'I got my period quite late – I was just past 16. My mum was the same and I was really athletic so we weren't concerned. I went on the pill straight away so that I could control my periods for my ballet.

'For a long time, I was fine. My periods caused me a lot of lower back pain, but I would brush it aside. What I now know, looking back, is that all the things I was going to the chiropractor for, the physio for, the acupuncturist for, all those points of pain – the signs of endometriosis were there. And when you're young, you don't clock that it's cyclical, so I would brush it off as scar tissue from dance injuries.'

Endometriosis

'I was on the pill for a good decade. I tried different types. In my early 20s, I had moved to the UK [from Australia] and was on a pill called Microgynon, which I had a horrific experience with. I came off hormones in my early 20s and all these symptoms kicked in. I asked my mum if she remembered my periods ever being particularly bad and she recalled that I had [previously] tried to come off [the pill] for a hot minute and "you nearly died", it was that bad. I have a very specific memory of getting cramps so bad I nearly hit the floor in a shopping centre. But I still hadn't connected it at all to my cycle. Massive digestive issues were misdiagnosed as IBS. I went to A&E. Was it gallstones? Was it my appendix?' There were no real answers forthcoming and things just kept getting worse and worse.

At one point, Rey's partner said, 'I don't think you realise how bad you are.' 'That's when I really started taking notice of what was going on, in 2015. But I didn't go to the doctor, because I thought they were just going to give pain meds and there was just too much going on in my life. 2018 was the last time I went to A&E, and after being sent home again, I thought there just has to be something. I had never heard the word endometriosis until I started googling my symptoms.' The information they found was 'conflicting and wishy-washy' and did not provide Rey with the level of information she needed. They joined support groups on Facebook and 'everything fell into place'. All their symptoms for the past 20 years aligned, and Rey was convinced that endometriosis was to blame.

By this point, Rey was bedridden for at least one week of the month, with daily nausea, 'chowing down on pain meds' and having panic attacks during ovulation. However, they still didn't have a solution. 'Birth control? Tried that, that just messed me up. My periods sucked, but they weren't heavy. I didn't want anything inserted into my body until I figured out what was happening.'

Rey went to the doctor 'armed to the teeth with guidelines' and told them they wanted a scan. 'My quality of life was in the trash.' So, they were sent off for a standard pelvic ultrasound, which unsurprisingly missed everything. It came back clear. Thankfully, Rey had a doctor who understood endometriosis enough to say that didn't rule out the disease. 'I got lucky,' they say, and they asked to be referred. I 'knew it had to be someone with experience with endometriosis, not a general gynae'. That information came from an online support group, not any of the UK's national resources. Rey was referred to the closest BSGE centre, which was in Scotland, 2.5 hours away from where they lived. No scan was performed before this first surgery other than that basic pelvic scan that missed everything.

'I just needed a diagnosis. I needed to know what was happening so that I could then make a plan for my treatment,' they explain. And they did receive a diagnosis. Their post-operative report says 'excised one small spot of endometriosis from pelvic sidewall; suspected adenomyosis'.

Rey asked for their post-surgical imaging, and in the photographs they could clearly see the presence of fibroids and that one of their ovaries was stuck. The adenomyosis and fibroids made their decision about their next steps easier for them. 'I never wanted children,' they say, so when they were given the option to take out 'this thing ruining my life', Rey was on board.

They knew that they wanted minimal surgeries, and that 'the next person I saw needed to be the best that I can afford, so that if any endo was left behind, they could take it out when they removed my uterus. The emphasis was on "best that I can afford".' Rey knew that to access the level of expertise they needed, they would have to look for a private endometriosis surgeon. The hospital fees in the UK, which make up the largest chunk of private healthcare bills, were just too prohibitive, so Rey started looking overseas. Travelling abroad seemed more affordable, with Bucharest looking like a great option. 'I was going to have to travel anyway due to where I live. But it's terrifying, and trying to convince your family that you need to travel abroad for surgery is a lot. But I had to go with my gut.' Rey is incredibly grateful for their supportive partner and family. It took a long time to come to the decision to travel overseas for surgery. 'No one wants to have surgery, but I got to a point where my quality of life was so bad,' they say, 'where I was a shell, I wasn't a human anymore. I wasn't living my life, I didn't recognise myself. My passion for anything, for life, was zero.'

After this surgery in Bucharest, Rey found out what was really happening inside their body. It was 'actually adenomyosis, fibroids, endometriosis on my left ovary, the base of my right ovary, uterosacral ligaments, spots around the pelvic cavity, rectovaginal pouch and sigmoid colon.' There were also adhesions as a result of the first surgery. This was a bit different from the 'one small spot of endometriosis from pelvic sidewall; suspected adenomyosis' reported after Rey's first surgery. 'I have no regrets about travelling, but I hate that I had to,' Rey explains. 'We're a G7 country, we have the NHS . . . It shouldn't be up to me to have to fight so hard. I shouldn't have to be reading research papers. I shouldn't have to be going to every doctor's meeting like I'm going to a negotiation. It shouldn't be that way. It made me angry and upset that I had to do it, and even more so that so many others won't get the chance to do it.'

Hysterectomy

We will talk more about hysterectomy in chapter 4, but for now it is important to know that a hysterectomy (the removal of the uterus) is not a cure for endometriosis. It was long believed that this major procedure would be the ultimate cure for the disease, the thinking being that if the reproductive organs were removed, a (wrongly believed to be) 'reproductive disease' could not exist without them. I honestly dread to think how many women had their organs and fertility removed under the belief and assurance that it would bring them lifelong relief. As I've shared previously, my mum was one of them.

It is true that some patients will feel symptomatic relief; never having to have another period again is a major perk of the procedure, and this alone can ease symptoms for many. If there are other conditions at play, such as adenomyosis or fibroids (which we will explore in chapter 4), a hysterectomy will permanently remove them, which is likely to bring some improvements to quality of life. However, a hysterectomy does not remove endometriosis, which will remain symptomatic and cause long-term issues. Sadly, we have not progressed very far at all in the 30 years since my mum underwent a radical hysterectomy (where both the uterus and the surrounding tissues are removed, including the fallopian tubes, part of the vagina, ovaries, lymph glands and fatty tissue) for her endometriosis. In 2024, a friend of mine was seen by a well-respected gynaecologist who confidently told her 'a hysterectomy is the gold standard cure for endometriosis. You won't have any issues once we remove your womb.' Doctors are still telling us to undergo life-changing surgery with permanent, irreversible consequences, despite us knowing it is not a cure.

That said, depending on a patient's specific circumstances and life goals, there are indications that a hysterectomy in conjunction with complete expert excision surgery can provide positive patient outcomes. However, it is imperative that the excision surgery be completed at the same time as the hysterectomy by a skilled endometriosis expert.

Hysterectomy jargon busting

There are multiple types of hysterectomy and, when you're in a consultation having medical jargon thrown at you, it can be a bit confusing and overwhelming. Figure 3.1 provides a quick reminder of some of the terms you might hear.

Figure 3.1: Hysterectomy – a brief biology recap

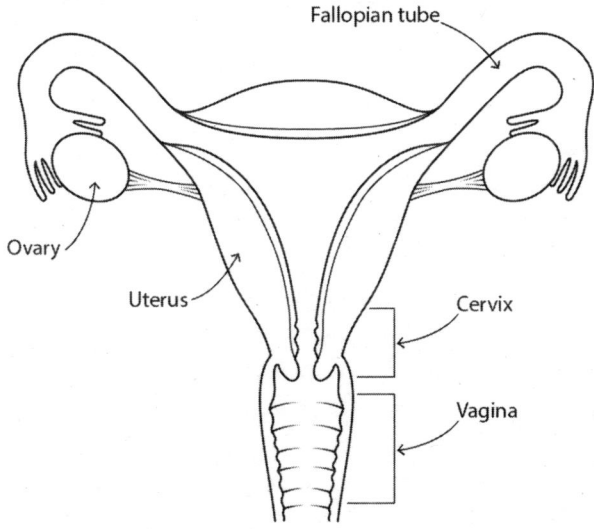

- Sub-total hysterectomy: Removes the uterus but leaves the cervix in place. Leaving the cervix in place does have risks associated, so make sure to talk these through with your surgeon. You will still need to have regular smear tests.
- Total hysterectomy: Removes the uterus and the cervix. This is usually the preferred method as the risk of developing cervical cancer at a later date is removed. You will not need regular smears (yay!), but you may need a vault smear.

A vault smear is similar to a cervical smear: a sample of cells is taken from the top of the vagina in someone who has had a total hysterectomy. The responsibility for this follow-up procedure rests with the treating gynaecologist, who should ensure the GP receives clear written guidance. You should consider a vault smear if:

- You have not had regular cervical smears (book a vault smear for six months after surgery).
- Abnormal cells were detected in the analysis of your cervix following your hysterectomy (book a vault smear for six and 18 months after surgery)
- Radical hysterectomy: Removes the uterus, cervix, fallopian tubes, ovaries and potentially part of the vagina and some surrounding tissue.
- Unilateral vs bilateral: Usually used in relation to salpingectomy and oophorectomy (*see* below). Unilateral means one side (one fallopian tube or ovary), whereas bilateral means both sides (both tubes or ovaries).
- Salpingectomy: Removal of one or both fallopian tubes.
- Oophorectomy: Removal of one or both ovaries. The removal of your ovaries will immediately put you into surgical menopause, so HRT and a management plan should be discussed before surgery. Usually, unless there is a clear reason to remove the ovaries, it is preferred to preserve them, avoiding surgical menopause and the associated risks. Please note that even if ovarian preservation occurs, the ovaries will have undergone significant trauma during surgery. There are no definite answers, but it is possible that ovarian function could reduce, cease earlier than usual or become a bit temperamental, as mine did. A plan should be put in place prior to the surgery for follow-ups and support such as HRT. If you have any concerns about any new symptoms after surgery, check with your doctor and ask about options.

A hysterectomy can be performed in one of three ways:

1. Laparotomy (open): The uterus is removed via a larger abdominal incision. This type of surgery has increased risks and a longer recovery time and will leave a large scar, but it may sometimes be necessary.
2. Laparoscopy (keyhole): The uterus is removed via small incisions made in the abdomen, but there is always the risk of needing to move to laparotomy. Laparoscopy an also be performed robotically, where the surgeon controls instruments from a console, allowing greater stability, precision and flexibility.
3. Vaginal: Removal of the uterus via the vagina, the least invasive option.

Your surgeon should discuss all options with you and suggest which route will minimise risks and maximise benefits in your specific situation.

What is an endometriosis expert?

My first surgery was ablation. Had I known what I do now, or had I managed to get hold of this book, I would have never gone ahead with it. It was performed by the first person who confirmed I had endometriosis. This simple fact, that he validated and confirmed what I had suspected for 22 years, meant I put my trust in him. He is a very well-respected and accomplished gynaecological oncologist, used to dealing with complex cancer cases. I trusted in his ability to help me too. However, he is not an endometriosis specialist. I now know that he used suboptimal techniques, missed significant disease and used outdated and debunked information to explain endometriosis to me. Had all of the information in this section been available to me, I would have chosen a different surgeon, even if that meant a further agonising wait. But how do we know in whose hands to put our bodies, our health, our lives?

'Diagnosing and managing endometriosis is uniquely challenging,' Mr Mikey Adamczyk, consultant gynaecologist and endometriosis surgeon, explains to me. 'Quite simply, not every gynaecological surgeon has the expertise to perform this type of complex surgery. It requires incredible hand–eye coordination and years of specialised training and fellowships to perform these surgeries safely and effectively.'

Most gynaecologists will say they can treat endometriosis because their medical training tells them that they can. There is no specific, formalised fellowship (specialty medical training) for this disease, so anyone can technically say that they have a 'special interest' in endometriosis or are an 'excision specialist'. Even being an expert in excision is not a guarantee of success if the individual in question is not entirely devoted to endometriosis and fully aware of all its presentations and manifestations. Surgeons can only remove what they see and recognise. 'I honestly don't think any clinician sets out to harm their patients,' Mr Mikey Adamczyk says, and, in all honesty, despite everything I have been through medically, I agree. 'But in medicine, especially among the older generation, we often rely on our experiences and on approaches that have worked for us in the past.' With endometriosis, though, as we have seen, this kind of thinking can create problems. 'I've seen it first-hand – how common myths and misinformation persist, like advising patients to get pregnant as a treatment or recommending hysterectomy for deep endometriosis, even when these approaches don't align with what we know now.'

'It's like going to a dentist with pain in a back tooth, and instead of addressing the actual issue, the dentist suggests pulling a front tooth simply because that's the procedure they know how to do. It doesn't make sense and, let's face it, it just would not happen. But due to a lack of prioritisation and funding leading to gaps in training and education, this is often what happens with endometriosis treatment advice.'

Use this list of questions in your consultation to determine your surgeon's approach to treating endometriosis and help you identify any red flags:

- Is endometriosis your sole specialty?
- Have you trained at a high-volume endometriosis centre that deals with complex cases? *They should have spent time at a centre specialising in endometriosis that deals with hundreds of surgeries annually, including complex cases.*
- How many endometriosis surgeries do you perform each month? *Remember that global experts and centres are performing hundreds each year – you need someone who is keeping up their surgical skills.*
- Which surgical method do you use? Why? *Excision!*
- Will you look for endometriosis on other organs? Which areas of the body do you check? *All organs should be checked for signs of disease, including behind the liver and the diaphragm.*
- Do you work with a multi-disciplinary team? *Endometriosis is a multi-disciplinary disease and a multi-disciplinary team (or MDT) is therefore needed to treat it, especially in cases of organ involvement such as the bowel or bladder.*
- Do you take biopsies for testing? *This is imperative for appropriate testing and diagnosis.*
- What steps do you take to preserve fertility?
- If there are endometriomas, do you drain them or excise them completely?
- Will you also check for adenomyosis, fibroids and cysts? What will happen if you find them?
- Will you perform the surgery yourself?

Understanding endometriosis care and surgery

- Will you take images and videos during the surgery? Can I have copies? *Always ask for full records, including imagery.*
- What are your complication rates? *These should be tracked and low. To give you an idea, a 2024 paper based on over 1000 surgeries at a globally recognised endometriosis centre showed a minor post-operative complication rate of 13.8 per cent and major complication of 1.5 per cent. There were no complications of the most severe kind.*
- What are your recurrence rates? *These should be tracked and low. As an example, one globally recognised endometriosis centre reports a 7–15 per cent recurrence rate post exicision surgery.*
- (For bowel involvement) What is your rate for stoma requirement? Can you perform resections? *A stoma is an opening on the abdomen that connects to your digestive system, allowing waste to be diverted out of your body and into a pouch. This can either be temporary or permanent. Stomas should not be a regular surgical requirement. In skilled hands, most bowel endometriosis can be carefully excised and a resection performed.*
- Do you do a pre-surgery MRI for optimal planning?
- What are your thoughts on hormone therapy for endometriosis? Do you recommend GnRH analogues? *Remember, no hormonal treatment cures or shrinks endometriosis lesions. There is some evidence emerging that progesterone treatments may be beneficial to prevent or slow the recurrence of endometriomas after excision surgery.*
- Are there any cases where you would not remove disease? Would you refer me to a surgeon with the required skills to remove it? *It is rare for there to be an area that cannot be excised by a specialist endometriosis expert, but it is also important that a surgeon does not operate beyond their limitations and capacity.*
- When will my follow-up appointment be?
- What is the plan for my ongoing pain management and aftercare? *Ideally, the doctor will recommend pelvic floor physiotherapy and monitoring of your symptoms and quality of life.*

Hopefully, the answers provided to these questions will give you a much better understanding of the surgeon and whether you would like to proceed to an endometriosis surgery with them. I know that asking questions and advocating for ourselves can be really difficult, especially when so many of us have been dismissed and belittled in medical settings for years. But this is your health, your life, and you deserve to have the correct care and treatment. A competent surgeon will be willing and able to answer any questions and be glad that you are well-informed and engaged. If you are nervous, take someone with you to your appointment and share these questions with them. They can then ask them with you or for you. And don't forget that you, or your support, can write down the answers for you to go over later.

Remember, who performs endometriosis surgery and how is the key to success and is ultimately up to you. Trust your instinct. Never be made to feel like you are being 'difficult'; you are a human being advocating for your body, your health and your future. You are the expert in this situation too. You are the expert in your own body, your own experience and how endometriosis impacts your life, shaped by your personal circumstances. Heather Guidone, Board Certified Patient Advocate, reinforces this: 'Often, the patient is the only expert in the room.'

Improving standards

As we've seen throughout the previous chapters, the state of endometriosis care is currently a bit of a mess. It is important that this book reflects reality, but that does not mean people are not working hard behind the scenes to raise the bar and improve the landscape for patients. One such effort is being undertaken by a group of endometriosis surgeons from numerous countries across Europe. Led by Mr Mohamed Mabrouk, endometriosis surgeon and president of the European Endometriosis League, this project seeks to create Europe-wide standardised accreditation criteria for endometriosis surgeons and high-quality endometriosis centres. Systems like the one being proposed exist for numerous other surgical specialisms, but not yet for endometriosis.

Mr Mabrouk explains that the list of accreditation criteria will be long and detailed, determined by a group of global expert surgeons, presidents and other representatives from endometriosis organisations across Europe, and patients. The aim? Raising, and holding, the bar for endometriosis patient care. Points will be attributed according to measures such as the structure of the clinic, the maintenance of an accurate database, the volume of surgeries performed, compliance to best practices, the rate of repeat surgeries and

Understanding endometriosis care and surgery

complication rates. Assessment of surgical skills and procedures will also form part of the process. Initially, this will be undertaken by an independent endometriosis specialist, but eventually, the idea is that artificial intelligence (AI) may be able to take over this part of accreditation. Mr Mabrouk likens the full process to a driving test, where there are major and minor faults. Some things will be 'instant failures' whereas others may lower a score. This process should create an educational feedback loop to surgeons and clinics to improve their care. A patient, he says, will be able to look at a website, check a clinic or surgeon and see their credentials and experience, find out who is in the MDT and what the complication rate is and then make a choice if they trust this person or team to operate on them.

The goal, according to Mr Mabrouk, is to make clinic- and surgeon-specific data 'transparent and accessible to patients', empowering them to make the right choice for their bodies. Mr Mabrouk says that if, for example, 'you log on and see that a surgeon has a 40 per cent complication rate for surgeries involving the bowel, you may not choose that surgeon'. Likewise, 'if fertility is a key concern, you will be able to see which clinics have a fertility specialist and that may inform your decision'.

The research and academic phase have just been completed at the time of writing, so next comes the hard work of implementing this independent network across Europe, then globally. If it comes to fruition, this could be a huge step forward for improving endometriosis care – something that, as we patients all know, we desperately need.

The reality of having no cure

I know that I keep stressing that endometriosis has no cure. That is the sad reality, despite what we are told by various doctors, media outlets and other well-meaning people trying to reassure us. Truthfully, it can be an extremely daunting thing to face. If that's where you're at right now, know that it is natural, and okay, to feel like that. I remember when it fully dawned on me that this is a lifelong condition. It was after my second surgery when I was still in persistent pain, caused by a variety of factors. That was two years into my endometriosis journey and was the moment I realised I needed to deal with this for the rest

> of my life. I cried. Probably for the first time since my diagnosis, I properly let it out. Because let's face it, it's rubbish and it can change your life completely. But please know that having a lifelong condition doesn't mean it's a life sentence. With the right medical care, a future-focused strategy and the right support at home, you can still lead a full and fulfilling life. It might look different from how you imagined – mine certainly does – but it is possible to reclaim your life while living with endometriosis.

Time for surgery

You've gone through years of trying to get someone to listen. You've had your scans. You've waited to see a specialist. You've confirmed that they are skilled in endometriosis excision. You've waited again on the list for surgery. And suddenly it's here: it's time for your endometriosis surgery.

Pre-surgery

Usually, you will either have a form to complete or a telephone appointment where you are asked lots of questions about your medical history. This is your chance to tell your doctor about any other conditions that you suffer with, any side effects you have had from anaesthesia and so on. You will then be asked to attend a pre-operative assessment. This is usually done a few weeks to a few days before surgery, depending on the clinic. You will have basic checks done, including your height, weight and blood pressure. You will also have a blood test, a urine test and possibly an ECG. Depending on your personal medical profile, you may have other tests too.

To aid recovery, most clinics advise taking some gentle daily exercise in the weeks leading up to surgery, as well as eating a balanced diet and getting regular sleep. Make sure you fulfil any prescriptions that you have so you are well-stocked with your medications.

Prepare the room in which you will be recovering at home before you leave for hospital. Trust me, you will not want to be waiting around to crawl into bed and get as comfy as possible. Change the sheets, clear away things that are not needed, get yourself a body pillow or a V-shaped pillow and set out anything you might like nearby while you rest. Sort out any distractions or entertainment you may want while you recover. Download podcasts or new audiobooks. Put some activities near the bed so you can easily reach them – whatever will make recovery easier for you. Make sure you arrange for someone to pick you up after surgery and stay with you for at least the first 24 hours after getting home. If this isn't in place then the hospital will not proceed with the surgery, so it's not something to skip.

Fill your fridge and freezer with easy meals that can just be reheated when you're back home. Go for lighter options, especially at first, but don't deny yourself any treats that you may fancy. My parents delivered two weeks' worth of meals for our freezer before my hysterectomy and it was honestly the sweetest gesture. It made my husband's life so much easier too as he took on the role of caring for me during recovery.

Packing for surgery

Your endometriosis laparoscopy may be done on a day-surgery basis, meaning you won't have to stay overnight, or you may be scheduled to stay at the hospital. This will depend on the complexity of your case.

Either way, I would 100 per cent recommend packing a full bag. You never know what will happen on the day and I promise you will be grateful to have everything on hand should you need it. This is the checklist I used for both of my endometriosis surgeries, so, let's get packing!

- Comfy, loose-fitting clothes
- High-waisted underwear in a larger size than usual
- Pyjamas, slippers and dressing gown
- Phone and charger
- Extra-long charging cable or power bank
- Entertainment (laptop, magazines, books)
- Toothbrush and toothpaste
- Hairbrush
- Baby wipes
- Lip balm
- Moisturiser
- Cooling face and body mist
- Handheld battery-powered fan
- Period pads or underwear

- Insulated cup with a straw to keep drinks cold
- All medications in their original boxes, as well as your prescription
- Throat sweets
- Mints and peppermint teabags for the gas pain (*see* page 135)
- Any paperwork associated with your surgery
- Pillow (for the drive home; *see* page 135)
- Any comfort items you may want to take (blanket, soft toy, pillow)

Surgery day

Make sure you follow all the instructions from your clinic and stop eating and drinking when they specify. I always try to make sure that last bit of food before being nil by mouth is something I love. For my last surgery, I ended up having homemade waffles and strawberries at 3 a.m. Before leaving for surgery, I also braid my hair to avoid it becoming a knotted mess. I say I braid it, but I'm terrible with hair so my sister-in-law actually comes and does it for me. Don't be afraid to ask for help from your friends and family.

Arrive at the clinic at the time you've been given, and you will be shown to your bed. You may have some further tests done, and you should be seen by your surgeon and anaesthetist, who will go over any last-minute questions. You will also be given consent forms to sign. Read these carefully and make sure you are happy with what you are consenting to before adding your signature. Patient advocate Rey, also known as @reythewarrior on social media, gives fantastic advice here. 'Literally write on that consent form, "I do not consent to ablation".' You are always in control of what treatment you receive; you are always in the driving seat. When it's time to go down to surgery, you will be taken to a room where the anaesthesia will be administered.

After your surgery, you will wake up in a recovery ward, where you will be closely monitored until the nurses are happy for you to be sent back to your ward. They will usually give you a sip of water and ask how you're feeling, but in my experience, you probably won't remember too much about this part as the anaesthesia will still be very much in your system!

When you come round from the anaesthetic, you may find that you are in pain or feeling sick. Make sure you call for a nurse and tell them so they can adjust any pain relief or supply nausea medications. During a laparoscopy, your abdomen is inflated with carbon dioxide gas so the surgical team can have a better view of your organs and tissues. After the surgery, this gas can become trapped, causing irritation and pain that is often felt up into the shoulder area and can last for several days. I wish I had been warned about this pain. I didn't have it at all after my first surgery, but after my second it most definitely made its presence felt. Tell your nurse if you are suffering with this pain; they will offer you a warm mint drink, which can help immeasurably. Have as many as you can! My husband also made me mint tea in between and brought some strong mints in for me to chew. Gentle heat can also help with this pain. Another great help is to, in the words of my nurse, 'have a really good fart!'

Before you leave the hospital, your surgeon should come and see you to tell you how the surgery went, what was found and what was done. You may still be groggy from medications at this point, so it is always worth asking them to write things down, having someone with you who can listen and make notes or asking to record the conversation on your phone to reflect on later. Make sure you also ask for the images and videos of your surgery. Before discharging you, the nurses may want to make sure that you are passing urine properly, take some blood tests and check that you can walk a short distance. If you and they are happy, you will be given a prescription for pain relief and discharged home. You may also be given a course of injections to administer yourself at home to prevent blood clots while you recover.

Don't worry about getting properly dressed if you don't have to. I usually just go home in my pyjamas, dressing gown and slip-on shoes. If you do have to get dressed, choose loose-fitting items that are easy to get on and off. Make sure you have someone with you to accompany you home, and have a pillow with you to gently press against the surgical site and protect against seatbelts. Make sure your driver takes it slowly, avoiding any bumps, potholes or sudden accelerations or braking.

Back home

Once you are home, it is time to rest. Rest as much as you physically can; your body has been through a lot and it needs time to heal. Recovery is not linear. One day you may feel like you can achieve a bit more, and then the next day you're back in bed. That's okay. It takes time. The important thing is to be gentle with yourself, remind yourself how much your body has been through and try not to compare your experience with that of other people. Your recovery will be as unique as you are.

Try to start gentle movement as soon as you feel able. Even a small walk around the house or garden will be hugely beneficial. If you are unsteady, have someone with you or use a mobility aid. Some gentle stretching after a few weeks can prove helpful as well, especially when it comes to reducing adhesion formation. This movement will also help move things along when it comes to your bowels.

Constipation can be a real struggle post-surgery, and you may find that your bowel movements are painful at first, but resuming regular movements as soon as possible is important. The hospital may provide you with laxatives, or you can take stool softeners to help manage this. I also fully recommend a 'squatty potty', or similar, to elevate your feet and maintain a more helpful posture. If you don't want to buy one, a box can work just as well! Eating a diet rich in fruits and vegetables and avoiding anything overly processed can also help, but don't deny yourself a treat too. You've been through a lot, so if you want some cake or some macaroni cheese, go for it.

The first couple of periods following endometriosis surgery can also be unexpectedly painful. My first period after my first surgery took me by surprise. I had experienced more than my fair share of painful periods over the years and was so hopeful that the surgery would help reduce that pain. However, no one warned me that the first few would be on a par with the most painful ones I'd ever experienced, in addition to the pain of healing from surgery. Make sure you're prepared and have pain relief and any other tools (heat, TENS machines, etc.) at the ready. Your surgeon may recommend a short-term dose of hormonal medication for a few months post-surgery to help manage this. It's entirely up to you whether or not you decide to use it depending on your experience with hormonal pharmacological options in the past.

When it comes to sex post-surgery, there are a few things to bear in mind. Your surgeon will likely say you need to wait for six weeks; as mine so delightfully told my husband, 'Don't worry. She will be good to go after six weeks.' Charming. However, it is entirely up to you. You may still be in discomfort from surgery. You may have dealt with painful sex for years previously and be nervous to explore your 'new normal'. If you are not ready after six weeks, then say so. It is always up to you – don't ever feel bad for drawing that boundary. You can use lube, pillows and toys if required to make yourself more comfortable, but the key part is communication. And remember, sex is more than intercourse. There are other ways to be intimate if you're not feeling ready.

You will have been told by your surgeon how long your recovery will take. This is usually six to 12 weeks depending on your disease type, location, extent and organ involvement. However, this length of time is for surgical recovery; it does not mean you will magically feel incredible by the end of it. Truthfully, it can take months, a year or even years to establish your 'new normal'. Think about how long you have been in pain. In my case, it was 22 years before my first surgery. That's a very long time for someone's anatomy to be under attack, to be irritated, inflamed, invaded and working sub-optimally. Then add the physical trauma of surgery on top of that. Recovery is going to take a lot longer than six to 12 weeks.

That doesn't mean you might not feel improvements quickly. Over the last couple of years I have spoken to hundreds of endometriosis patients who have undergone surgery. Some patients report that they can almost immediately feel relief after expert excision surgery. Others say it took a few months before they started noticing that their daily pain levels were lower than before and they were able to do more and enjoy their lives. Others still say that they remain in considerable pain, months, even years post-surgery. This is why comparing our experiences is helpful only to a point. We have to remember how individual we, our lives and our endometriosis experiences are.

You should have a follow-up appointment with your surgeon, usually 6-12 weeks post-surgery, to check how you are healing and how you are doing. This is your opportunity to ask as many questions as possible about your surgery, what was found, how it was treated, what the histology samples came back saying and what the plan is for your care going forward.

Asking for support

It is very easy to say 'make sure you rest for as long as you need', but in reality, our life circumstances may not always permit this. Maybe you are a single mum who needs to look after your children, or you need to get back to work within two weeks, not 12, or you have elderly parents who need caring for – the potential scenarios are endless. If you are in

> this category, please ask for as much help as you can. Whether it's from work, friends or family, please use any support network available to you as much as possible. Try to prep things like meals before your surgery to ease that burden and, if you do have to return to work, ask about flexible working or adjustments such as different seating.
>
> Remember, we are all doing the best we can at any given point in time with the resources available to us. No one can judge you for that.

What if no endometriosis is found?

Endometriosis and adenomyosis were identified on surgical imaging before both of my surgeries. Despite that, I was still paranoid that I would come round from the anaesthesia to be told that 'nothing was found' and 'everything was normal'. It became so much of a worry that I genuinely had nightmares about it in the weeks leading up to surgery. It sounds odd, doesn't it? That you're hoping for the doctors to find disease, not to tell you that everything is fine. It was a contradiction that I used to be ashamed of. Of course I didn't want to be ill, but I also couldn't take being told, again, that nothing was wrong when it so very clearly was. And I know I'm not alone. I hear from so many endometriosis patients that they also have these fears. If you think about it, it makes sense that we worry about this. We have spent years being told nothing is wrong. Even scans can inaccurately tell us that everything is 'normal'. It is therefore perfectly natural to worry that, after all this time, pain and distress, it may have been for nothing. Maybe it was all in our head after all? Most of the time, we wake up validated, with disease confirmed and the next steps agreed upon – but not always. So, what happens if you do come round from your surgery and hear the words 'we couldn't see any endometriosis'?

First, it's okay to feel disappointed to not have an answer for your symptoms. When I've talked to patients who were in this position, the words 'lonely', 'confused', 'exhausted', 'angry', 'crushed' and 'felt like giving up' have all come up. Allow yourself to feel whatever emotions arise for you without feeling guilty or ashamed. The most important thing right now is to focus on recovering from your surgery. Your pain and symptoms are real and deserve answers, but right now you need to heal.

What happens next ultimately comes down to the skills and experience of your surgeon. Are you confident in their ability to look for and recognise all aspects and presentations of this disease? Remember, lesions can even be transparent in appearance. Did they check all organs and structures? Extra-pelvic endometriosis (*see* pages 22–23) is not as rare as once thought, but it is only rarely looked for. If you have any doubts at all, consider seeking a second, third or fourth opinion. You can ask your GP to refer you to an endometriosis specialist centre (*see* pages 111–113), citing persistent symptoms, or you could select a specialist yourself. Really do your research when deciding who to go to. Make sure you gather all your records and images from your previous surgery, along with any scans. Use the questions for surgeons listed earlier in this chapter (*see* pages 128–129) and make sure you're happy that they fully understand the complexities of endometriosis. Unfortunately, this often means private healthcare, which is inaccessible to many patients.

Either way, being told that no endometriosis was found should never mean the end of your care. Make sure you ask your surgeon the following questions:

- Were there signs of any other conditions such as adhesions, adenomyosis, fibroids, cysts or polyps?
- Did you take any biopsies and send them off for analysis?
- Did you take photos or videos and, if so, can I have a copy?
- What is the next step to investigate the cause of my pain?

Depending on your symptoms, you may find that you are referred to other departments, such as to a colorectal specialist if you are dealing with bowel symptoms.

Don't give up. As exhausting as it is, you deserve answers.

Surgery is step one

Surgery is not a cure for endometriosis, not even excision performed by the most experienced and skilled endometriosis surgeons. This means an excision surgery is not the end of your endometriosis journey. In fact, in terms of the rest of your life, it is step one.

Before I had my second surgery, I had an expectation in my head of how life would be afterwards. That I would be pain-free, able to do whatever I wanted and live life fully and carefree. Now, for some people, that is what happens. Some people get halfway there and, let's be honest, any improvement is something we will gladly and gratefully accept. But I still live in daily pain and, at first, it spiked my anxiety. Was the endometriosis 'back'? Was some disease missed? Had I done something to cause it? By the way, the answer to that last one is always, always no. Each one of us will have an entirely unique experience with pain after surgery.

Why do some of us still experience pain after excision surgery? It's to do with something that was once described to me as the 'pain puzzle': a jigsaw puzzle made up of pieces representing the issues potentially causing you pain. Could it still be due to endometriosis lesions? Yes, possibly. If your surgeon is not experienced enough to recognise and remove all disease, persistent endometriosis could absolutely be causing your symptoms. However, your pain may not have solely been down to endometriosis. Several issues and conditions can cause us pain, even after expert excision. My second surgery removed adenomyosis, fibroids and all visible signs of endometriosis, but the continuing pain indicates that other pain generators are still very much active. Some of these 'puzzle pieces' could include the following:

- Long-term inflammation
- Numerous other chronic conditions, such as adenomyosis, fibroids, painful bladder syndrome and fibromyalgia
- Damage to the pelvic floor tissues after years of hypertension
- Altered anatomy due to organ removal
- Bladder and bowel symptoms
- Central sensitisation (*see* page 141)

This pelvic pain puzzle will be completely unique to you and your experience, and is as individual as your fingerprint. You and your care team need to identify the pieces of your own personal pain puzzle and develop a treatment plan for each one. To give you an illustration, Figure 3.2 shows you what my pain puzzle currently consists of. All of these contribute to my pain and require their own management strategies, including physical therapy (both pelvic floor and musculoskeletal), pain management, surgical interventions and lifestyle changes. What does your current pain puzzle look like and what can you do to manage each piece?

Figure 3.2: My current 'pain puzzle'

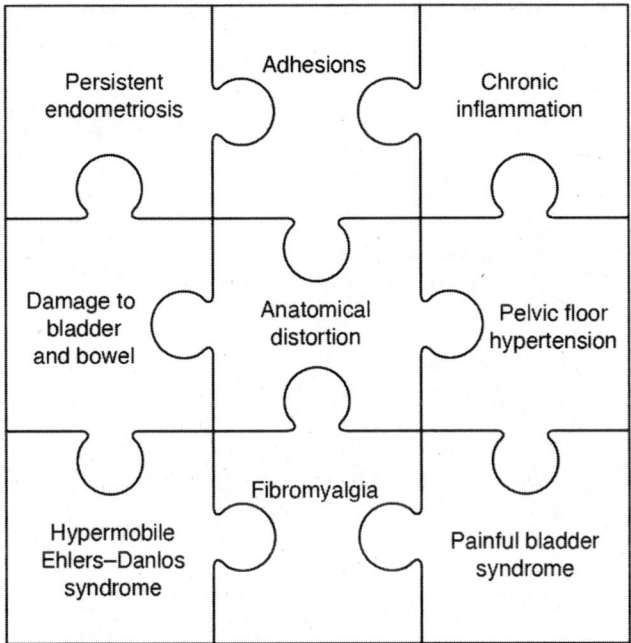

Central sensitisation

Central sensitisation refers to the process where our nervous system changes how it responds to pain, particularly when it is experiencing pain over the long term. These changes can make us more sensitive to pain over time as our body learns to constantly anticipate it. Pain management services look to 'down-regulate' the nervous system, rewiring the brain to not be in continual flight-or-fight mode, expecting pain. If you have been suffering with chronic pain, you can ask about pain management services. Physical therapy can also be a very useful method for this 'desensitisation' process.

Remember, pain may be 'created' in the brain, but that does not mean it is 'in your head'. It is a very real, physical sensation. Central sensitisation should never be used to dismiss your pain or terminate investigations.

Pelvic floor physiotherapy

Pelvic floor physiotherapy has long been known to help endometriosis patients, yet it remains shockingly underused by healthcare professionals. I knew when writing this book I wanted to talk about pelvic floor physiotherapy so I contacted Clare Bourne, specialist pelvic health physiotherapist and author of the book *Strong Foundations*. She explained that 'the role of a pelvic health physiotherapist for someone with endometriosis is largely misunderstood'. The current Western model of medicine is 'what is the problem and how can we fix it?', but, as Clare describes, 'physiotherapy is not directly treating endometriosis or adenomyosis; we're not going in and changing the fundamental issue'. That said, she believes, and many patients agree, that pelvic floor physiotherapy can hugely support endometriosis sufferers in managing symptoms and their overall pain puzzle, which we discussed earlier. 'We're coming alongside to support the patient and maximise their recovery.'

Clare describes the pelvic floor as a bodyguard that is at the core of us. It's there to shield us and our organs. 'Naturally, when you have pain in an area, repeatedly, probably for years, you've probably been gaslit, probably been told that it was in your head and that your body's designed to protect you,' as a result of that pain your muscles tighten up and wrap around the site of injury. 'It's a subconscious process that occurs in the body, to protect you. If someone is going to come up and punch you in the belly, what are you going to do? You're going to recoil, to tense up. That process is happening over months and years in an endometriosis patient. Eventually, the muscles start to behave in a different way.' As we saw when discussing the pain puzzle, some of our symptoms may not be directly related to endometriosis itself. Some of them may be down to your body adapting and your muscles tensing and behaving in a way that, although designed to be helpful, is actually causing issues.

We know that surgery is not a silver bullet nor a miracle fix for our quality of life. Clare says that she sees many endometriosis patients in this situation. A 'surgeon thinks, "tick, removed it", but the patient is still in pain, they still can't have sex, they still struggle with bladder or bowel issues. Yes, it's great that the endometriosis is removed, but there's all this other stuff that means quality of life is so far from where it needs to be. We find that a lot of women also have other symptoms: bladder symptoms, bowel symptoms or relating to intercourse. As physios, we work with the pelvic floor muscles, which are foundational to the bladder, bowel and sex.' A pelvic floor physiotherapist can help bridge the gap between medical intervention and the rest of your life. This physiotherapy support may include pelvic floor muscle rehabilitation, internal and external manipulation, exercises focused on the mobility of the muscles around the pelvis and hips, breathwork to relax the pelvic floor and advice on education about pain.

Sounds great, right? So, why isn't pelvic floor physiotherapy part of the care pathway for every endometriosis patient? Sadly, as Clare explains, 'it comes down to money. The prioritisation is not there. Our current medical model focuses on survival, not necessarily quality of life.' There is no mention of pelvic floor physiotherapy in the NICE guidelines for endometriosis management, even in the 2024 update. Despite there being a section devoted to 'non-pharmacological options', pelvic floor physiotherapy doesn't get a single mention.

Within the last three years, Clare says that pelvic floor physios are seeing more and more endometriosis patients, with a significant increase over the last year. However, this increase in interest is coming from 'word of mouth from patient to patient. I can't think of a single doctor referral that we have seen for endometriosis.' She sums up what seems to be the case for so much of endometriosis care: 'a lot of the interest is coming from the endometriosis community educating themselves and supporting each other'.

When we spoke, I told Clare about my recent experience with a pain management clinic. I asked about pelvic floor physiotherapy and stressed that I was very interested in exploring this option. 'You do know that all they will do is teach you how to tighten your muscles and help with any bladder incontinence? Do you have bladder incontinence?' was the reply I was met with. Clare's reaction is a mixed one: part disbelief, part frustration, part not sure whether to laugh or swear. 'There is such a confusion about what physiotherapy actually is and how it can help,' she delicately puts it. 'Even in my own physiotherapy degree, I was not taught about the pelvic floor. It was an obscure reference in a module called "women's health", because some people still don't realise that men also have a pelvic floor.' This was only 15 years ago. For this reason, Clare has 'slightly given up' on trying to extol the benefits of pelvic floor physiotherapy to clinicians and is instead reaching out directly to patients. 'We need top-down change, but we could wait decades for it. We need to empower women now,' she says.

Endometriosis

We talk about the idea of surgery being the first step, and Clare poses an interesting challenge. 'I disagree,' she says. 'Pelvic floor physiotherapy should be step one, then surgery.' She argues that we would see even 'better results from surgery if we did some work beforehand', comparing it to knee replacements, where physiotherapy is conducted prior to surgery 'to optimise recovery and results'. However, she appreciates that this will be an even harder sell to those in charge of hospital budgets.

Clare believes, and I am inclined to agree, that pelvic floor physiotherapy would help every single endometriosis patient. 'Anyone who has been in pain for that long will have adaptations in their body,' she continues, 'and there are definitely things that we can do to help and support through that process'. She 'can't promise the road will be easy', but she sees the results every day in her clinic.

Clare Bourne's top tips

- Educate yourself. Understand what your pelvic floor is, where the muscles are and that the pelvic anatomy is super close together. Organs are sandwiched together and work as a team. Our organs never work in isolation, struggling with one can affect another.
- Learn how to do diaphragmatic breathing. Breathwork can be really powerful to support your body, organs and pelvic floor.
- Look up pelvic floor health resources that can guide you through gentle exercises such as body scanning, stretches and relaxation techniques
- Avoid anything that tells you to tighten your pelvic floor. When you have been in pain for so long your muscle tone (tightness) is likely to be very high. The last thing you need is to increase it.
- Access support in your local area, ask about pelvic health physiotherapy, particularly those with experience in endometriosis.

While many doctors don't yet understand the full benefits of pelvic floor physiotherapy for endometriosis patients, endometriosis experts generally do. Mr Mikey Adamczyk, consultant gynaecologist and endometriosis surgeon, goes so far as to call it 'absolutely crucial' for quality of life in the long term. Some BSGE endometriosis centres (*see* pages 111–113) do now have pelvic floor physios as part of their MDTs, or you may be able to get a referral from your GP. It is always worth asking. If not, you can find some incredible resources from people like Clare.

Mr Mikey Adamczyk's top tips for navigating the healthcare system at any stage of your endometriosis journey

When trying to get a diagnosis:

- Trust yourself and listen to your body – you know it better than anyone else.
- Take the time to educate yourself about your symptoms and options.
- Bring a friend with you to your consultation for support and perspective.
- Make sure you're seeing an expert.
- Never hesitate to seek a second opinion if you feel it's needed.

When discussing endometriosis with a consultant:

- Do your research and ask questions, especially when it comes to surgery. I can tell you, as a surgeon who does a lot of endometriosis surgery, we don't get offended by questions. In fact, I love it when patients ask about my surgical numbers, complications and experience. I truly believe that every surgeon should have their numbers available for patients to see, no questions asked. So, ask how many surgeries they do per week, month or year.
- Don't assume anything – you need to differentiate between excision specialists and those who perform ablation. I'd like to think ablation isn't really a thing any more, but still, ask.
- Ask about the complications, ask about the MDT and just ask. It's your body, your care, and you should be getting all the information you need to feel confident and informed. Ask away!

Living with endometriosis long term:

- First, make sure your surgery is with an expert – someone who genuinely knows how to find and excise the disease properly.
- After that, it's all about recovery. Here's the thing: even with all the endometriosis excised, sometimes there's still some lingering pain. That's because, after years of living with pain, the body doesn't always just let it go instantly. Those pain signals can stick around, and it takes a bit of time for them to fade. On top of that, when we're in pain, we tend to tense up, and that constant tension can lead to weak, tight muscles. That's where physiotherapy comes in, and it's absolutely crucial.
- Beyond that, I can't stress enough the importance of a healthy lifestyle. A holistic approach – things like balanced nutrition, acupuncture, yoga or Pilates – can be incredibly valuable for recovery. All of it together plays a big role in helping you truly heal.

Chapter 4

The evil step-sisters – associated conditions

'Adeno ... sorry what?! Is that a real condition? Could you spell it for me?' – GP

Endometriosis is not the only pelvic pain generator that we may be facing. While it can and does exist in isolation for some patients, many others find that they may also have at least one other associated condition. Truthfully, we don't much about the relationship between endometriosis and these other conditions, known as 'comorbidities', but there have been attempts over the years to investigate whether endometriosis could be linked to everything from polycystic ovary syndrome (PCOS), painful bladder syndrome (aka interstitial cystitis), IBS, postural orthostatic tachycardiac syndrome (POTS), asthma, autoimmune disorders and even cancers. Some tentative links have been made, proposing that endometriosis increases the risk of other chronic diseases, but we simply do not have enough data to prove it – and we must always remember that correlation does not equal causation.

There are, however, a couple of conditions that I wanted to spotlight in this chapter. To be honest, they could each be their own book, but their prevalence in and relevance to the endometriosis population means that their inclusion here is also necessary. So, let's take a closer look at adenomyosis and fibroids.

Adenomyosis

(add-en-oh-my-oh-sis)

Once thought to just be endometriosis inside the uterus, or 'endometriosis interna', we now know that these are two completely separate conditions. Adenomyosis is characterised by the presence of endometrial-like stroma and glands within the myometrium tissue of the uterus (*see* Figure 4.1). Stroma are cells and tissues that support organs, glands or other tissues, made up of connective tissue, blood vessels, nerves and lymphatic vessels. Glands are structures that synthesise, transport, and/or secrete substances such as hormones. In other words, adenomyosis occurs when cells and tissues infiltrate the muscular wall of the womb, causing an enlarged or 'bulky' uterus.

Figure 4.1: The myometrium and adenomyosis

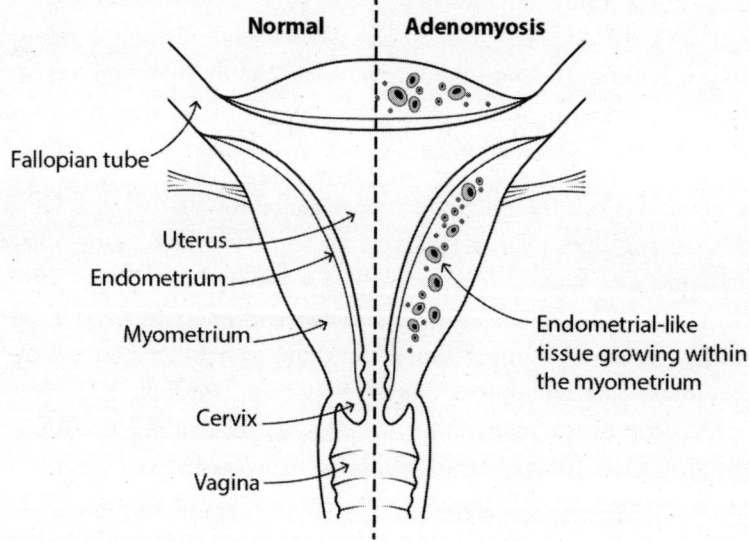

Adenomyosis is a condition that we know very little about. If you think endometriosis is misunderstood and under-researched, just you wait. A quick search on PubMed, an online searchable database of medical research, in November 2024 revealed 36,402 articles for endometriosis and a paltry 4,201 for adenomyosis. To put that into further context, diseases with similar population numbers bring up 228,648 (asthma) and a whopping 1,020,217 (diabetes). It was only in 2023 that adenomyosis received its own page on the NHS website; previously, it was only mentioned on the hysterectomy page. At the time of writing, NICE does not have a clinical guideline for the diagnosis and treatment of adenomyosis. Again, these points may seem trivial, but, as founder of The Adeno Gang, an adenomyosis and menstrual health organisation, Tanya Simon-Hall perfectly sums up when we speak, to

The evil step-sisters – associated conditions

those suffering 'it is not semantics when you are actually trying to figure out what is wrong with you . . . you are not a tick box.'

Adenomyosis is thought to impact one in 10 women but, like endometriosis, it is surrounded by myths and misinformation that mean the true incidence is relatively unknown. Depending on the study, the definition and diagnostic criteria, the prevalence of adenomyosis ranges from 5 to 70 per cent, with most recent reports suggesting around 20 per cent, or one in five. This lack of clarity highlights just how little confidence we have in our knowledge of this disease. We do, however, know that the incidence of adenomyosis is disproportionately high among Black patients. It is thought that adenomyosis can occur in anywhere between 20 and 80 per cent of endometriosis patients, but that does not mean you have to have one in order to have the other. What it does mean is that if you have been told you definitely do not have endometriosis, or if you have persistent pelvic pain after surgery, adenomyosis could be the cause and should be investigated.

Endo vs adeno – the key differences

Endometriosis	Adenomyosis
Full-body disease	Uterine disease
Endometrium-like cells	Endometrial tissues (glands and stroma) are found in the myometrium (the wall of the uterus)
No cure	A cure exists
Hysterectomy is not a cure	Hysterectomy is a cure
Definitively diagnosed during laparoscopy	Definitely diagnosed after hysterectomy
Do not need a uterus to have endometriosis	Only occurs in those who were born with a uterus

Unlike my experience with endometriosis, I had never heard of adenomyosis before my diagnosis. Even then, it was very much a throwaway comment when my doctor was reviewing my ultrasound. 'Think of your uterus like a cake,' I was told. 'Adenomyosis is just where the layers and filling have become a bit squashed together and mushy.' Yum.

Adenomyosis is not a well-known disease, even among the medical population. It is even less well-known that there are three different types of adenomyosis: focal, adenomyoma and diffuse (*see* Figure 4.2):

- Focal adenomyosis occurs in a particular site or location of the uterus.
- Adenomyoma is a form of focal adenomyosis, but it is more extensive, resulting in a uterine mass or benign tumour. The structure of an adenomyoma makes it different from a fibroid.
- Diffuse adenomyosis, unlike the other two types, spreads throughout the uterus.

Figure 4.2: Types of adenomyosis

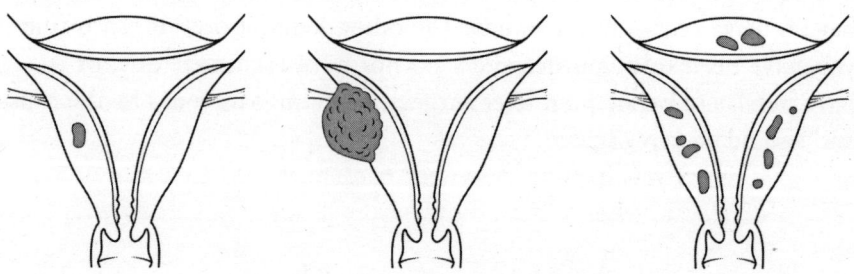

It is really important to understand the difference and to know which type you have; as adenomyosis advocate Tanya Simon-Hall explains when we speak, 'there are different clinical pathways depending on which type of disease you have'. If you are reading this having been diagnosed with adenomyosis already but are not sure which type you have, make sure to ask your doctor as it may help inform your treatment and management options. Tanya says she really had to advocate for herself to find out this information. The first doctor she asked admitted that she didn't have the expertise to discern that information but, in a move I wish more clinicians would be bold enough to make, brought in someone who did: Mr Joel Naftalin, consultant gynaecologist and @gynaescanner on Instagram. He performed an ultrasound on Tanya, who recorded the whole process for educational purposes and posted it on her page @theadenogang. Mr Naftalin was able to diagnose Tanya with an adenomyoma.

Adenomyosis symptoms, which we delve into in a moment, will likely seem very familiar as there is a large overlap with the symptoms of endometriosis. If you have both, it can make it difficult to decipher which

The evil step-sisters – associated conditions

symptoms are attributed to which condition. I didn't know it at the time, but adenomyosis was an enormous part of my pain puzzle (*see* pages 140–141). I would describe a feeling of a bowling ball sitting in my pelvis, trying to break my bones from the inside. At the time, before my diagnosis, I just attributed it to endometriosis. However, once adenomyosis was identified and I started learning about the condition, I realised just how much it was impacting me. My first surgeon told me that 'adenomyosis doesn't cause that much pain; it simply doesn't do that' and suggested psychotherapy instead. Less than a year later, the instant post-hysterectomy relief from that metaphorical bowling ball proved just how wrong – and dangerous – his opinion was. Adenomyosis was a huge factor influencing my quality of life, and conversations with others highlight that it is for them too.

Tanya Simon-Hall was 17 when she first went to the doctors complaining of her symptoms. She complained for years and, sadly, had a miscarriage in 2014. By 2019, she says that the symptoms were so extensive that they were affecting her job: 'my contract was not going to get renewed if I didn't attend, but I couldn't, I was in pain.' She went back to the doctor's that year and pushed for a scan, where she was given a diagnosis of endometriosis. Then the pandemic came and her investigations were put on hold. Later, in 2020, Tanya had two scans. One picked up endometriosis, the other adenomyosis, but neither picked up that she had both. She received her results in 2021. She was called and told 'you've got something called adenomyosis, but it's nothing to worry about.' She remembers thinking 'adeno . . . what?' so took to Google to try to understand the condition. She couldn't find much on the NHS website or more widely.

'I went on Instagram and found advocate Nat Blake and her community, Sunday Sips. I told my story there and decided in 2021 to open up my own page. I was looking specifically for women with adenomyosis, because at the time I was under the assumption that this thing couldn't exist in many people . . . not many people talk about it.' She started a global campaign, with participants from as far away as Australia and Canada, called 'I Have Adenomyosis', with various women showing that none of us are alone. 'It still wasn't really making much sense to me, so I started researching more.' Tanya was led to believe that despite having both adenomyosis and endometriosis, it was only the endometriosis causing her issues. 'It wasn't . . . it was based on the fact that more people know about one [endometriosis] over the other [adenomyosis].' Despite causing 'excruciating pain', the adenomyosis was dismissed. 'I tried to find out as much information as I could and listened to the stories of other people.' That's when Tanya decided to advocate for increased awareness and education around adenomyosis.

Adenomyosis symptoms

When someone has heard of adenomyosis, they often picture painful, heavy and irregular periods. While these are very common symptoms, it is important to note that not everyone with adenomyosis will experience them. In fact, it is thought that approximately one-third of adenomyosis patients have no symptoms at all. Unfortunately, for others, myself included, the pain and other symptoms caused by adenomyosis can greatly impact our lives. Like endometriosis, adenomyosis is a spectrum, and most patients will fall somewhere in between the two extremes. Here are some common adenomyosis symptoms:

- Extremely heavy blood loss during menstruation
- Bleeding and/or pain outside of periods
- Irregular cycle
- Extremely painful menstruation
- Passing large and/or frequent clots
- Anaemia
- Heaviness in pelvic area
- Pain on urination and/or bowel movement
- Lower back pain
- Fatigue
- Bloating
- Uterine contractions (like labour pain)
- Pain during or after sex and orgasm
- Fertility issues and miscarriages
- Nausea and/or vomiting
- Constipation and/or diarrhoea
- Pain in hips and legs
- Urgency to pass urine

As with endometriosis, adenomyosis symptoms may be encountered cyclically, or throughout the whole month. Don't forget, you can have some,

The evil step-sisters – associated conditions

all or none of these symptoms and still have adenomyosis. Lots of these symptoms overlap with endometriosis, but it is important to remember that they are two separate diseases with different pathologies.

Diagnosing adenomyosis

Historically, adenomyosis has been both under- and misdiagnosed. A definitive diagnosis of adenomyosis is currently made by the microscopic study of a sample taken from the uterus following hysterectomy. This is obviously a very radical surgery to undertake in order to obtain answers. As such, many adenomyosis patients receive a 'working diagnosis' via one or more of the following:

- Medical history
- Physical examination
- Ultrasound
- MRI
- Surgical findings

The problem with all of these methods, as with endometriosis, is that they rely heavily on the education, skills, expertise and empathy of the clinician involved. As we've seen, adenomyosis can present with a huge number of different symptoms, so medical history alone is rarely used for diagnosis. Due to this broad constellation of symptoms, adenomyosis is often misdiagnosed at the GP stage as IBS or other bowel and bladder conditions. Sadly, due to the uterine nature of adenomyosis, its symptoms are also often downplayed and/or dismissed as 'just a bad period'. That's if the doctor has heard of it at all. One GP asked me to explain what adenomyosis was and if I was sure I had the name right.

During a physical exam, a clinician who understands adenomyosis could look out for certain signs. For example, a patient might be experiencing iron deficiency, or even anaemia, due to heavy menstrual bleeding (a classic but not essential symptom of adeno) or have a very tender abdominal and pelvic area. Neither medical history nor physical examination is likely to provide a diagnosis of adenomyosis on its own; however, they can be very useful in combination with imaging and/or surgical findings and should therefore never be ignored.

As with endometriosis, the features of adenomyosis can be seen on ultrasound and MRI. The sensitivity of transvaginal ultrasound to detect adenomyosis can be higher than for endometriosis, ranging from 65 to 81 per cent, if the person performing and reading the scan knows what to look for. Signs that might be present include thickening of the uterine walls, an irregular, bulky shape to the uterus, spots or patches within the myometrium (the wall of the uterus), cysts in the myometrium, widening of the junctional zone (between the endometrium and myometrium) or increased blood flow in the area. Pelvic imaging can provide an accurate diagnosis, but – and it's a big but – it hugely depends on who is performing and reading the scan. For this reason, a clear scan cannot rule out adenomyosis.

Laparoscopic surgery, for example during endometriosis surgery, can reveal clinical signs of adenomyosis. These are usually referred to as a visually bulky, boggy, enlarged, asymmetric or lumpy uterus. If you spot any of these phrases on your medical notes and it hasn't been brought up with you, make sure you ask about the possibility of adenomyosis.

Worryingly, the accepted gold standard for diagnosis, and the only way to 100 per cent definitely confirm adenomyosis, remains testing of a sample following the removal of the uterus. In my opinion, adenomyosis could, and should, be diagnosed through much less invasive means than an irreversible organ removal. However, as Dr Susanne Johnson was quoted earlier in the book, the fact remains that if 'clinicians do not know what to look for, they will not find it'. This hinges on the knowledge, skills and expertise of clinicians, highlighting the need to improve education at every touchpoint.

Adenomyosis myth-busting

- **Adenomyosis is not an 'older woman' disease.** In most medical literature, adenomyosis is described as a disease found in patients between the ages of 30 and 50. However, we have to remember that a definitive diagnosis is made following hysterectomy and patients are likely to make this choice after 'completing' their family or later in life, skewing the data in a harmful way. You are not too young to have adenomyosis.

The evil step-sisters – associated conditions

- **Adenomyosis does not only affect women who have given birth.** I get this question in my inbox almost every week: 'My surgeon says it cannot be adenomyosis because I haven't given birth. Is that right?' This is another myth perpetuated by skewed and outdated data focusing on patients later in life, which prevents access to much-needed treatment for patients who have not given birth. N.B. you may see on your notes the following terms: multiparous, meaning having borne more than one child, primiparous meaning one child and nulliparous meaning never having given birth.
- **Adenomyosis does not always cause heavy, irregular periods.** You can have a 'textbook' period and still have adenomyosis. You can have all the symptoms of adenomyosis, some of them or none of them, and still have the condition.
- **Adenomyosis is not just endometriosis inside the uterus.** Endo and adeno are two separate diseases with different pathologies. It's not just about the location, and it's not just semantics. Getting the definitions right has huge implications for access to treatment pathways.
- **You do not have to have endometriosis to have adenomyosis.** While endometriosis and adenomyosis often co-exist, this is not always the case. In a 2014 study, the prevalence of endometriosis in adenomyosis patients was 80.6 per cent and the prevalence of adenomyosis in endometriosis patients was 91.1 per cent. They clearly are (painful) bedfellows but you do not have to have both. You might have endo, adeno or both.
- **Adenomyosis is not rare.** Truthfully, we do not have an accurate rate for the disease; the reports all show different results. But we do know that adenomyosis is not rare, although access to diagnosis and care is.
- **Adenomyosis can cause pain.** Adenomyosis is a spectrum. While some patients will experience mild or even no symptoms, for others the condition can be completely debilitating, causing a huge amount of distress and disruption.

Managing adenomyosis

When it comes to adenomyosis management, there is yet another overlap with endometriosis in that the options can be split into lifestyle, medical, hormonal and surgical. We looked at lifestyle and medical options earlier in the book (*see* chapter 2) and they mostly apply here too:

- Non-medical methods: Heat, baths, TENS machines, balanced lifestyle and diet, avoiding personal triggers, stress reduction, sleep, pelvic floor relaxation, gentle stretching, physiotherapy
- Non-hormonal medical treatment: Over-the-counter pain relief, prescription NSAIDs (anti-inflammatories), prescription codeine or opiates, tranexamic acid (for blood loss), iron tablets or infusions, nausea relief
- Hormonal treatment: Hormonal pills, progestin treatments such as an IUD or GNrH analogues

Depending on your individual case, your doctor may suggest a combination of the above. For some people, these methods manage their symptoms and minimise disruption to their life. The winning combination for you is likely to be different from what works for someone else so, as always, try not to compare and do what works for you. Unfortunately, these methods, even in combination, may still not be enough or may not be desirable (due to side effects, for instance), in which case surgical options will be discussed. Tanya, the adenomyosis advocate we met earlier in the chapter, is a perfect example of the individuality of patient care. After a stroke at the age of 21 and the presence of a blood-clotting disorder, she cannot have hormonal interventions as they could quite literally risk her life. Tanya is also at high risk of severe complications from surgery, making her choices limited and a difficult balance. Once again, we're seeing how care for conditions such as adenomyosis and endometriosis cannot be a simple, blanket algorithm.

If you've researched adenomyosis management after being diagnosed (or suspecting you have the condition), and the topic of surgery comes up, your first thought is likely a hysterectomy. We will cover this later in the chapter. However, there are other options available to patients, especially those wishing to preserve fertility or to avoid major surgery. As with any treatment, your doctor should take time and care to explain all of the options, including any associated risks. Informed consent is key, so make sure you are with a specialist who can help you come to the best decision for your body.

The treatments you may be offered are detailed below.

The evil step-sisters – associated conditions

Pre-sacral neurectomy (PSN)
This procedure is carried out under general anaesthetic and involves the removal of the pre-sacral plexus, the group of nerves that conduct pain signals from the uterus to the brain.

Laparoscopic uterine nerve ablation (LUNA)
LUNA involves the destruction of a small segment of the uterosacral ligament, which carries nerve fibres within the pelvis. This procedure is normally performed under general anaesthetic.

Uterine arterial embolisation (UAE)
This procedure is performed by a specialist called an interventional radiologist and is less invasive than surgery. Tiny particles of polyvinyl alcohol, PVA, are injected into the blood vessels, aiming to create a blockage, cutting off the blood supply to the womb and therefore the adenomyosis. This treatment is usually only explored when surgery is to be avoided but fertility does not need to be protected. The evidence on success rates varies, but some studies have shown symptom improvement. On the flip side, recurrence rates appear quite high. UAE is currently only in the NICE guidelines as a treatment option for fibroids, but recent reports suggest that for adenomyosis 'UAE should be offered to women as an alternative to hysterectomy, as many case series (detailed groups of patients undergoing similar treatments) have demonstrated the safety and effectiveness' of the procedure.

Endometrial ablation
This is not recommended for adenomyosis, as it destroys the endometrial layer of the uterus, usually using heat. Unfortunately, some doctors do still suggest this procedure for adenomyosis; I am including it here so you can recognise it as a red flag if this procedure is offered to you.

Usually, the first step is to take a biopsy during a procedure called a hysteroscopy. If the results show that the procedure is suitable, for example where no adenomyosis is present and no future pregnancies are desired, a device is placed inside the uterus and the lining is destroyed. This is a very quick procedure and can work effectively for heavy periods. However, it is not recommended for adenomyosis patients, especially where pain is a factor. Studies report that adenomyosis patients can often develop worsening pain after endometrial ablation, so if you have, or suspect you may have adenomyosis, avoid endometrial ablation.

Excision of adenomyosis/adenomyoma
Also known as an adenomyomectomy (try saying that three times faster), this is a surgical procedure similar to that for removing fibroids (*see* pages 160–168). It can be used to remove adenomyoma or focal adenomyosis and is usually performed laparoscopically, but as with all surgery there is a risk of needing to move an open surgery, called a laparotomy, where a large incision is needed.

This procedure highlights the importance of knowing which type of adenomyosis you have. It is not currently suitable for diffuse adenomyosis. Some surgeons are investigating its use in this context, so in the future it could be a viable option and alternative to hysterectomy, even in diffuse cases. This would help counter the negative impact adenomyosis can have on fertility, increasing the chance of conception and decreasing adverse pregnancy outcomes when performed by an expert surgeon. However, as with all surgery, there are risks and complications that should be discussed in depth with your surgeon.

Hysterectomy
A hysterectomy is the complete removal of the uterus and, as a result, the adenomyosis contained within its muscular wall. It is currently the only 'cure' for this disease, if we take cure to mean the removal of all disease and zero chance of recurrence. A hysterectomy is not a decision to take lightly, and it is irreversible. If fertility is not a key concern for you – perhaps you do not want children, or you have completed your family –a hysterectomy may be an option for you. Before my own hysterectomy, surgeons would repeatedly tell me that one in four women end up regretting the decision. However, some studies show this 'regret rate' to be as low as 2.8 per cent. The only person who can make this decision is you, but making sure that it is absolutely the right decision for you, your body, and your future is imperative. You can find more information about hysterectomy, including the different types, on pages 124–129.

Whichever type and whichever method of hysterectomy you are discussing with your surgeon, make sure that you are fully aware of all the risks and implications. This is a major surgery, even if it leaves minimal scars, and has

The evil step-sisters – associated conditions

lifelong consequences. Make sure you are prepared for that and are sure it is the right decision for you.

Sadly, I speak to far too many patients who have been denied a hysterectomy, despite them understanding the procedure fully and deciding it is the right choice for them. The reasons have ranged from 'you might change your mind', 'you're too young' and 'you might meet a husband one day who does want children and then what will you do?' to the frankly disgusting 'you're not married, and no one will want to take you if we do this surgery now'. This is even more prevalent in communities where a woman's worth is heavily intertwined with her fertility. One patient I spoke to, who requested to remain anonymous, explained: 'In my culture, and in many others around the world, fertility is currency. The more fertile you are, the more attractive you are to potential partners and their families. Even the idea that you may have an issue affecting your fertility is a huge taboo. Adenomyosis was destroying my life, and I knew I wanted a hysterectomy. My quality of life was more important to me than my childbearing ability. Thankfully, I have a wonderful partner and family who supported that decision fully. But the doctors declined. They insisted that because of my cultural background it would not be appropriate.'

Please know that if adenomyosis is severely affecting your quality of life and you have made the decision to pursue a hysterectomy, that is your choice. If you understand all the risks and all the alternatives, and decide this surgery is the right option for you, your quality of life cannot be held ransom to your fertility. It is your body. Your treatment plan should always be based on knowledge of all options, informed consent and, vitally, your personal preference and choice.

This cultural nuance extends beyond fertility and can be found at every level of talking about diseases like adenomyosis. However, advocates such as Tanya Simon-Hall are leading the revolution. 'I will keep talking about periods and the things that I'm not meant to, if you listened to my community, because no one deserves to suffer this pain.' She works tirelessly to champion those with adenomyosis, including at a parliamentary level, advocating for increased, dedicated research on adenomyosis.

Tanya does believe things are slowly improving. 'There is more information out there than when I first started researching adenomyosis,' she says, 'but it's still not good enough'. She cites the NHS only adding adenomyosis to its website in July 2023 as an example. 'It's there, but it's not good enough.

It doesn't even tell you that there are different types.' Tanya believes, and I agree, that it took BBC television and radio presenter, newsreader and journalist Naga Munchetty to open up about her own experiences with excruciating adenomyosis symptoms, live on her radio show in May 2023, to really raise the profile of the disease and to get people to start paying attention. I was part of that, and subsequent, shows, describing my own experience and the issues we face as adenomyosis patients. Naga's openness created a buzz and a shift in awareness of the disease among certain parts of the population.

Something else that Tanya and I agree upon is that when we step into rooms where policy and strategies designed to address the healthcare of women and those assigned female at birth are being discussed, adenomyosis is still neglected. As Tanya recalls, at one event the person delivering the speech, positioned as the expert on 'women's health', could not even say adenomyosis. What's on Tanya's wish list for adenomyosis policy? 'Collaborative approaches', 'more data on the experiences of Black women', who we know are disproportionately affected by menstrual conditions such as adenomyosis, improvements in medical imaging and 'dedicated research'. 'I want adenomyosis to be taken just as seriously as endometriosis,' she explains. 'I understand that endometriosis can be in vital organs, causing objectively "worse" outcomes, but to be honest, the effects on quality of life can be just as bad from adenomyosis and, at times, worse.'

I couldn't agree more. Adenomyosis is not rare, but it is rarely understood. There is so little that we know about this disease. To give you a very clear example, we have always considered that adenomyosis grows only into the myometrium (the muscular layer of the uterine wall). But one guest on Naga Munchetty's BBC Radio 5 show described how, following a total hysterectomy, analysis showed that the disease had also infiltrated her cervix. We desperately need to know more about this disease.

Fibroids

When I received the results of the lab tests performed on my uterus after my hysterectomy, I learned something that I had never previously been told. Not only did I have endometriosis and adenomyosis, I also had fibroids. I had, apparently, been hit by an evil trifecta of conditions that can cause debilitating pain and bleeding. This was news to me, as the fibroids had

The evil step-sisters – associated conditions

never been picked up on imaging, nor during my first surgery (potentially confused with the existing patches of diffuse adenomyosis). Even when I did receive the diagnosis, I was not told how many fibroids were present or their size.

Fibroids:

- Are the most common gynaecological condition – so really, we should all be aware of them
- Can cause a huge amount of debilitating symptoms
- Often co-exist with endometriosis

And, shock horror, there is nowhere near enough research and information about them.

A uterine fibroid is a benign (non-cancerous), slow-growing tumour formed of smooth muscle and connective tissue that can develop in the uterus. You can have more than one (towards the end of this chapter we will hear from a patient who had 18) and the size can vary greatly, generally from 1cm to 20cm – the size of a melon. In rarer cases, they can grow even larger; in 2018, doctors in Singapore removed a fibroid from a 53-year-old patient that weighed 28kg. The largest recorded fibroid, which was only discovered upon autopsy, weighed a staggering 63.3kg.

Fibroids are extremely common: according to the NHS, around two in three women will develop at least one fibroid at some point in their life. But, as always, women are not a homogenous category. When we dig into the data a little bit more, we find that fibroids disproportionately affect Black women. It is thought that more than 80 per cent of Black women will develop fibroids.

Types of fibroids

There are thought to be four types of fibroids, depending on where they are found (*see* Figure 4.3), and they can develop as singular fibroids or 'clusters':

- Submucosal fibroids grow just under and into the inner lining of the womb.
- Intramural fibroids grow within the myometrium (the muscle layer in the wall of the uterus where adenomyosis is found).

- Subserosal fibroids grow on the outside of the womb and into the peritoneal cavity (the space within your abdomen that contains most of your abdominal organs, including your stomach, intestines and liver).
- Pedunculated fibroids attach to the womb via a narrow stalk.

Figure 4.3: Types of fibroids

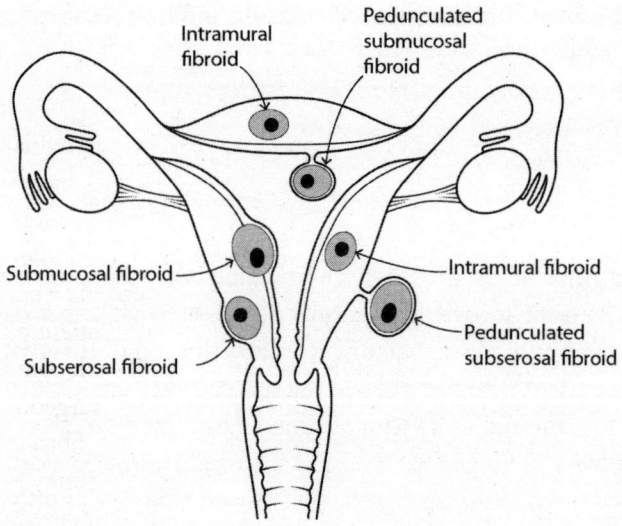

Despite being the most common gynaecological condition, fibroids are hugely under-researched. We do not even know exactly what causes fibroids. We do know that they are influenced by the hormones oestrogen and progesterone, the two main drivers of our hormonal cycle, meaning that symptoms can often be worse during periods. Studies suggest that post-menopause, when levels of these hormones drop, fibroids may shrink and cause fewer symptoms. However, menopause is not a cure. If you are taking HRT, your fibroids may not shrink as much or at all, and even without HRT, the ovaries are not the only hormone-producing part of the body. HRT is not thought to contribute to the growth of new fibroids but, in some women, it has been shown to increase fibroid size. This should not put you off trying HRT if you wish to, but if you are concerned and are experiencing symptoms, it may be wise to ask for periodic scans to monitor any changes. Again, much more research is needed.

The evil step-sisters – associated conditions

Symptoms of fibroids

Symptoms of uterine fibroids can include heavy, painful periods, stomach pain, lower back pain, bloating, urinary issues, bowel issues, pain during sex and fertility issues. As with endometriosis and adenomyosis, the impact on quality of life varies from no symptoms at all to completely debilitating, and everything in between.

Diagnosing fibroids

Fibroids are usually diagnosed via an abdominal and/or transvaginal ultrasound scan (*see* page 49), but can also sometimes be felt (palpated) via a vaginal exam or even as a mass protruding through the abdomen. As with endometriosis and adenomyosis, a scan is not always accurate. The results depend significantly on who is performing and reading the scan, and how. Fibroids were completely missed on all my scans and during both my surgeries. Patient advocate Rey tells a similar story. They had an ultrasound that came back completely clear. After their surgery for suspected endometriosis, the surgeon mentioned endometriosis and adenomyosis but said nothing about fibroids. However, Rey asked for their surgical images and, lo and behold, 'chunky fibroids were staring me right in the face'. It was confirmed later, during a second surgery, that Rey had multiple fibroids, including one the size of a strawberry.

Treatment of fibroids

Treatment for fibroids largely depends on a combination of the following:

- Your symptoms (both type and severity)
- The size and location of the fibroids
- Your fertility goals

For example, if you are able to manage your symptoms (or maybe do not even have any) and the fibroids are small and not likely to impact your fertility, you may be happy managing them with pain medication and lifestyle measures. However, if you would like to have children, have symptoms that impact your quality of life and/or the fibroids are large, medical or surgical intervention may be required.

Endometriosis

Most of these methods will be very familiar after reading previous chapters. Tranexamic acid is prescribed for blood loss, while anti-inflammatories, pain relief and hormonal interventions (an IUD, the hormonal contraceptive pill or even GNrH analogues) are also all common options. If these methods are ineffective or undesirable, or cause side effects, surgical options are usually then offered. When it comes to surgery, sadly, I hear from so many fibroids patients who are told a hysterectomy is their only option. This, as you can imagine, is not something that most of us would like to hear, especially as there are now many other options available if a hysterectomy is not something you wish to pursue. Some of these include the following:

- UAE: As discussed in the adenomyosis section (*see* chapter 4), this is performed by a specialist radiologist who blocks the blood vessels to the uterus, with the aim of shrinking fibroids. While this is a non-invasive option and can improve quality of life, its effects on future fertility are not yet fully understood.
- Myomectomy: In this procedure, the fibroids are removed while preserving the womb. Depending on the size and location of your fibroids, a myomectomy may be performed via laparoscopy or laparotomy.
- Hysteroscopic resection: If you have submucosal fibroids (inside the womb; *see* page 161) you may be offered a myomectomy via hysteroscopy, where the fibroids are removed via the vagina.
- Morcellation: You may also see this term in your notes; it refers to the fibroids being cut up into smaller pieces before being removed.
- Endometrial ablation: As with adenomyosis (*see* chapter 4), this is not recommended for fibroids patients, particularly if fertility is a concern. Some fibroids patients have reported more severe or prolonged pain following this procedure.
- Hysterectomy: As we've discussed, this is the removal of the uterus and possibly other reproductive organs (*see* pages 124–127). This will undoubtedly remove the fibroids and mean they will not come back. However, it is major surgery and has significant, irreversible consequences. If you decide that a hysterectomy is the best option for you, that is fine; but please don't feel like it is the only option that you have.

The evil step-sisters – associated conditions

There are emerging methods that seek to destroy fibroids using laser or ultrasound energy, guided by MRI or ultrasound. When performed by an expert, there is some suggestion that this method could provide short- to medium-term symptomatic relief, but research is still being undertaken and the data on efficacy and long-term outcomes, especially on fertility, is very limited.

Unless there are very clear reasons, a hysterectomy is not your only option for fibroid removal. While a hysterectomy might be the only option that removes the risk of recurrence, it is not the only way to drastically improve your quality of life. The type of procedure that is most suitable for you depends on your goals and the location, size and number of your fibroids. Each option varies in terms of invasiveness, risks and its potential effect on fertility. So, as ever, discussing your options with an expert is paramount.

Dawn Heels, fibroid campaigner and founder of The Guidance Suite, a fibroids community, education and advocacy group, tells me her experience of fibroids started when she was 14. 'I had my first period, which was very heavy and painful.' She spoke to her mum, who told her 'that's how it is in our family', a generational response that I'm sure many of us will have heard. When the pain and heavy bleeding persisted, Dawn and her mum went to the doctor. 'I was told it was "very normal", "very common", and that "that's just what happens when you're a teenager."' She was told not to worry and that her periods would 'peter out' as she aged. Her pain continued and when she was 17 she started taking the progestin contraceptive Cerazette, which stopped her periods and allowed her to 'live her best life', period-free. But in her 30s, Dawn wanted to have children so came off the pill and was 'met with the most horrendous periods, really heavy, even worse than before'.

At 33, she started to get a severe pain in the left side of her abdomen that persisted over the next few weeks. Her doctor said it was probably to do with her cycle and to take ibuprofen, but Dawn couldn't shake the feeling that 'something was not quite right'. She asked to see a female doctor, who suggested that it might be a cyst on Dawn's ovary. A scan showed that Dawn had two fibroids, 4cm in size. She was sent back to the original doctor for answers, but he dismissed her, saying, 'They're very normal, very common, nothing to worry about.' She was told to deal with the pain with a hot-water bottle and ibuprofen.

For the next six years, Dawn experienced every fibroid symptom listed on the NHS website, and more. She was in 'top-to-toe' pain, suffering with 'very heavy, clotty, prolonged periods', leg pain from her thigh down to her toes, butt-cheek pain, lower back pain, pelvic pain, abdominal pain, nausea, vitamin D deficiency, iron deficiency, headaches, extreme fatigue, painful sex and she then noticed that her stomach was actually protruding and could feel 'a massive lump, right at the front'. Throughout this time, the doctor's response was depressingly the same: 'There's nothing to worry about, fibroids are normal, common, you need to stop worrying'.

But Dawn *was* worried. On top of the huge list of symptoms, she was also 'thinking about having a child, and it just wasn't happening'. A friend then mentioned transvaginal ultrasounds to Dawn, and eventually she persuaded her doctor to send her to a gynaecologist. It was confirmed that her fibroids had grown to 6cm and 7cm, but there was no discussion about management. Instead, the gynaecologist told her, 'I see women get pregnant all the time with fibroids; you just have to get on with it.'

This back-and-forth went on for six years. The pain was so excruciating that on one occasion Dawn went to A&E. During an examination, a clinician told her, 'It feels like you're pregnant in there.' Dawn replied, 'One hundred per cent I am not pregnant, I am in pain.' 'Oh, but your uterus is really bulky,' countered the clinician, telling Dawn to 'wait a few weeks, you're definitely pregnant'. Once again, Dawn had sought medical help for pain and was dismissed.

Then the pandemic hit. She remembers working from home and thinking, 'I cannot do this anymore.' A colleague reminded Dawn that they had private medical insurance through their company. The consultant she saw 'changed my life'. After talking him through everything, he ordered a new transvaginal ultrasound, which showed she 'actually had six fibroids, the largest being the size of a grapefruit', which was the protruding lump that Dawn and her mum could feel. The consultant advised that she needed major surgery (an open myomectomy) to remove the fibroids. During the procedure, the consultant actually had to remove 16 fibroids, which Dawn describes like the solar system, 'all varying in size'. Two fibroids were left to give her the best chance of conception, meaning that she actually had had 18 fibroids in total – 'the balls of hell that had destroyed my entire being'. The recovery was long and difficult, but six months after her surgery, Dawn found out that she was pregnant with her daughter.

The evil step-sisters – associated conditions

'If I had continued seeing that original doctor, who kept fobbing me off... I can't even imagine what would have happened. I wasted six years of my life, and I'm still not over it.' She now collaborates with medical professionals to increase education about fibroids but also to bridge the gap between doctors and patients, and holds offline and online support groups that combine education and community, something that she feels was missing from her own journey.

Calling herself 'the accidental advocate', Dawn also campaigns for change in the way fibroids are seen and managed. 'This was never the plan', but she insists that 'if I can help, I will help.' So, what would she like to see changed in the management of fibroids? 'I don't know why women have to fight so hard for that first scan,' she says. 'There needs to be an emphasis on doctors believing us and sending us straight to the scan. After that, we tend to see that diagnosis can happen quite quickly, but then things fall apart afterwards. We're just dismissed and told it's normal.'

'There needs to be a proper management plan put in place that the two people – the consultant and the patient – have come together to decide upon.' Even simple things like information sources for patients don't really exist for fibroids. 'We have to educate ourselves,' Dawn says, 'but there's just no signposting, no information'. 'It would be such a relatively simple fix,' she says, and she and her Guidance Suite team are driving this forward. Unlike adenomyosis, care pathways do exist for the management of fibroids. However, various guidelines say slightly different things. 'We need unification of guidelines,' Dawn tells me. Otherwise, doctors end up picking and choosing and there 'is no consistency' in the care of patients.

I have no way of knowing whether fibroids were a factor in my own suffering, because I didn't know I even had them until after my uterus was removed. However, for other women, like Dawn, fibroids take over their whole lives. I asked her how it feels, knowing that fibroids are the most common gynaecological condition but that there is nothing really at the national level the way that there is for endometriosis. 'Who does it affect most?' Dawn asks me. The answer is Black women. 'If it affects a population you don't really care about, why would you bother?'

Dawn often partners up with The White Dress Project, a fibroids campaign group in the United States that has received multi-million-dollar funding. 'This is what we need in the UK,' she says: dedicated research into fibroids, dedicated education, dedicated spaces for patients. Too often, the topic of fibroids is just tagged along under endometriosis or heavy bleeding. We also need more research into why these conditions affect Black women disproportionately because right now, that data does not exist.

What has struck me, speaking to Tanya and Dawn, as well as advocates such as Rey, Katie and Heather throughout the rest of the book, is how much of the work falls to patients. We are not simply expected to live with these potentially debilitating conditions. We are also expected to educate ourselves on these topics, often to a level beyond that of the trained medics in charge of our care. And then, on top of that, it falls, time and again, to patients to push for change. To stand up in rooms and relive their traumas over and over. To push back against misinformation and educate others so future generations do not have to suffer like we did. It shouldn't be like this. Having to live with these conditions should be enough of a burden. However, as US-based Board Certified Patient Advocate Heather Guidone says, 'If not us, who? If not now, when?'

Chapter 5

Living with endometriosis – the art and the science

> *'Oh! I totally know what you're going through. I hurt my elbow playing tennis last week.'* – gynaecology surgeon

We are starting to grasp that endometriosis is a full-body disease. However, it goes further than that. It is a full-life disease. There is not a single area of my life that has not been irrevocably touched and altered by endometriosis.

The impact of endometriosis is so much more than the biochemical factors creating vessels, nerves and pain. It is so much more than the medical perspective. 'From a human perspective,' Mr Mikey Adamczyk, consultant gynaecologist and endometriosis surgeon, tells me, 'it's a real enigma.' He continues, 'It's heartbreaking to see how this condition affects so many lives.' The 'impact on people's lives is profound – it can destroy families and ruin careers, and even marriages. It can lead to divorce and prevent couples from experiencing intimacy, making it incredibly isolating.' I'll be honest, Mr Adamczyk's answers took me by surprise. It was possibly the first time I felt that a clinician really, truly grasped the extent to which endometriosis can impact a patient's life. 'Many people with the condition miss school or work because of it. It robs people of their youth, their middle age, and even their post-menopausal years.'

Nothing in the realm of endometriosis is black and white, and nowhere are there more shades of grey than when it comes to actually living your life with the disease. Hopefully, in this chapter you will see how to take the knowledge you have learned so far and apply it to your own reality. I have focused on four areas that all of us tend to deal with at least once, in some capacity:

- Relationships
- Work and studying

- Special occasions
- Day-to-day life

Relationships

Endometriosis has a significant impact on quality of life, not just for those of us with the disease but also for those who are closest to us and care for us. I met my now husband when I was about to turn 21. By then, I had been on the pill for nearly 10 years and had become (semi) used to the routine of three weeks of feeling okay and then a week of feeling like I was dying. He, however, had never experienced anything like it, despite growing up with three women in the house, and it was never a 'thing' in his previous relationships either. So, when we first got together, while he was incredibly supportive of my needs and would do anything to help, he definitely thought I was being 'a bit dramatic'. And that was about it for 12 years. By the time I received an endometriosis and adenomyosis diagnosis, I had just turned 33. The 18 months before that were the turning point where he really began to see that this was not 'just a bad period' and that something was very seriously wrong. Every part of our relationship has changed over the last few years. Sex, intimacy, social life, household responsibilities, freedoms, goals and dreams, financial responsibility . . . all of it is different. But different doesn't always mean worse. It just means different.

Our relationships are as individual as we are. Yours is likely nothing like mine or any other person's. That's fine. However, I am hopeful that this section can help both you and your partner navigate the changes that endometriosis can bring to a relationship, remembering that not all relationships are romantic. Obviously, the sex part might lead in that direction, but the boundaries, expectations and helpful and unhelpful things to say or do can apply to any relationship in your life.

When I am asked how to navigate endometriosis in a relationship, I always start with the same advice: communication. It's a cliché, but it truly is the bedrock of any solid relationship, with or without the involvement of chronic illness. You and your partner will both be learning so many new things about yourselves and your relationship during this process. However, neither of you is a mind reader. Tell them your worries, thoughts, feelings and ideas and, just as importantly, ask them for theirs. When I first started my Instagram account, I realised that our partners and those supporting us closely were very often left out of the conversation. You could argue that it's our bodies. Endometriosis is happening to us, and we have to bear the brunt of the disease and its effects. But your partner's life will very likely change too, and that's something they will also have to navigate. I started talking to my husband about this and realised he felt lost, useless and out of his depth in how to help the person he loved. It opened up a channel of communication for us that strengthened our relationship, even after a decade of being together.

I decided to interview him for my page and share the answers, the idea being that it would help other endometriosis patients either understand the perspective of a partner or encourage them to ask their own partners the same questions. I repeated the questions when writing this chapter, now that we are a few years into this journey, and his answers revealed just as much as the first time. Before I share the questions and my husband Chris's answers, I can't stress how much I encourage you to do this with your partner. However, you both have to go into the exercise feeling safe to share openly. It can get emotional. I definitely cried. You need to remember that their feelings are also valid when navigating the absolute overwhelm that is life with endometriosis.

Interview with my partner

Me: What kind of menstrual health education did you have when you were younger?
Chris: None. There was nothing at school beyond 'girls have a period once a month'. School separated the boys and girls. When the girls came back, they told us that we hadn't missed out – the only thing they were shown was a tampon in a glass of water. My two sisters didn't talk about it that I remember. I knew what a tampon and pad were and what they were for, but that's about it.

Had you heard of endometriosis before me?
Only when you started talking about it.

We were together for 12 years before I was diagnosed. What did you think about my periods during that time?
I knew you struggled and suffered, but at the start I didn't really know too much – you kept it to yourself a lot. To be honest, I thought you were being a bit dramatic for a while. I'm ashamed to say it now, but I didn't really listen.

I just thought I was meant to offer some comfort food and a hot bath. I didn't understand, but at the same time I was trying to be sympathetic. I could see you were in pain but thought, 'How bad can it be?'

I first noticed something was unusual when we lived together and you started your corporate job, and I noticed you were bedridden for a few days at a time and missing work. At times I thought it was more to do with mental health than your menstrual health. Earlier on, I probably even just thought you were a bit lazy, but I didn't understand anything then.

We had a few more conversations as our relationship progressed, but it wasn't until you came off the pill and everything went spiralling that we started talking really openly.

How did you feel when I got a diagnosis?
Initially, not a lot because I didn't know what it was. But then, when we started talking about it and I started looking up what it was, I was weirdly pleased for you. It gave us direction and a sense that we could fight this and even overcome it. I didn't realise then just how long and up and down it would be.

When did you realise that this was lifelong?
After the second surgery. Before surgery one, I was naive and hopeful. After that surgery, I was really deflated and sad. I thought that the second surgery was going to be a miracle fix. When you still had symptoms after the second surgery, I was broken but had a much deeper understanding of just how serious this disease is. I had all sorts of thoughts about what our lives and futures would be like. Would we end up living separate lives? Would we ever be able to do the things that we wanted to? I didn't deal with it very well. I'm starting to accept it, but it really is just shit. I don't think I've fully accepted it yet and understood what it means for our life. I've given up trying to second-guess it and have probably become pretty numb. I don't know what our future looks like. I try to just take it day by day. I just know I want to spend it with you.

How has my endometriosis affected your life?
Stopped it, put it on hold, took it over. We couldn't go on holiday. It's changed the way I think about the most basic of tasks. Even the simplest things now require a thousand considerations. Have we got your painkillers? Are they due? Will you get a flare? What will we do if the pain flares while we're out?

It turns a simple task into a military operation. When you had to give up work, it made me the sole breadwinner in our household. That financial responsibility fell completely on me. I also do most of the tasks in our house, so the practical burden is also there. Truthfully, I'm permanently exhausted.

How has endometriosis changed our relationship?
It has slowed things down. I now swap between husband and carer. It hasn't changed the way I see you, but it has put a filter over how I view our lives. It populates everything; it feels like most conversations include it, even if they don't really. The way it infiltrates your body is the way it infiltrates our life. Our food, our social life, travel, shopping, intimacy – it's always there. There's not a single aspect of our life that doesn't warrant a consideration of endometriosis. Take when we went to the fireworks display on Bonfire Night. Instead of just attending a display, I was thinking, 'Have you been in pain all day? Will we make it? Will we park close enough for you to walk across? Will the food trigger you? Will you be able to stand long enough for the display? Will it make you suffer the next day?' It puts a lot of strain and stress on a relationship and can take the enjoyment out of the most basic things.

How does it feel when you see me in a flare?
I hate it. I hate the fact I can't help you. It's like having to sit and watch someone you love being tortured and not being able to do a thing. I feel powerless and useless, especially when we've exhausted all the things to help and you're still in pain. And then I feel guilty because I'm thinking about how it affects me. I just want to hold you, but I don't want to hurt you.

What do you wish endometriosis sufferers knew about their loved ones?
That we mean well. We want to help you, but we don't understand. We need your help to understand and to know what you need. We're not mind readers, so if you're able to tell us what you need, that would be amazing – although I do understand it's not always easy or possible in the depth of a flare. It's exhausting for us too, physically and emotionally.

What has been helpful for you in terms of navigating life since my endometriosis diagnosis?
Getting over that thing, that all boys are taught, that periods are gross and nothing to do with us. Being able to talk openly and honestly with you,

without judgement, and you being patient with me when I don't understand. You understanding that it takes a toll on both of us has been a huge support.

The internet was really useful for educating myself and suggesting practical things that could help me support you. When you send me social media posts and say, 'I didn't know how to explain this before, but this is exactly what it's like', it's really helpful for my understanding.

What do I do that isn't helpful?
Tell me you're in pain without telling me what will help. You push yourself too hard. I want you to rest and pace yourself because I've seen how much you suffer, but I also get that you don't want to miss out on things. It's hard to help you balance living versus dealing with your symptoms. It can sometimes feel like I have to parent you and ask if you need to rest or if you're sure you want a dessert at dinner, for example. It probably looks controlling from the outside, but I just want to try to help you avoid a flare.

How have we managed to keep intimacy in our relationship?
We've always been a close couple and enjoy making time for moments together. We've always been quite physically affectionate. Endometriosis has changed things a bit, of course, but rather than feeling like we have had to give things up, we try to look at how we can adapt to our current circumstances. Understanding that intimacy is so much more than sex has helped. One thing that we have always done, since the beginning of our relationship, is take a bath together. Maintaining something like that has helped.

Has endometriosis changed our sex life?
It has changed it. Without a doubt. It is less frequent and is more about being comfortable and choosing positions that will not cause you pain. I constantly worry about hurting you, and for a long time it stopped me initiating things. I used to take you turning down sex personally and felt a sense of rejection. But that's where our ability to have those open conversations comes in. I understand a lot more now and we try to come up with ways to keep that part of our relationship fun.

Does sex feel different after my hysterectomy?
No. Even if it did – for example, if you had gone straight into menopause and suffered with dryness – we would have just worked around it. The

only thing I worry about is causing you pain. Everything else we can deal with.

How has my infertility affected you?
Truthfully, I don't think it has. I think there's been maybe one time in the 18 months since your hysterectomy that I've considered having children in the future. Your hysterectomy was always ultimately your choice, but I am grateful that you included me in the conversation. I never really wanted children, so if it came down to keeping your uterus versus removing that side of your pain, it was a clear choice for me. If we later decide to start a family, we can look at the options open at the time and go from there.

How has endometriosis strengthened our relationship?
It's hard to wrap my head around considering anything positive coming out of this experience when I still see you in pain every day. It has changed a lot of our dynamics; some have held us back, but others have been a driving force and productive. It's given you a purpose in life, and it has encouraged me to step up and push forward in my own career to get to a point where I can be flexible with my time and financially support us. I feel like we communicate in a way that I've never been able to do before.

What have you noticed when you come to my appointments?
It's really mixed. I want to be there to support you and help you. I also want to hear what they say. But then there's part of me that dreads it each time. It's a weird rollercoaster each time, but I try to remember that if someone hadn't listened to me for 22 years, I would want back-up too. I see my role as somewhere between carer and interpreter. I try to listen and take notes in case you're overwhelmed and also try to remind you of any questions that you wanted to ask.

I'm always dumbstruck when I'm spoken to instead of you. Coming to these appointments was the first time that I really started to understand the medical gaslighting you go through. Like when we asked if your cervix would be removed, and the surgeon started reassuring me about my sexual pleasure . . .

I don't believe doctors are out to hurt people. I'm sure ego is involved, but I do believe they want to help. And after listening to thousands of the same stories, it must become easy to be blasé and make assumptions. But I do sit there and think that if they just stopped and actually listened and thought, 'Hang on, that's not right', then how different could that patient's life be? I'm definitely angry at the medical system that has failed you in so many ways.

When you look back over the last few years, how does it make you feel?
Sad and ashamed. I wish we had done things differently. I wish I had pushed earlier. I wish I had listened to you more and had more consideration when you said you were in pain beyond offering you a hot-water bottle and some pasta. I've had days where I'm terrified that I'll come home from work and you'll no longer be here. I worry that the pain has become too much and that you've either taken too many pain meds by accident or that the toll of everything has become too much. I start mentally preparing for what I might walk into when I get home. Sometimes, I can't quite believe we're in that position.

How do you see our future?
Endometriosis has made me re-think things, but I still see us and the future we always dreamed of. You're still my Jen. But it does feel like we're in a threesome with endometriosis. When you're in the trenches, it's hard to see beyond the pain and issues. But when we look back, I believe we'll see how much we've done together and all of our memories. I just hope that we never give up trying. I love you and I'm proud of you.

What are three words to describe your experience with endometriosis?
Exhaustion, frustration, paralysis.

What are your tips for anyone supporting someone with endometriosis?
- Remind yourself they didn't choose this.
- Try to educate yourself about this disease and what it does.
- Listen to them.
- It's okay to step away for a minute if things are getting too much.
- Know your own limitations. Be honest and make sure you're not pushing yourself to breaking point.
- Asking what helps and what doesn't before a flare hits. Then, when it inevitably does, you have a starting point.

- As bad as flares get, remember these spikes are temporary.
- Take the pressure off. If you have to cancel or change plans, do it. It's okay. And don't feel like a good day has to be crammed full to make up for lost time.
- Have your own coping strategies, your own toolkit for dealing with this. A hobby, whatever it is – something to immerse yourself in that is for you and gives you that time out.
- Show interest in them and their day. Don't just assume you'll know the answer. Listen to them. Ask what was good about their day too.
- Go with them to their appointments and help advocate for them.

This was an incredibly vulnerable experience for us both, which is never easy. I choose to be exceptionally open about my life publicly; Chris absolutely does not. He barely has social media, let alone uses it. However, there is power and strength in vulnerability, which can bring you closer together.

Disclosing chronic illness

Chris and I had been together for a long time before I received my endometriosis and adenomyosis diagnosis. But what if you are in a new relationship? What if you are dating or looking to start dating? Do you disclose your diagnosis to this person? The answer to this is that there is no right answer. It is entirely up to you.

There is no 'correct' way or time to tell someone about your endometriosis. The best thing you can do is go with your gut and share that very personal information when you feel the time is right. Maybe you want to include it in your profile on a dating site. Maybe you could include a mobility aid in one of your pictures. Or you could mention it while messaging, or on the first, second or third date. The important thing to remember is that you do not 'owe' somebody that information, and there is no hurry to disclose endometriosis. Just wait and see where it comes up naturally and, importantly, whether you like the person enough to share the information.

I do not have experience of this part of dating life, so I asked Gemma, who also has endometriosis and adenomyosis, how she deals with this.

'It was terrifying to me! I was so worried that a potential partner would only focus on my disease, not me as a person,' she says. 'There was no formula for if or when I would tell dates about endometriosis. The only time that I felt I really should tell them was when the subject of children came up and I personally felt I should warn them that I had a condition that might affect my fertility . . . But to be honest, the ones I really liked were all really kind, interested and supportive. I haven't ever really had a disastrous experience with telling someone about my conditions, but there have been some awkward encounters. To be fair, I wouldn't want to be with someone who couldn't handle my reality anyway. Telling people was scary the first few times, but once I realised that I'm so much more than my endometriosis, I relaxed. There are far more interesting things about me.'

Dating with endometriosis

Whether you're newly dating someone or having date nights in an already established relationship, dates can be a bit of a minefield when you're dealing with endometriosis. As my husband mentioned in the interview earlier in the chapter, even a simple trip out of the house can feel like a military manoeuvre, which doesn't necessarily create the most romantic ambiance. However, there are ways to support yourself before and during a date and allow you both to enjoy your time together:

- If you are in the early stages of a relationship, choose the time, day and location yourself to make sure it will be comfortable and accessible for you. For example, if you know that you have limited mobility, are suffering with pain and fatigue and burgers and alcohol are flare triggers for you, you are not going to want someone to lovingly plan a rock-climbing date followed by burgers and cocktails. Remember that this doesn't have to be forever. Once a partner knows more about you and how endometriosis affects you, they will be able to plan dates that accommodate your symptoms. However, at the start, retaining that control can take some of the anxiety away for you.
- Make sure you are comfortable when you get there. Wherever 'there' is, make sure you are able to find a comfortable spot. My husband is

amazing at doing this for me now. If, at a restaurant, we're directed to a table with hard chairs, which will undoubtedly make my hip pain worse, he won't sit but instead asks for somewhere more comfortable or a cushion. Simple things like that are so validating, and I wish I had had the confidence to do them for myself over the years rather than suffer needlessly. If you're going on a casual date, you can always get there a little bit ahead of the meeting time to make sure you can be comfortable before your date arrives.

- Have a flare-up kit. I don't go anywhere without my flare-up kit now (*see* page 45), whether it's a date or not. Try to think about your most common symptoms and make sure you have something to help in case they spike while you are out. If you are on early dates and not yet ready for a big conversation, this could be as simple as mints for nausea, a menthol strip for your abdomen or back and a painkiller.
- Think creatively. Dates do not have to revolve around meals and drinks, which can be a nightmare if you're suffering from dietary triggers or bowel symptoms with your endometriosis. There are so many options for dates now and there is bound to be something you will enjoy without triggering flares (as much as we can ever prevent them!).
- Please, and this is a rule for life, do not ever feel pressured to drink alcohol if you have decided that you do not want to or if it triggers your symptoms. Alcohol is pretty much an instant, guaranteed flare for me, and so it is one of the very few things that I have cut out entirely. I have never received pressure from my husband, but I have definitely felt it from others. They thought I was 'being dramatic' and told me 'one won't hurt' or 'it can't be that bad', and it did make me think about early dating life and how many meals are shared over wine and how many cocktails are drunk in bars. Research places that do amazing mocktails if you still want that vibe without the pain, and never feel pressured to drink alcohol, no matter your reasons for avoiding it.
- Even if you're on early dates and you are not ready to talk about your diagnosis yet, don't try to hide your reality. It will not be sustainable, and you will likely cause yourself to flare up anyway. Do not be afraid to be who you are, right now. You are more than good enough and deserve a loving relationship as much as anyone else.

Ways to support a loved one with endometriosis

If you're reading this part of the book because you want to help a loved one, whatever their relationship to you, through their journey with endometriosis, then thank you! This disease can be incredibly isolating and knowing that someone wants to help can be hugely supportive by itself. We are all unique, so this list will never replace open communication with your loved one, but from conversations with thousands of endometriosis patients, these are the things that keep coming up:

- Validate their feelings – no toxic positivity here, please. There are lots of ways to do this in the section on 'Helpful (and not so helpful) things to say to an endometriosis patient' (*see* overleaf).
- Do some research. Educate yourself on endometriosis and its impacts.
- Know that they are more than their illness.
- Encourage them to never hide their bad days from you.
- Offer to help with simple things such as cooking.
- Never stop inviting them to things, but try to give them notice so they can allocate their energy accordingly. It's not just about the time of the event itself; the build-up, event and recovery can leave us flaring or exhausted.
- Be understanding if they need to cancel last minute or leave early.
- Be as accommodating as possible with their needs.
- Listen, don't assume.
- Check in with them regularly.
- Advocate for them – start conversations, correct misinformation and go with them to medical appointments.

If you are supporting someone with endometriosis, it is important that you also look after your own wellbeing and mental health. You must engage in open dialogue about what's working for you, what's not and what you need. When talking to Dr Sula Windgassen, a health psychologist specialising in chronic illness, she stresses the need for 'clear communication and compassion'. 'Don't push yourself to the point of burnout, which then often leads to "withdrawing" from the relationship and feelings of resentment and frustration. Give yourself permission to look after yourself too.' What that looks like will be unique to you. It could mean taking up or reigniting a hobby, setting aside some time to accomplish your own tasks, spending time with your friends – whatever nourishes you. You need to recognise and honour your own needs as well as those of your partner or the person for whom you are caring. Finally, remember that therapy can be hugely beneficial for partners and carers as well as the person suffering from endometriosis. The changes this disease can bring are huge, wide-reaching and long term. It is absolutely okay to seek help and advice for how to navigate that.

Helpful (and not so helpful) things to say to an endometriosis patient

Helpful
- I believe you.
- I love you.
- I researched endometriosis and I found . . . is that your experience?
- It must be so difficult to be in pain all the time.
- I'm here for you.
- You're not alone.
- You're not a burden.
- You don't need to apologise.
- Endometriosis is not your fault, nor your choice.
- You deserve to be believed.
- It's okay to set boundaries, rest, use mobility aids and so on.
- I know I can never truly understand, but can you help me understand a little better?
- I value you exactly as you are.
- What you're capable of today is more than enough – you don't have to push yourself.
- I know you're doing your best.
- How can I best support you?
- Can I get you anything?
- Do you want advice or to vent? I'm happy with either.
- (If an invitation is declined): I completely understand. Let me know if I can do anything.
- (If an invitation is accepted): Is there anything I can do to make you more comfortable? If you're flaring on the day and have to cancel last minute, I understand.
- I wish I knew what to say, but just know I am always here for you.

Not so helpful
- 'Get well soon.' Something more empathetic would be, 'I hope this flare eases soon.'
- 'It could be worse; at least it's not . . ..' This is hugely invalidating. Say something like, 'That sucks; I'm so sorry you're dealing with that' instead.
- 'But you look great!' We hear this a lot as chronic illness patients. While on one hand it is always nice when someone compliments you, that sneaky 'but' at the start can also make you feel like your reality is not being taken seriously. Some of us have even been told this by doctors as a reason to deny investigations. Try saying, 'You look great, but how are you really feeling?' instead.
- 'But didn't I see you out a few days ago?' Endometriosis can vary drastically day to day, even hour to hour. We might have been able to do something this morning but be bedridden in the afternoon. Just because you saw us doing something a few days ago, it doesn't mean we weren't still suffering, even if it looked like we were enjoying ourselves.
- 'So, you're better now you've had surgery, right? It's all fixed?' Surgery is not a cure for endometriosis. Endometriosis has often been part of our lives for years, even decades prior to surgery. There's a lot of damage in there that will take a lot of time to heal. Try saying 'how is your recovery? I hope the surgery brings you some relief'.
- 'Why are you using a mobility aid? You're not disabled.' This comes down to internalised ableism as a society. We do not question someone's need for glasses because their prescription is lower than someone else's.
- 'Oh yeah, I totally get it; I'm so tired too.' When we are trying to explain our fatigue, please know that it is very different from being tired – even very tired.

Again, we are all different. Some of these might not be as relevant to you as others, and that's where communication comes in again.

The sex talk

Sex and endometriosis are intimately connected. Dyspareunia (diss/pah/roo/nee/ah) may not be a word you have come across, but if you have endometriosis, adenomyosis or fibroids, you may well have experienced it.

Dyspareunia means painful sex. Other causes could be a tilted uterus, pelvic inflammatory disease, pelvic floor dysfunction, adhesions, menopause, cysts, vaginismus or vulvodynia; in other words, a lot of us likely have dyspareunia, but very few of us talk about it or even realise that it is not 'normal'. As you can see from the list above, painful sex is not rare, but it could be a symptom of something that needs treating and is therefore a topic that we need to get comfortable talking about.

The most common symptom is pain with intercourse that occurs at the vaginal opening or deep in the pelvis. It can be a distinct pain in a particular area or widespread across the pelvic area, and can be a sharp, burning or throbbing pain or a general feeling of discomfort. I also experienced deep ripping sensations, which, it turns out, were the adhesions following surgery.

Dyspareunia can occur during or after sex. For a long time, I did not realise that endometriosis and/or adenomyosis were causing dyspareunia because my pain happened after sex, not so much during it. Sometimes, it could be 30 minutes afterwards. It was only when I began thoroughly tracking my symptoms that I started noticing the pattern. But why the connection? Endometriosis can lead to painful sex as a result of the irritation and aggravation of endometriosis lesions, cysts, adhesions and scarring. The pain can vary based on the location and extent of this endometriosis tissue. For example, pain is more likely if disease is located around the pouch of Douglas (*see* page 21) or the cervix, or if the vagina is adhered to the rectum. As with many symptoms of endometriosis, the severity of dyspareunia can vary during your cycle. You may find the pain more intense around ovulation or menstruation, or the pain may be present the whole month through.

First things first: painful sex is not normal and you should never be expected to tolerate it. Sadly, these myths persist even among some medical professionals. One patient, who wishes to remain anonymous, told me that sex was incredibly painful for her, and it was starting to impact her marriage. Her GP's reply? 'And?! It doesn't matter if sex is painful for the woman.' Another endometriosis patient, in Wales, mentioned painful sex to her gynaecologist. The response was a very dismissive 'Just push through it'. A third told her gynaecologist that she and her husband were unable to have sex without it causing extreme pain. Despite knowing this couple's desire to have a baby, the gynaecologist responded with, 'Just stop having sex then.' Please, never normalise painful sex or this kind of comment. If you are experiencing painful sex, see a doctor, and keep seeing doctors until one listens.

If painful sex is being caused by endometriosis, there are numerous ways to manage it and regain some control over this part of your life and relationship. Open communication is key, before, during and afterwards. No one who loves or respects you wants you to be in pain. Try different positions and different times in your cycle, and track your symptoms. There are also numerous products designed to help. One company leading in this area is The Pelvic People, who describe it as 'their mission to end painful sex'. They share lots of free resources on their website and social media and also work with clinicians to understand painful sex more deeply (pardon the pun). Lube can also be your best friend, so don't be afraid to experiment and see what works for you. Remember, sex is not just your traditional cis-heteronormative, penis-in-vagina stereotype. There are myriad ways to bring intimacy and pleasure to your relationship, so if that type of sex is too painful for you right now, have some fun exploring other ways to connect.

The most important thing of all is to go at your own pace. Take your time and communicate with each other. You do not owe anyone sex.

Sex after surgery

After surgery, your surgeon will likely tell you when you can resume activities, including sex (*see* pages 136–137). Follow their advice, but take it as a minimum. If you're still not feeling ready after the six weeks (for example), that is fine. Maybe sex has caused you pain for years and the thought of it is causing you anxiety. Maybe you had some complications after surgery and are not quite ready. Whatever your reasons, the timeline given by your surgeon should never be a mark on the calendar for when you will actually feel ready. It just means that after this point, sex shouldn't cause any post-surgical healing issues.

Always remember that sex is more than intercourse. Take it at your own pace, be open with your partner and experiment with what works for you. If you're particularly anxious, you can always explore your post-surgery body solo before introducing your partner again.

The impact endometriosis can have on our sex life goes beyond pain or bowel flare-ups. Endometriosis, or any chronic illness, can change your relationship with your own body. The symptoms, scars, hot-water bottle burns and weight changes (up or down) can leave us feeling anything but sexy. However, that does not mean you are not sexy. It does not mean you do not deserve pleasure, nor that you are not capable of giving it. Communication comes in here again. The more we are able to be open about our insecurities and issues, as well as our wants and desires, the better sex we will all have.

Ultimately, whether it is about sex, dating or relationships in general, whether you have been with your partner for decades or are just starting out, the best advice I can give is to have the confidence to do what is right for you. Even if it seems different from what everyone else is doing, your personal experience with endometriosis and how it impacts your life and your relationship will mean that approaching things in an unconventional manner might just be the best way forward. It's okay if you're struggling with pain at night and need to spread out so your partner sleeps in a different bed. It's okay if your sex life doesn't include 'traditional' intercourse. It's okay if your relationship doesn't look like that cheesy, romantic Christmas movie (whose does?). And, thinking about relationships more broadly, it's okay if you don't join in big family occasions every single time. It's all okay. Finally, just in case I haven't said it enough already, communication is key. It can be scary to be vulnerable and open ourselves up to people, especially when fears of being a burden or not being enough come in. The truth is that it's not easy, but with practice it gets more natural and it can lead to the strongest relationships, romantic or otherwise.

Work and studying

Endometriosis can impact every part of our lives. Seeing as the average human spends one-third of their time at work, of course it makes sense that our work lives are not left unscathed. In 2020, the All Party Parliamentary Group on Endometriosis released their first major report, and the statistics about work were pretty stark:

- Fifty-five per cent of respondents have often or very often had to take time off work due to endometriosis.
- Thirty-eight per cent are restricted in the work they can do.
- Thirty-eight per cent have had difficulty pursuing the career they want due to endometriosis.

- Twenty-seven per cent believe they have missed out on a promotion due to endometriosis.
- Thirty-eight per cent have often or very often have concerns about losing their job due to endometriosis.
- Twenty-eight per cent have had to change or leave their job due to endometriosis.
- Thirty-five per cent have a reduced income due to endometriosis.
- Eighty-seven per cent believe endometriosis has impacted their long-term financial status.
- Endometriosis costs the UK economy £8.2 billion per year in treatment, healthcare costs and loss of work.

Another study shows that one in six of those with confirmed endometriosis have lost their job due to the demands of the disease and its management. Dearbhail Ormond, founder of frendo, is part of that statistic, losing her job when she returned to work from endometriosis surgery. frendo is an app for those with diagnosed or suspected endometriosis, providing a community, resources and symptom tracking. Their research found that 20 per cent of endometriosis sufferers 'feel their workplaces are unsupportive of chronic health conditions', and while almost a quarter (24 per cent) of workplaces provide employee support for people experiencing fertility issues, 'there is very little support in the workplace for endometriosis'. Dearbhail believes this is caused by the 'long-standing stigma and deep misunderstanding' of endometriosis, and the frendo research backs this up. They found that more than a quarter (26 per cent) had felt shamed or pressured to return to work when taking time off due to their health issues. As we've been saying throughout this book, endometriosis education needs to improve at every single touchpoint – not just within the care pathway but in wider society too.

Driven by Dearbhail's experience and their research findings, the frendo team established frendo@work, which aims to tackle some of the challenges we face in the workplace by 'providing organisations with the resources they need to support their employees with endometriosis'. Dearbhail explains that these resources are wide-ranging, covering 'company workshops, self-management tools, informative expert panel discussions and guidance for line managers to help them support and communicate with staff members affected by the disease'. Staff members themselves also gain access to the frendo app, itself a wealth of knowledge for endometriosis sufferers, covering nutrition, fertility, pain management, communication, symptom tracking and community support. 'It needs to be a collaboration,' Dearbhail says. Endometriosis affects every single area of our lives, 'so we need open conversations with all relevant parties.'

Huge companies have started signing up for frendo@work, including Salesforce, Slack and Indeed. This multi-disciplinary approach to endometriosis support in the workplace is refreshing to see and something I hope is adopted by many more companies of all sizes, prioritising staff welfare and wellbeing, reducing absences and leading to improved engagement and performance. Too many of us face embarrassment, shame and stigma about our symptoms, particularly around heavy bleeding, and I know from my time in a corporate office that my male counterparts had no such worries discussing their bowel movements in depth – sometimes with photographic evidence. Now, I am not saying we should all embrace quite that level of openness in the workplace – there are extremes and limits to everything – but a middle ground where health conditions are taken seriously should be found for us all, regardless of sex and gender.

The impact endometriosis will have on your work life will be as unique as every other aspect of your experience with the disease. There will be some who are able to work without it impacting them at all – remember, 30 per cent of patients are asymptomatic. Then there will be some who attend work but are not able to function at their best, known as 'presenteeism'. Some people will need to take absences to deal with symptom flares, appointments and surgeries, known as 'absenteeism'. Others still will have to reduce their hours to part time or become self-employed to manage their workloads and schedules with more flexibility. And then there will also be some who cannot work due to the severity of their symptoms. You may find yourself in one of the categories at a certain point in your endometriosis journey but in a different one another time.

How to ask for support

There are ways to support yourself through working with endometriosis, and it's important to make sure that you are making the most of the support that exists. If you are struggling with endometriosis at work, here are some tips for how to navigate conversations about support:

- You are under no legal obligation to disclose endometriosis, or any disability or illness, at interview stage. There may be benefits to doing so – for example, if a company is signed up to the Disability Confident Scheme, you will be guaranteed an interview. However, there is undeniably still stigma around long-term health conditions, so this choice is yours.
- That said, if you would like support with your condition or any adaptations to be put in place, your company cannot do this if they do not know about your endometriosis. They may expect you to undertake tasks that are not accessible or manageable because they do not know. This disclosure can happen at any time, so if your symptoms become more unmanageable over time, please do not feel that you cannot bring it up with your manager or HR department because you didn't say anything when you joined.
- As with anything to do endometriosis management, think about what symptoms you are struggling with and then come up with ideas or suggestions that would help you at work for those issues. The box on work adaptations (*see* overleaf) will give you some ideas
- The Equality Act 2010 enshrined certain rights in law, including the legal right for 'reasonable adjustments' to be put in place for you at work to help you manage chronic illness, including endometriosis. Depending on the size of your company, ask to speak to Occupational Health, HR or your manager.
- Try to read your company's policies about health, welfare, absences and adaptations in advance so you are informed about the process and what they currently offer.
- Before approaching your employer, think about what your goal is. Would you like practical adjustments? Increased awareness? A new role that accommodates your symptoms? Different working hours? Remember that the result will likely be a compromise, but it is always helpful to go into these discussions with an idea of what would be most beneficial to you.
- Bear in mind that levels of endometriosis awareness and education are generally low, and this is likely to be the case at your workplace too. It can be helpful to print out accurate resources about endometriosis and take them with you to any discussions to provide context about why it can be so debilitating. You can also ask your GP to complete a

'fit note' for you to use, highlighting what you struggle with and how that may impact your duties at work. For example, a flare-up may make commuting difficult or even dangerous, so working from home that day would be the doctor's recommendation. While this can be very helpful, bear in mind that the contents of the fit note are recommendations only and your employer is not obligated to follow them.

Work adaptations for endometriosis

We are all so different, as are the jobs we do and the symptoms we suffer from. Therefore, rather than trying to think of every eventuality, I asked the endometriosis community for some of the adaptations their workplaces have put in place for them that have helped them at their jobs:

- 'I am allowed to come in a little later as I struggle with fatigue and pain first thing.'
- 'I now work solely from home. It's a slightly different role, but it works so much better for me.'
- 'I have flexible working, so while I go in to the office as much as I can, I can also work from home on flare days.'
- 'When I'm flaring, I let my manager know. They either give me extra time to complete tasks or, if it's more urgent, they assign someone to help me.'
- 'I work in a really small team in a very small company. They made me a pain scale board so I could display how my symptoms were doing and if I needed some help or to be left alone. I don't think it would work in larger, more formal companies, but I love it.'
- 'My team know I struggle with bloating and nausea and make sure I'm always stocked with mint tea.'
- 'I asked to have my workstation moved closer to the bathrooms so I'm not always running through the entire office.'
- 'When I told them about my endometriosis, they asked if there were any resources to help them understand more. The management team then had a learning session and a "lunch and learn" for staff to increase awareness and education.'

- 'I asked for a more comfortable chair as I really suffer with back and hip pain.'
- 'They've made sure that our weekly strategy session was moved to after lunch. It used to be in the morning, when I would suffer from more pain and brain fog, so I felt like I wasn't contributing.'
- 'My work allows me to keep a spare change of clothes at work in case I bleed through.'
- 'They allow me time off for medical appointments and surgeries without making me feel like I'm dossing or shirking off.'
- 'My manager has never once made me feel like I'm exaggerating or being dramatic. Turns out her sister has crippling endometriosis too, so she understood. We're working together on a project now to raise awareness in the company.'
- 'I remember very clearly that one time I was upset when a pregnancy announcement was made. I desperately wanted children, but endometriosis had other plans. My manager noticed and now will always check in on me whenever announcements like this are made. When someone brought their newborn into the office, my manager pre-warned me and asked if I would like to take a break or stay.'

You can see that there is a huge range here, from major changes to how you work to things as simple as a more comfortable chair. Others are more based in empathy, particularly around pain or fertility. Others may seem trivial but provide a sense of validation and being seen. Consider what might help you and see what can be put in place.

Self-employment

Even if you are self-employed, do still think about what adjustments you could make to your working environment and practices. Symptom tracking can be useful here. Do you notice that your symptoms are always worse at a certain point? Factor that into your schedule. Does your pain spike after sitting at your laptop on those admin days? Look at your set-up; what might help? Are you getting enough breaks? Hydrating enough? Making sure you give yourself enough time to complete tasks?

Studying

If you are still at school, or perhaps if you are advocating on behalf of a teenager with endometriosis, all of the workplace recommendations apply in this setting as well. Make sure you tell the school that you have endometriosis, even if it is only suspected, and set up a conversation to discuss how they can best support you. Maybe that's an understanding that extra bathroom breaks may be required or that certain activities will not be accessible. Have you had a flare-up this week and need a little longer to complete an assignment? Looking back now, something I think would have been a huge help to me as a teen was a relatively simple adaptation – being allowed to wear trousers instead of the school regulation skirts. The comfort and peace of mind that would have brought teenage Jen would have been huge. Think about the symptoms you are struggling most with, then think about what could help you better navigate school life for each of those symptoms. Approach the school and enter an open dialogue with them. They might not be able to offer all of them, but there may be ways they can help that you have not even thought of.

As with workplaces, schools are unlikely to be up to date with what endometriosis means and how best to support someone who is suffering. This means that, at first, you might have to take on the burden of education – ironic, I know. Take in accurate materials for them, take in this book, direct them to people and organisations who can come in to schools for this specific purpose. While bringing it up to the school might be your responsibility, the burden then shifts on to them. You are an adolescent, trying to cope with all the stresses of school and manage a life with a chronic illness. The school should be supporting you with this in the long term, not the other way around.

Special occasions

These special occasions will vary depending on your life, your culture and your situation, but could be anything from Christmas, other celebratory holidays, weddings, birthdays, travelling and vacations – anything that is out of the ordinary 'day to day' of our life. There is no time off from living with a chronic illness like endometriosis, so it is really important that you find and implement strategies that help you manage your endo but still allow you to enjoy yourself.

Endometriosis

Generally, I find the following to be really helpful things to remember during these occasions. Don't get me wrong, I still have to remind myself every time because I get too excited and want to do everything, or get serious fear of missing out (FOMO). Don't beat yourself up if these do not come naturally to you, especially at first:

- Do not overcommit. It is more than fine to say no to some events to make sure you have time to rest. If you do attend and start flaring, please speak up. You don't have to find a microphone and make a grand announcement, but don't suffer in silence. Tell a trusted someone that you are struggling. Your loved ones do not want you to be in pain. Remember, it is also okay to leave earlier than intended.
- Avoid your triggers. This can be so incredibly hard when it comes to special occasions. Who doesn't want that slice of birthday cake, some champagne to toast the newlyweds, or that feast at Christmas time? But do try to identify and avoid any personal triggers. Know which ones are complete no-goes and which ones you can have a little bit of. I know how tempting it can be, but is it really worth the flare-up?
- Stay comfy. I still struggle with this one. I feel like since my endometriosis really ramped up, I live in the comfiest clothes I own and all of my beautiful pieces have been relegated to the back of the wardrobe. So, of course, when I'm invited to something and I actually have the energy to go, I desperately want to dig out something that makes me look my best. But the importance of comfort cannot be overstated, particularly around the waist and abdomen. Try to choose clothes that make you feel fantastic but are also comfortable. Before my second surgery, endo belly (*see* page 38) was a huge challenge for me, which meant jeans or anything with a tight waistband were just non-starters. They simply weren't worth the agony. Again, this is about knowing what symptoms you suffer with and finding a combination that works for you, while keeping your personal style.
- Pack a flare-up kit. The contents will vary depending on your situation, but as an example mine includes medication, water, mints, a TENS machine, a heat pad, menthol strips, a folding walking stick and (before my hysterectomy) period products and fresh underwear.
- Set boundaries. If you need to leave early, do. If you don't want to talk about your fertility status, then you do not have to (a rule for life, not just

special occasions!). If you need to use a hot-water bottle to make yourself comfortable, go for it (just be careful with burns; see pages 93–94).

- Make a list of the things you would like to do and prioritise them. Create a 'must-have' list, a 'nice-to-have' list, and an 'only if we have extra time or energy' list, and be flexible if plans need to change last minute. Try to spread things out as much as possible so you don't spend the second half of an event, trip or holiday season in a flare after going too hard too early.
- Order medications. If you're going on vacation or have lots of plans over the holidays, make sure you have enough of your medications and place repeat prescriptions early to make sure you don't run out. Remember that doctors, pharmacies and shops may be closed on public holidays so this may take some planning.
- Avoid comparison. It can seem as if everyone else is having a magical time at Christmas or living their best life on a beach holiday. Seeing those images or hearing those stories while you're curled up in a pain flare can sting and make you feel like you are missing out. However, humans are exceptionally complex beings and we can hold more than one emotion at the same time. It is okay for you feel happy for a friend who's on a beautiful holiday but also sad at your current situation. It doesn't make you a bad friend. Try to remember that, by and large, social media is not real. It is the tiniest snapshot of someone's highlights. Stay in your own lane and do what you can, when you can. Try to find the small moments of everyday magic, and don't forget you can always unfollow any accounts that make you feel worse.
- 'No, thank you' is a complete sentence. You do not have to justify yourself or provide any reasoning beyond that.
- If your plans involve some travelling, especially on something like a train or a plane, make sure you look into what schemes are available at the station or airport. If you are a passenger with a disability or reduced mobility, you are legally entitled to support. This could include special assistance, priority security at airports, special lounges, closer parking and lots of other accommodations, and it is well worth researching before you travel.
- Car journeys are obviously not limited to special occasions, but they can become longer and more frequent with family events, holidays and

gatherings. With seatbelts pressing exactly where my pain is, bumps in the road, potholes, roundabouts, sudden braking and twisty country roads, car journeys are not an environment that my endometriosis likes. Keeping a stash of medication in the car (be very careful about taking medication if you're driving), building in time for regular breaks, not overfilling your bladder, packing flare-friendly snacks, wearing comfy clothes, communicating honestly with the driver and using heated seats can all help you navigate car journeys, especially longer ones. If your car doesn't have heated seats, you can buy heated mats designed for the car seats to put behind your back. Do not drive if your judgement or concentration is impaired.

Coping with flares in hot temperatures

Whether it's summer, a heatwave or you're lucky enough to be heading on holiday to a warm location, rising temperatures can play havoc with our symptom management. Again, this works on a case-by-case basis and some people find they feel better in the summer heat, but for many of us it can make dealing with certain symptoms even more difficult and even put us at risk of serious heat-related complications. Here is what you can do to help:

- Check your medications: Certain medications can put you at higher risk of heat-related illnesses such as dehydration, heat strokes and heat exhaustion. These include antidepressants, beta-blockers, certain anti-histamines (including some anti-nausea medications), benzodiazepines and more. Check with your pharmacy or doctor and, if you are on these medications, take extra precautions against the heat.
- Keep hydrated: Water is important, yes, but don't forget you can also get hydration from certain foods too, like cucumbers, watermelons, strawberries, salads and anything fresh and juicy. Avoid alcohol as it can increase dehydration.
- Fans: I cannot live without my fan. Pain makes me really hot anyway, so chuck in extra heat from the environment and I am cooking. We have fans around the home, and I always have at least one portable fan with

me, either electric or an old-school one for when I need to be quiet or have run out of battery. I used to be so self-conscious getting them out in public, but I really do not care any more and, to be honest, most people wish they had one too.
- Clothing: Choose loose-fitting clothes made from natural fibres like linen, silk or cotton. Try to avoid anything too restrictive or tightly fitting. Summer dresses are usually endo-belly-friendly too, which is always a bonus. Wear a hat to protect your head and face.
- Protect your scars: Unfortunately, if you have had invasive surgery, you will have scars. They are nothing to be ashamed of and, while they can impact our body image, they do not need to be a reason to hide away during hotter temperatures. However, they do require some extra protection. Scars are very sensitive to sunlight and can burn easily, so use a good sunscreen with a broad-spectrum SPF of at least 30 wherever you have scars to protect them. If your scars are still healing or are new, cover them with either clothing or a dressing.
- Ice therapy: If you are dealing with endo pain, you are likely pretty attached to your hot-water bottle or heat pad. But in hotter temperatures, these methods aren't always desirable or helpful. Try some cold therapy instead by wrapping ice packs in towels (always making sure to protect your skin).
- Warning signs: Having a chronic illness such as endometriosis can make you more susceptible to heat-related complications, which should never be taken lightly. Learn the warning signs of dehydration, heat exhaustion and heat stroke as well as some basic first aid to help.
- Be flexible: Be as flexible as you can with your schedule and try to avoid exertion in the hottest parts of the day. I realise that this is not an option for everyone, but if you can add in even the smallest amount of flexibility – running an errand before work instead of at lunchtime, for instance – your body and health will thank you. Go easy on your workouts too.
- Check in on your chronically ill friends: They might not be aware of these extra risks, so just ask how they are doing and if they need anything.

Day-to-day life

All of the strategies we've covered in the 'special occasions' section above are also great for day-to-day life. Setting boundaries, being on top of prescriptions and avoiding triggers will help you in everyday life too. But what about some other things you can do for those 'normal' days, whatever that looks like for you? The answers will be personal to you, your life circumstances, the stage of your endometriosis journey and what you are currently struggling with. However, there are a few key things that I think are helpful to know for all of us:

- Pacing
- Available support
- Hobbies and interests
- Connection

Pacing

Does this sound familiar to you? You wake up one day and realise you're having a low, or lower than average, symptom day. So, you think it's the perfect day to get through that massive to-do list that's been building up. Maybe you'll also arrange to meet a friend for a last-minute catch-up – why not? But by the end of the day, you are really struggling. Your body is angry at you, you have had to up your pain relief and you are exhausted. In other words, you're in a flare-up. Now you've got to rest to recover, which also means you might have to rearrange the appointment you have tomorrow or the next day too. And so, you rest, you apply your full symptom management arsenal and, eventually, the flare eases. Then you wake up, realise that you're having a low, or lower than average, symptom day, and the cycle continues.

There are many different definitions of what pacing actually is, but, broadly speaking, pacing is the balancing of activity and rest. The aim, as described by occupational therapist Kathryn Jamieson-Lega in a 2013 study, is 'for the purpose of achieving increased function and participation in meaningful activities'. It's the fine art of managing your days to allow you to accomplish what you need and want to do without causing a flare of your symptoms. The idea is that we move out of the boom-and-bust cycle in which so many of us with endometriosis find ourselves.

Living with endometriosis – the art and the science

Learning this balance is one of the hardest things I have had to train my brain to do and, to be honest, it does not always work. Life inevitably throws things up (negative or positive) that are unavoidable. Sometimes, you just don't want to miss out on opportunities that arise; you want to live your life. All of that is okay and understandable. However, having a grasp of the basic concept of pacing has definitely been helpful. I once opened up to a pain management specialist about my frustrations with pacing, particularly when endometriosis is inherently unpredictable in nature. She gave me some great advice: 'No one, whether they have endometriosis, another chronic illness or are in perfect health, can pace 100 per cent of the time. Aim for a certain percentage of the time. What that percentage is will be up to you to decide, but maybe you can increase it if you find it is helping.' She suggested I started with 75 per cent of the time, which I don't always meet but is much better than putting that unrealistic aim of 100 per cent on myself.

Assuming that pacing means doing all or nothing is harmful in more ways than one. Take our initial example of tackling your to-do list and heading out for a coffee. You might still be able to do both, even while pacing, but you might instead prioritise a few things off the list instead of the whole lot, and you might suggest meeting your friend at home or asking them to pick you up, for example. Pacing doesn't have to mean giving things up; it means thinking about the who, what, where, when and why of your daily activities. Let's be honest, this can be pretty exhausting in itself. It's okay if you find it challenging or even frustrating. I resisted it for years. It is truly a process of trial and error, and the best way to feel its benefits is to give it a go.

If you recognise yourself in that boom–bust cycle of activity versus flare, I encourage you to look further into pacing and experiment with it. There is lots of information available online, but you can also ask your GP for a referral to your local pain management clinic, which will be able to guide you through the process. Some multi-disciplinary endometriosis teams even have pain management specialists as part of the clinic, so it is always worth asking.

Available support

We've discussed support that may help at work, school or at home, but there is also wider societal support available if your endometriosis symptoms are having severe effects on your quality of life and mobility. Two that I'd like to briefly touch upon in the UK are Personal Independence Payments (PIP) and Blue Badges.

PIP is a type of benefit that 'can help with extra living costs if you have both:

- A long-term physical or mental health condition or disability
- Difficulty doing certain everyday tasks or getting around because of your condition'

The application process is extensive, requiring you to gather as much medical and supporting information as possible, but it is available to endometriosis patients whose symptoms are severely disrupting their lives. As with most societal bodies, the level of understanding about endometriosis can be low, so be prepared that you may have to appeal an initial decision. Sadly, there is seemingly little consistency across how awards are given, with different endometriosis patients telling me the following:

- 'I was declined but won at appeal.'
- 'I was turned down completely.'
- 'I was awarded the higher rate straight away.'
- 'I was awarded nothing but then the appeal awarded me the higher rate.'
- 'I was given the standard rate.'

It really will come down to you, your personal experience with endometriosis and its impacts on your life. You can get PIP even if you're working, have savings or are getting most other benefits, so please don't let this put you off applying if you think you meet the criteria. The Citizens Advice Bureau offers help and guidance for those applying for PIP if you would like some more support.

The Blue Badge scheme is not a financial one but can be a life-changer for those whose endometriosis causes mobility issues. It allows you to park closer to your destination, either as a passenger or a driver. You apply online and, at the time of writing, they cost £10 in England, £20 in Scotland and are free in Wales. In Northern Ireland there is a slightly different process, but if you search 'Blue Badge scheme' and your location, you should be directed to the relevant information. Lots of people say to me, 'Oh, I don't think I'm

Living with endometriosis – the art and the science

"bad" enough for a Blue Badge' and I always reply with the same thing: there are people whose job is to assess these applications and decide whether or not you meet the criteria. If you think it might help you, apply, be honest about your situation and see what happens.

Hobbies and interests

For a while, whenever I was asked what my hobbies were, I would joke and say 'endometriosis' because it felt like my whole life revolved around this disease. Understanding it, researching it, educating others about it, managing my own, advocating for myself at endless medical appointments – I lived, breathed, ate and spoke endometriosis. Then a gentle conversation, initiated by my husband, made me realise I was losing 'Jen' amid the endometriosis. A huge part of who we are, the identity that we create for ourselves and portray to others, is made up of our interests and our passions, and we don't have to lose that because of endo. You might have to give up certain hobbies (it is perfectly okay to feel rubbish about that, by the way), you might set some aside for now but find that with time and treatment you can pick them back up, you might have to adapt some and you might discover new ones that are more accessible to you.

Try to think about your hobbies and other topics that interest you. How can you adapt them or bring more of them into your life? Could you find a way to access your hobby from a more comfortable location, especially during flares? Are there any adaptations that can be made to allow you to continue? Is there something you've always been really interested in that you'd like to explore more? Remember, hobbies don't always have to be active. Gentle hobbies for days when you're flaring or particularly fatigued are great too and keep our mental health from plummeting. If you like reading fiction or learning about topics but can't concentrate during a flare, you could try audiobooks, for example. Think about hobbies you can pick up and put down as required without much effort or hassle.

I wish I could list out a whole bunch of hobbies that might work for you, but our symptoms, lives, interests and capabilities vary so much. If nothing else, I hope this small section encourages you to hold on to your interests and not become consumed by endometriosis. I've been there – many of us have – but your energy is precious and limited. Try, where you can, to spend it on things that bring you something positive, whether that's enjoyment, distraction, fun, accomplishment, mental health benefits or connection.

Connection

Endometriosis is a very isolating disease, largely because it is so misunderstood and dismissed but also because it is so individualised. While there are clear patterns in the stories of endometriosis patients around the world, our individual experiences with the disease are completely unique, shaped by our individual biophysical situation, culture, work situation, financial independence, culture, country of birth, religion, relationship status, access to information, mental health and too many other factors to name. We often end up feeling alone. Connection to other people who are also going through their own endometriosis journey can be hugely validating and supportive for many people. It is up to you what this looks like. It could be through in-person or online support groups. It could be setting up a page on Instagram or TikTok to share your journey. It could be starting a book club specifically for endo patients who love reading, or a gaming group or running club – the list is endless for what connection with the endo community might look like. Having a network of people who truly 'get it' can be a lifeline for so many. Have a search for what's out there based on your needs and what you would like to achieve, and see how it goes. If you find that it's a bit much, step back. Finding it helpful? Lean in. Go with your gut and what is working for you in the moment.

Balancing endometriosis and your life can be overwhelming. Even when you think you are in a bit of a rhythm and figuring things out, something will usually crop up that throws it all out again. Communicate your needs clearly and allow your loved ones to help you. Be kind to yourself. You are not a burden. You deserve loving relationships and a life full of wonderful memories too.

Chapter 6

Not all endometriosis pain is physical

'You know, if you're happier, you feel less pain. Have you thought about being happier?' – thoracic surgeon

This chapter contains references to suicide and suicidal ideation. If you are in crisis and need urgent support, please call 111 or use the resources at the end of this book (see pages 288–290).

When you've been diagnosed with a physical condition such as endometriosis, it is very easy for your mind to go straight to supporting your physical health. However, the body and the brain are not two separate entities. Endometriosis can impact mental health in more ways than I could possibly fit into a single chapter, and we must prioritise supporting our emotional wellbeing as well as our physical. Managing your mental health is as much a part of your multi-disciplinary toolbox for endometriosis as anything else and should not be underestimated.

Before we get stuck into this chapter, I want to make something clear: acknowledging the brain's role in pain and the effects that endometriosis has on mental health is *not* the same thing as saying your pain is in your head or that you're making it up. You can adopt all the strategies in the world and still have endometriosis. Being in constant pain is going to impact your mental health. The two are linked and *both* must be addressed. A positive mental attitude is not going to treat your endometriosis, while toxic positivity, as you will see shortly, is an instant red flag. Mental health strategies, however, can absolutely help us cope with the pain and all of the other mental traumas that living with this disease inflicts. This chapter could quite easily be an entire book – to be honest, most of the chapters could – so please know that mental health is a vast and hugely nuanced topic. What works for one person might not work for you, but something will.

The impact of endometriosis on mental health

While each patient experience is unique, endometriosis can be extremely demanding, both physically and mentally. Years of being gaslit, constantly explaining yourself, relationship breakdowns, fertility worries, isolation, losing your self-identity and worth, losing your financial independence, constant medical admin, repeated medical traumas, losing opportunities and mobility, all on top of the physical symptoms of a disease like endometriosis, often result in mental distress. It is not uncommon for patients with endometriosis to also suffer from anxiety, panic, depression, PTSD or even suicidal ideation (having thoughts about the possibility of taking your own life).

In fact, a 2020 report revealed that 95 per cent of endometriosis sufferers said that their wellbeing has been negatively impacted by the disease. A staggering 81 per cent said endometriosis had impacted their mental health negatively or very negatively, while 89 per cent reported feeling isolated due to their endometriosis. In a heartbreaking study by the BBC and the charity Endometriosis UK, around half of the respondents said that their endometriosis had led to suicidal thoughts. None of us should ever feel like death is the only way to escape our pain. Despite these heartbreaking statistics, and an increasing understanding that living with this disease can also harm our mental health, 90 per cent of endometriosis sufferers were found to have wanted access to psychological support but were not offered any. We cannot treat endometriosis effectively without also bringing mental health, and the trauma our minds have also endured, into the conversation.

Health psychologist Dr Windgassen, aka @thehealthpsychologist, explained during our conversation that 'endometriosis patients have so much to balance. There's the high mental load, depleted physical capacity, and a really difficult context of the healthcare system and society. It's unreasonable for anyone to expect you to be able to navigate that by yourself.' Driven by her own health experiences, Dr Windgassen specialises in the interplay between mental health and chronic illness. While she suffers from bladder issues rather than endometriosis, she notes that there was a common 'lack of clarity and a heavy burden to advocate' for herself that is mirrored across so much of women's healthcare. 'So much of that journey makes you feel like you're going to be stuck in that amount of suffering forever,' which had a massive impact on her 'wellbeing, mental health, psychology' and her perception of herself. 'I didn't really recognise myself at all.'

Not all endometriosis pain is physical

Her father, a psychiatrist, suggested she try mindfulness techniques. 'I had the same reaction that so many of us do when we hear the word "mindfulness". People don't understand how physical this pain is.' Her father's partner was a psychologist in a clinical health setting and helped Dr Windgassen see that her father was not proposing to change her physical experience through mind control but rather that the body and brain are hugely interconnected. 'Working with the brain might not change the physical mechanisms happening in your body, but looking at mental health aspects can make living with the condition less miserable.' This message, Dr Windgassen says, was 'really hopeful to me' and encouraged her to start exploring and engaging with these ideas. 'Obviously, my physical symptoms didn't disappear, but it changed my experience with those symptoms.' This led to Dr Windgassen setting off on an impressive academic and research career, focusing on the interaction between psychological therapy and physical health, particularly in chronic illness. 'It's not about making people less stressed; it's about helping people navigate what's happening in their bodies.' The more we try to oversimplify the message, 'the more we risk gaslighting and dismissing people'.

Sadly, this dismissal is all too common in journeys with endometriosis. Instead of being supported via the interplay of physical and mental health, many endometriosis patients see their experiences of mental health used to dismiss or devalue their physical struggles. I remember after my first surgery in 2022, I was still in the same pain, and I made that known to the surgeon. His reaction to me was he had 'done [his] job', 'that this is probably psychosomatic now', and that I should investigate therapy – psychological of course, not physical – and 'be aggressive with pain medication'. A few months later, it was shown on MRI by an endometriosis expert that there was still considerable endometriosis left in my body, including some that was endangering my vital organs.

My experience is not an unusual occurrence. Every single patient I have spoken to through my campaigning work and while writing this book has their own version of the story:

- 'I was told it was just stress and to calm down.'
- 'The doctor said if I didn't stop coming in to talk about periods then people might start thinking I was obsessed and paranoid.'

- 'They said to calm down and that it's only feeling this bad because I'm getting this upset.'
- 'My symptoms were blamed on PTSD relating to childhood trauma.'
- 'He said to try not thinking about the pain and that would help.'

Dr Windgassen says that her work reflects these experiences. She sees so many people having mental health weaponised against them in their quest for answers and treatment. 'They're told, "it's just stress; have you tried mindfulness?", so of course, when you try to introduce the topic of psychological support, an endometriosis patient may well think, "Here we go again, another person telling me it's all in my head".' Dr Windgassen says that overcoming this hurdle is often the first step when she's working with endometriosis patients, especially those who have experienced prolonged medical gaslighting. She is 'always clear that my model is not just to make you less stressed and then your endometriosis will be better. It's much more nuanced.' She uses a bio-psycho-social model, saying, 'We have to take into account what is going on with your biology, and we know that there are very specific biological processes occurring with endometriosis that we have to be aware of. It's not about "curing endo". It's about lightening the high mental load of a life with that disease. It's mitigating the extra layers that accumulate on top of your endometriosis.'

The bio-psycho-social model

This model takes into account the various factors – biological, psychological and social – that can influence our health and our experience of our health (*see* Figure 6.1). This approach suggests that health is made up of all three of these factors. In 2023, researchers highlighted that 'psychosocial factors such as stigma also play a role in mental health distress among endometriosis patients'. It is not a perfect model, with emphasis sometimes placed on one segment with the others neglected, but it's the one that the NHS uses, including NHS pain management and psychological services, so it's worth knowing and understanding it.

Not all endometriosis pain is physical

Figure 6.1: The bio-psycho-social model

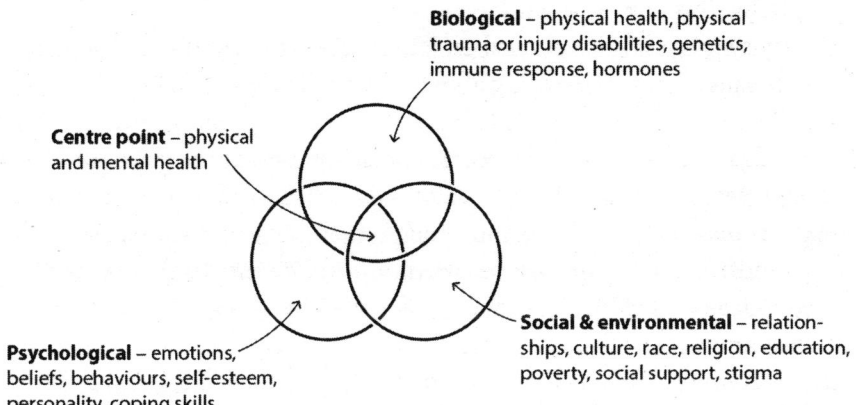

'We do sadly see some healthcare practitioners veer into victim-blaming language and patterns,' says Dr Windgassen, especially in conditions as misunderstood as endometriosis. 'They say things like, "You need to get a handle on your stress", but it places too much guilt and burden onto the patient – that they haven't done enough, that they're not managing their life with the disease "correctly".' Experienced repeatedly over time, this medical and societal gaslighting 'deeply embeds core ideas about ourselves and how others might perceive us. That maybe we're weak. Or lazy. Or bringing it on ourselves. It can be extremely distressing, eating at our self-esteem and our self-worth. This then leads to low mood, making it even more difficult to manage our symptoms and lives.'

The effect of appallingly long diagnosis times on our mental health is bad enough. The internalised gaslighting, the uncertainty, the draining fight to be heard and believed – none of it is conducive to balanced mental health. However, we often forget that the fight doesn't stop after diagnosis. The effort to access sustained treatment is a battle in its own right. While writing this book, the first endometriosis clinic appointment I should have had since spring 2023 was cancelled. Again. First June, then August, then October. No explanations, no new date offered, despite having recently received an MRI report showing disease impacting multiple organs and sites.

Frustrated, I rang the clinic. The phone call that ensued went along these lines:

Jen: Hi, I'm calling because my appointment has been cancelled for the third time and no new date has been given.

Clinic: Yes. The consultant is leaving so everything has been cancelled and moved.

Jen: Permanently leaving?

Clinic: Yes. So you will go back on to a waiting list and receive an appointment in due course.

Jen: Do you have any indication of when that might be? I'm in a lot of pain and should have been seen back in June. I've not been seen since for 17 months despite ending up in A&E and having an MRI show disease present.

Clinic: No, there's nothing more we can do for you, but you are still in the system. *hangs up*

clinic calls back

Clinic: Good news! The consultant isn't leaving, he's just going on holiday.

Jen: Oh, great! So, if it's a diarised absence, can I please have a new appointment date?

Clinic: No.

Jen: *getting upset* Please, I know it's not your fault, but is there nothing you can do? What am I meant to do? I'm in a lot of pain and haven't been seen for such a long time.

Clinic: If you haven't heard back in two weeks, you could always call back.

Jen: Will they be able to book an appointment, though, if we couldn't today?

Clinic: Probably not, but it might make you feel better.

Jen: . . .

After the call, I burst into tears. I don't really know why other than pure frustration and exhaustion. Living with endometriosis feels like you're clinging to a buoyancy aid in an ocean. Sometimes the water is rougher, and sometimes it's a bit calmer, but you're always clinging on. When I hung up the phone after that call, it felt like someone had ripped that buoyancy aid away and wouldn't tell me if help was on the horizon. The mental exhaustion of that uncertainty is something I don't see talked about publicly, yet everyone I speak to personally understands and experiences it.

I called my husband, who was at work, and talked him through what had happened. The whole time, all I could think was that if that conversation had happened 18 months previously, when my pain was at its unbearable

Not all endometriosis pain is physical

worst, I would genuinely have considered whether I could carry on living in that state. Being in that much pain and being made to feel like you're on your own puts you in a very dark place. You start to think, 'What if this is what the rest of life is going to be like? I can't live like this. I can't be in this pain forever.' It made me wonder how many of us are having conversations like this, then hanging up and deciding they can't carry on. It broke my heart.

If this strikes a chord with you, if you are in that darkness right now, please know that you will not feel like this forever. Focus on one day at a time and please reach out, whether it's to a trusted person in your life, to your medical team or to one of the resources listed in the back of this book. You are not alone. You are so much stronger than you know. I'm just sorry that you have had to be so strong for so long. I'm sending you love and compassion.

The state of endometriosis waiting lists in the NHS, and worldwide, is causing untold harm – not just physically, but mentally too. In fact, some patients believe that navigating the medical system causes more psychological distress than dealing with the disease and its effects. In a very casual Instagram poll on my page in 2024, the fight for diagnosis, dismissal, constant self-advocacy, self-education, stigma, misogyny, chasing appointments, scans, cancellations, waiting lists and surgery cancellations all came up as significant challenges.

Endometriosis challenged my mental health in ways I didn't realise until it was almost too late. Two decades of trying to be believed followed by an extremely intense two years of constant, agonising pain, the loss of my mobility, the never-ending explanations of 'what is wrong' with me, the changes it wreaked on my body, the loss of my career and financial independence – I could probably fill this chapter with a list of the ways endometriosis pushed my mental health to breaking point. At my lowest, I described the feeling as literally not being able to see a life beyond pain. I tried to look forward, but pain was all I could see. I couldn't even see how far I was slipping beneath the waves until my husband came to me and explained how worried he was. 'I've reached the limit of how I know how to help,' he told me. For a man who prides himself on being practical and finding solutions to any of our problems, I knew how much it took for him to admit this to me. We decided that I would contact the GP the next day and ask for mental health support. Again, this is absolutely not the same as someone saying, 'Your pain is psychosomatic, you need therapy'. This is admitting that the impacts of your illness are a lot to carry, and it is more than okay to ask for support with that.

Having limited space in a single chapter in a single book, it is impossible to cover all the ways in which endometriosis and negative mental health feed each other. I have therefore tried to cover a few different categories in this chapter. There will be overlaps, and there will be areas that I haven't covered. Just know that whatever you're feeling, it is valid.

Comparison

As human beings, we compare ourselves to each other. It's one of the ways in which our brains make sense of the world around us and our place within it. However, the saying 'comparison is the thief of joy' is true. In fact, when it comes to chronic illness, there is even a specific term: 'comparative suffering'. This is the practice of trying to make sense of your pain by comparing it to the pain of others. Put even more simply, it is when you, or someone else, judges you for feeling pain you don't think you should be feeling or feeling as intensely.

This is a perfectly human response, which has been strengthened by social media and the abundance of human stories we now have access to. See if you can relate to any of the following statements:

- Why can they do that when I'm stuck here in pain?
- They 'only' have stage 1 or 2 endo – they can't be in as much pain.
- Oh wow, that person has stage 4 endo – they must have it so much worse!
- How can that person run a marathon with endometriosis?! Am I lazy?
- They have endometriosis and are smashing it at work. Am I being weak?
- I have endometriosis and can do that; surely they're milking it a bit?

Don't feel bad if you recognise any of these statements. Hopefully, after getting to this point in the book, you will understand why you might have thought them and will now be giving yourself, and other endometriosis patients, a bit of grace. But if you do relate to the statements, you've likely engaged in comparative suffering. These thought patterns are not just unhelpful; they can be harmful to our mental health, leading to feelings of shame, fear, frustration or loneliness and resulting in us invalidating and downplaying our own pain. This can stop us from reaching out for help or even showing ourselves basic empathy.

The current staging system of endometriosis (*see* pages 18–20) is the perfect nurturing ground for comparative suffering, particularly when it is used to invalidate our own or others' experiences. The truth is, we simply cannot tell who 'has it worse' – and it really does not matter anyway. All of our pain is real and valid. We are all worthy of support and relief from endometriosis.

Remember, your experience with endometriosis is as unique as you are. If you notice yourself slipping into comparative suffering, here are some things to remember:

- You can express gratitude for your privileges without slipping into harmful invalidation habits.
- More than one thing can be true at once; you can be grateful and upset at the same time.
- Empathy is infinite – giving empathy to yourself does not mean you won't have enough for someone else too, and vice versa.

It is so easy for me to write, 'Just don't compare yourself and your journey to others', but it is so incredibly difficult to do. I still find myself comparing myself to other people. We encourage each other to share our stories to increase awareness. We find networks and communities to reduce the isolation that endometriosis brings. We trade stories about treatments, surgeries, symptom management options and surgeons. We know that nothing in endometriosis is black and white, but at the same time, comparing our story to those of others in similar positions is the way so many of us find out about new information and feel seen for the first time, often in decades. It's a fine balance, but being aware of comparative suffering is sometimes enough to know how to recognise the signs and pull yourself out of the practice. Do something that you enjoy to distract yourself, try to plan something fun (but manageable) and, as always, be kind to yourself and go at your own pace.

Body image

I touched briefly on this during the previous chapter, but I wanted to bring it up here too. Body image is more than feeling good in your appearance.

Your body will have changed so much thanks to endometriosis – both inside and outside. Over the last few years, endometriosis has meant I have put on 20kg, gained six new scars, suffered hot-water bottle burns (erythema ab igne; *see* page 92), had to reconcile using mobility aids in my 30s, lost organs and irreparably damaged others. Some of these experiences have meant I have had to tackle society's and my own internalised prejudice about weight gain and ableism around the use of mobility aids (that is, that they are only for those with a specific type of disability or a stereotypical image of what 'disabled' looks like). Both of these things are largely seen in society as negatives, so when I started noticing weight gain or realised that a mobility aid would actually really help me, they became negatives to me too. At first, I was incredibly reluctant to try a walking stick, despite endometriosis and adenomyosis quite literally making me fall to the ground in public on numerous occasions owing to the pain in my uterus, pelvis, back, hips and legs. Still, I resisted. My husband hatched a plan. He went to his family home, borrowed one of his stepfather's walking sticks and started taking it with us wherever we went. No matter how long it took, his plan was to carry it everywhere himself, knowing that at some point I would give in and admit that I needed it. It didn't take that long. The next day, we were walking around the supermarket and I needed the stick.

Unpicking my assumptions and prejudices about what disability is has taken time. I still struggle with it, especially when I get stares when I'm out with my walking stick because I 'don't look sick'. Someone once even came up to me in a shop and kicked my stick away from me. 'You obviously don't need that,' they said. 'I bet you're one of those benefit frauds who fleeces the taxpayer.' That day was the first time I had gone out alone with a walking stick. I had been stuck in the house for weeks prior and finally felt well enough to go somewhere and have a look at what was new in the shops. After that incident, I came straight home and cried, then refused to go out again without my husband for two weeks. Even then, he had to encourage me to use the mobility aid that actually helped me manage my symptoms, purely because I was so nervous about attracting that level of vitriol again.

I still get looks and comments. But now, I will not let anyone make me feel ashamed or embarrassed for using something that helps me live my life with slightly more freedom or in slightly less pain.

Not all endometriosis pain is physical

> ### What are mobility aids?
>
> Endometriosis can cause a lot of debilitating symptoms. Mobility aids are anything that help you move around more easily or with less pain. The most common types are wheelchairs, walkers, crutches and walking sticks. If you experience any of the following, it might be worthwhile having a look into mobility aids:
>
> - Pain, especially when standing or walking
> - Dizziness, especially when standing up for long periods
> - Fatigue (*see* pages 35–36)
> - Apprehension about terrain such as steps or uneven ground
> - Reluctance to go somewhere due to potential symptoms
>
> It is important to remember, especially when discussing conditions such as endometriosis, that disabilities are often dynamic. This means that from week to week, from day to day or even from hour to hour, your symptoms and their impact on you can change. One day you might need an aid, and the next day you might not. One day you might find a stick the most useful, another day a wheelchair is what allows you to live more freely. A wheelchair does not always mean that a person cannot walk, and using a walking stick one day but not the next does not mean a person is 'fixed'. Be careful not to slip into comparative suffering (*see* pages 208–209).
>
> We need to give mobility aids a rebrand. If you are reading this and wondering if a mobility aid might actually be quite helpful for you, you would probably benefit from one. There are no criteria or tests to pass before you can use a mobility aid. If you feel like one might help, just try using one and see.

My understanding of body image, and my relationship to my own body, has changed so much over the last few years. It used to mean, in an admittedly very shallow way, my size, my outfit, my make-up and how sexy I felt. I then felt so incredibly disconnected from my body in a way that took me completely by surprise. All I saw was pain and the impacts of that pain. I felt like my body was a traitor, that it hated me and had sold me out to the demons that were endometriosis and adenomyosis. It betrayed me and was, system by system, failing me. Clare Bourne, the pelvic floor physiotherapist we heard from earlier in the book (*see* pages 142–144), confirms that 'this is something we see so often, particularly with endometriosis patients . . . this sense of total disconnection from your body' and says that pelvic floor therapy and relaxation techniques can really help. Coming back to a more positive relationship with my body is taking time – emphasis on present tense, because it is still ongoing. I would say we have a fairly neutral relationship these days, still with negative moments but with more positive ones too.

Endo emotions

You might experience any number of emotions at various points in your endometriosis journey. Some you might expect, some you might not have expected to come up at that point and others might surprise you entirely. There is no right or wrong. You may relate to all of this section, some of it or none of it, but I wish I had known earlier about the maelstrom of emotions that can occur when living with endometriosis. Let's have a look at some of the more commonly identified emotions and why they might be showing up for you:

- Exhaustion: Chronic pain itself is exhausting, as is constantly battling symptoms, gaslighting and medical admin. Endo life can feel relentless.
- Confusion: There is so much information out there about endometriosis, most of it conflicting. Historically, we have not even been able to trust 'official' sources such as doctors, the NHS or charity resources due to the lack of education or dissemination of updated information.
- Disappointment: Whether it's missing out because of a flare, not being able to achieve what you'd hoped or yet another 'clear scan', disappointment is a commonly expressed emotion when discussing living with endometriosis.
- Boredom: Whether from the monotony of the relentless routine of seeking medical help, clear investigation results and being sent home with no answers or the physical boredom of being stuck at home in bed recovering from flares or surgeries.
- Uncertainty: Around what's going on in your body, when a flare will hit, how long it will last, how you may feel in the future when you want to try to plan something or whether a doctor will believe you.

- Frustration: At your body for not allowing you to achieve what you want to, at people for not understanding and at the systems that don't prioritise endometriosis care and research.
- Guilt: For not being able to keep commitments, for 'letting others down' or disappointing them, for not being to keep the pace you used to or do as much and for feeling like a burden to others.
- Grief: Grieving the life you thought you would have, the loss of your abilities and life before your symptoms, as well as fertility-related grief.
- Anxiety: What if the pain never goes away? What if this is as good as it gets? Will you ever be able to have a baby? What if it gets worse? Will you ever find someone who understands? Will anyone ever believe you?
- Anger: At everyone who ever dismissed you and your pain, at your body, at the systemic misogyny that led us here and at the fact that nothing is changing.
- Irritation: At the constant pain, the unpredictability and people not listening or understanding.
- Despair: At the first realisation that endometriosis has no cure and is lifelong.
- Relief: That someone has finally listened to you and believed you, that you know that it wasn't all in your head and when you find something that helps with symptom management.
- Hope: That treatments, medications or surgeries will help ease your pain and improve your quality of life, and that things will change.
- Gratitude: For the clinicians who are amazing and really 'get it', for the people in your life who support you and for a treatment option giving you enough freedom to achieve something you wanted.

There are so many more, but I hope this gives you a sense of how complicated the relationship between endometriosis and emotions can be. Emotions are not a one-at-a-time thing either. Human beings are hugely complex, and part of that is being able to hold more than one emotion simultaneously. I'll give you an example of an endometriosis situation that highlights this complexity perfectly: diagnosis. When I was diagnosed after 22 years, my body didn't know whether I should smile or cry. For the next couple of hours, and even the following days, I swung between so many different emotions. I was relieved that it wasn't all in my head. Angry that it had taken 22 years. Validated that I had been right and something was indeed wrong. Worried about just how wrong things were. Grateful that someone had finally believed me and found out what was going on. Sad that my pain was not over yet. Hopeful that the treatment plan they had put together would help give me my life back. Fearful about the major surgery being proposed. Confused about how we had even got to this point. Terrified of what it would all mean for me and my husband. Shame for being relieved to have a diagnosis – why did I 'want' to be sick? Obviously, I didn't want to be sick, I just wanted an answer for my suffering, but my brain was quite clearly spiralling by this point.

Some people find journalling helpful for navigating these conflicting emotions. Other people express themselves visually in artistic ways. Others swear by therapy. Most people will find that a combination of methods will help. Early in 2024, I found a deep rage building inside of me. By this point, and after two rounds of therapy, I was managing to identify and deal with most of my emotions quite successfully. I think that as I delved more into campaigning work and starting really seeing the injustices faced by endometriosis patients up and down the UK, as well as across the globe, I was becoming increasingly angry. My husband took me to a rage room. In case you've not heard of these, you are literally let loose in a room with a baseball bat or a scaffolding pole, a bunch of crockery and household items that were otherwise headed to landfill, some safety gear and a playlist of your choice. And you let loose. Now, I'm not saying that this is necessarily the most productive way to manage anger in the long term, but I felt so incredibly light after our time there. It might have sent me into a bit of a pain spike afterwards – to be fair, it was the most vigorous exercise I had done in a good while – but the release was incredible.

As with other endo symptoms, your emotions also have triggers. You can identify what these triggers are and take steps to minimise your exposure to them or find ways to soothe them if they are activated. For example, if you know that fertility topics likely trigger feelings of sadness, know that it is okay to decline an invitation to a full-on baby shower.

On the flip side of mental health triggers are something called 'glimmers'. The term is fairly new to me, but it's one I really love. A glimmer is a small moment of pleasure or joy that happens during simple, everyday moments. They're a micro-moment of happiness, calm, gratitude, peace or connection.

They have even been shown to soothe our nervous systems, moving us away from the inherent bias that our brain has to focus on the negatives. Glimmers will be completely personal to you. Some of my recent ones have been playing with my cats, cuddling with my husband while we play video games or find a new series to enjoy, putting up our Christmas decorations, laughing at the memes my best friend sends me, my baby niece's laugh at a puppet I bought for her, spotting wild animals when driving around . . . the list goes on.

I encourage you to start noticing the glimmers in your day. It could be the warmth of your bed, relaxing in a hot bath, the refreshment from a cold drink or listening to your favourite song. It doesn't matter if they make sense to anyone else or not. Glimmers are yours. You can start tracking your glimmers, jotting them down, putting them in your Notes app or just recalling them at the end of each day. You could even share your glimmers with others, online or in person, to help you build that habit. We are wired for connection, and sharing the positives can be a great way to achieve that. When you start noticing what your glimmers are, try to actively bring more of them into your life. Noticing glimmers is obviously not going to change your endometriosis, but it can help you manage the impact of endometriosis on your mental health by reducing the overwhelming feeling the disease can have across your whole life and the hopelessness that can bring.

Toxic positivity

Conversations around mental health and strategies to improve or protect it can very quickly veer into toxic positivity, and this is especially true when it comes to how our mental health is impacted by illnesses such as endometriosis. Toxic positivity has numerous definitions but can be boiled down to the assumption that we should always maintain a positive outlook, even if we are in emotional or physical pain. The result is often the opposite, with a negative mental health impact created by the pressure to be unrealistically optimistic at all times.

Positivity can be brilliant, but toxic positivity is a pattern of behaviour that leads to invalidation or dismissal, two things I think we can agree endometriosis patients do not need more of. The avoidance and rejection of negative experiences associated with toxic positivity can take the form of denying your own emotions or someone else denying your emotions, instead insisting on 'good vibes only'.

When you are experiencing endometriosis, examples of toxic positivity will be flung at you from all quarters – from yourself, well-meaning friends and family, teachers, employers, those looking to sell you dubious cures and even medical staff. This is a small sample of the toxic positivity examples that the endometriosis community has shared with me:

- 'Oh, my friend has endometriosis and she was cured by XYZ.'
- 'I read about endometriosis. You can just take a pill to fix it, right? It's not that big a deal any more, from what I've heard.'
- 'Other people have it so much worse though, so at least you're lucky.'
- 'You should try being a bit more positive.'
- 'If you haven't tried XYZ, then you don't know it's not a cure.'
- 'If you worry about it less, you won't notice the pain as much.'
- 'Your endometriosis is caused by your diet or lifestyle – but great news, I can show you how to cure it.'

All of these examples are invalidating and lead to increased feelings of shame, guilt, confusion, sadness and isolation. Know that you never have to listen to or accept toxic positivity, and that while dwelling on 'negative' feelings is not advisable, neither is denying them or dismissing them as nonsense. Your experience is as valid as anyone else's.

When I asked for her advice, Dr Windgassen, health psychologist, suggests 'getting to grips with the idea of assertiveness'. Assertiveness is naturally equated with aggression, particularly for women and marginalised communities. 'But there is a middle ground,' she explains. 'Assertiveness is such an important quality to nurture when you live with endometriosis. Not only will it help you when advocating for yourself in the doctor's office or asking for adjustments at work, but also when you encounter those unhelpful messages in your daily life.' Standing up for yourself and setting those boundaries 'doesn't mean you don't have to call everyone out, but you have the choice, instead of always feeling stifled and dismissed'.

Dr Windgassen's favourite way to practise this assertiveness in the face of toxic positivity is to ask a question back. 'If someone, for example, says to you, "It could be worse – at least it's not cancer," you can reply, "That's interesting; why do you think that?"' She explains that toxic positivity does not always come from a place of malice or dismissal. Sometimes, Dr Windgassen says, 'people just say dumb shit'. Often, these statements come from a well-meaning place, where lack of awareness means the person is not sure how to help, 'so they try to reframe the situation and, in their mind, make it more positive'. Challenging their toxic positivity with kindness and compassion can then open a dialogue that can encourage them to reflect. Practising assertiveness is difficult, and even more so when you are emotionally and physically depleted. 'You are under no pressure to do this,' Dr Windgassen concludes, 'but it can be really helpful to know that it's okay to challenge these statements.'

The following things are not 'being negative':

- Being honest about your symptoms, your limitations and your boundaries
- Talking about your experience with endometriosis
- Opening up about your mental health
- Debunking misinformation, particularly around 'new cures' or 'new hope on the horizon' articles
- Calling yourself disabled or chronically ill
- Saying that endometriosis is chronic and incurable

Fertility

Struggling with fertility undoubtedly impacts mental health. From issues with conceiving to miscarriages, ectopic pregnancies and stillbirths, there is a well-documented and clearly understandable link between negative mental health and fertility. Given the links between endometriosis and adverse fertility outcomes, I felt it deserved its own space here in this chapter too.

When we talk about fertility, we often talk about two extremes. We either think about the couple who desperately want a child and will do anything to try to achieve that dream, or we think about those who are child-free by choice, who know they do not want children and that this is simply not part of their life plan. However, life is not so black and white and, as we have seen throughout this book, for 99 per cent of us, 99 per cent of the time, life happens in the varying shades of grey between these two extremes. Fertility is a sliding spectrum for most of us, and my husband and I were no exception. He was perhaps more on the 'I'm okay never having children' side, and I was very much on the 'maybe one day, but not right now' part of the scale. But I always thought I would have the option to choose.

By the time I found out just how bad my adenomyosis had become, my only thought was a hysterectomy. I could not carry on in the amount of pain and suffering that I was in. Obviously, it was ultimately my choice, but my husband and I had numerous conversations about what a hysterectomy would mean for our future, particularly with regard to fertility. We decided that my quality of life was more important to both of us, and my surgery was booked. However, I didn't quite realise just how much I valued having choice over my fertility until it was removed. It was something that I had taken for granted as a White, Western, well-educated woman, then suddenly the option to choose 'later' was gone. The door was firmly closed. That doesn't mean I regret my hysterectomy; I would make the same decision again in a heartbeat. It just means that I wish I had been a little bit more prepared for the emotional turmoil that was to follow.

Something that I did not expect to happen was for my sister-in-law to conceive her daughter pretty much on the day of my hysterectomy. We are very close, in terms of both relationship and location, and witnessing her pregnancy progress was surprisingly difficult. I was overjoyed for her and excited to be an auntie again, which I truly adore. But suddenly, a whole bunch of emotions that I didn't realise were simmering came to the fore. I needed to excuse myself from the baby shower when it became overwhelming. I cried in a shop buying baby outfits for my newborn niece. I let out what I can only describe as a primeval howl when I got back in the car after holding her for the first time. On the first Father's Day that rolled around, I felt a heavy sense of guilt that the surgery that had removed my adenomyosis also took away my husband's chance of being a father. Despite him saying he doesn't want to be one, and me believing him, it remains true that he would have been a wonderful one, and I felt that my illness had robbed him of that opportunity. Time has worked wonders, and it is now pretty rare that I catch myself thinking 'what if?' But sometimes it does still creep up on me. I used to berate myself for that, thinking, 'I should really be over this now', but something my mum shared with me really helped. She told me about her aunt, my great-aunt, who was also unable to have children. Even now, she still has moments where it hits her and she gets upset. However, she has led a wonderful life, full of love, joy and memories. For me, there might well be times that trigger these emotions, but they will get fewer and further apart. And life will expand to fill the time in between.

I don't really feel like I relate to childlessness, as I was never desperately maternal or knew for sure that I wanted children. I don't really relate to the child-free by choice camp either, because I don't really count infertility caused by multiple chronic illnesses a choice. My hysterectomy didn't feel like a good choice; it felt like my only choice. When talking to others who had been in a similar situation, I stumbled across a term that I felt suited me much more: 'child-free by circumstance'. This covers so many areas on the spectrum of fertility: maybe chronic illness took the choice away, or maybe you were just never in the right circumstances. Having this terminology really helped me make sense of my mental health and feelings after my hysterectomy, and I hope it helps some of you who may be in a similar situation too.

Something else that really helped was taking note of the things I do have in my life that bring me joy, or that I want to try, and actively doing more of those. Accepting that my life might not be the one I grew up expecting or hoping for is an ongoing process, and I needed to grieve for that because the loss of an expected life is absolutely something valid to grieve. But reclaiming the idea that I have the rest of my life ahead of me to shape and play with has been powerful.

Whatever your situation with fertility and your mental health, please know that you are not alone. There are organisations and groups out there to support you if you feel that is something you would like to explore. As we saw right at the start of this chapter, not nearly enough of us are offered mental health support for endometriosis and its impacts, but it does exist. Ask your GP for a referral or search online if there are self-referral processes for your area. You can also find wonderful people, like Dr Windgassen who specialise in mental health with chronic illness and who share so many free resources as well as their clinical work. You can find a list of support resources in the back of the book.

Grief

Grief is a surprisingly common emotion among endometriosis patients, for numerous reasons. There is the clear link between grief and baby loss or infertility, but there is also a wider aspect of grief that is 'uniquely relevant to chronic illness,' says Dr Windgassen. Letting go of part of your life, or a life that you hoped to have, can create strong feelings of grief too. 'It's great that we're identifying this as grief, as opposed to giving it a blanket label of depression,' Dr Windgassen adds. 'There's power in calling it grief. It gives you permission and space to process it, because letting go is not a light thing.'

Endometriosis can mean we have to let go of so many things. Hobbies, our physical capabilities, our energy levels, the time we've lost to flares, surgeries and chasing answers, our careers, our relationships, triggers, our future hopes and goals, our fertility dreams – depending on the severity of your symptoms, endometriosis can certainly wrench you from your previous existence and cut off your future plans. And that is a lot to process. 'I think people are really unfair on themselves with how quickly they expect to transition from this loss, especially when things like fertility can be taken off the table before you even have a chance to consider them properly,' says Dr Windgassen. 'Grieving for something you never even had the chance to want is super hard. It's not something that you can just process and move on from. It will be re-presented at different points in life at different life milestones.'

These unarticulated expectations for life are something that I feel very deeply. Despite making progress with the grief that has developed over the last few years, somewhere I still struggle is comparing myself to my friends and peers of a similar age. I see them reaching milestones that I used to dream of. Pregnancies, births, career progression – whatever the milestones are, it can be heartbreaking to feel like you are watching from the sidelines while your friends and family move forwards. Just remember that you can be ecstatic for your friend and sad for yourself at the same time, and that moving at your own pace is also progress. Where you are right now is enough. You are enough.

When I first started referring to what I was feeling as grief, the healthy-bodied people in my life were generally confused. We are so used to equating grief with death that they couldn't see where I was coming from. But when I started talking to other endometriosis patients and chronically ill people, the reaction was instant. Some immediately related, and for others it was like a lightbulb went off above their head as something clicked into place for them. Dr Windgassen says this is perfectly understandable: 'If you've not had personal experience of chronic illness and something being permanently closed off to you and your future, for reasons beyond your control', it is a tricky concept to grasp.

Not all endometriosis pain is physical

If you recognise these feelings of grief in your own endometriosis journey, know that it is very common and perfectly natural. The conversation with Dr Windgassen reminds us that mental health support is much more than pills or formalised therapy, although they may also be helpful for some. 'Connection and community' can also be supremely helpful, especially when it comes to navigating these complex emotions.

Dr Windgassen warns against blanket approaches to supporting our mental health. 'There are lots of people peddling lots of different things,' she says, especially on social media. Every day, my social media algorithms highlight courses, products and protocols promising to 'fix' my mental health, if only I follow these five steps, seven steps, 10 steps of whatever it may be. Some of them even message me offering money if I share their product with my followers, without my ever having followed their process (I have always declined). Therapy in the context of health conditions is exceptionally nuanced and needs to be tailored to each individual. Dr Windgassen advises to 'really think about what stage you are at, and what your goals are. Do you need space to process all the changes? Do you need practical advice to help navigate life with endometriosis? Do you need to work on maintenance or improving your mood? This will help identify which approaches are most suited to you right now.' She believes that one-size-fits-all approaches are harmful – 'they're too generalised and lead to a chronic illness patient thinking, "What's wrong with me? Why didn't it work for me? I must be more complex. Maybe I did it wrong." It can really do a number on hope for an endometriosis patient.'

Endometriosis has undoubtedly done a number on my mental health. From the undiagnosed teen dealing with medical gaslighting that made her question her sanity, to the years wondering if there was any point in continuing this life, to the crisis in identity and body image, to the coming to terms with infertility, to the 35-year-old woman writing this book who still feels searing anger for a system that has allowed all this to be normalised, it feels like endometriosis is as relevant to my brain as to any of my pelvic organs. It's been affecting it for just as long and just as deeply. However, on the reverse, endometriosis has also made me more understanding of others. It has made me more compassionate. It has caused me to stop and consider what challenges somebody might have that we just don't see. It has opened my eyes to the extra layers of systemic issues that people who don't have my privileges face. It has taught me to listen to my body, to understand and respect what it needs. It has shown me how strong I am, but that I don't always have to be the strong one – that it is okay to vocalise my needs and allow myself to be supported. It has reminded me that I always had a voice, but that now is the time to use it, for myself and for others.

Some reminders for harder days

- You are not a burden.
- Your pain is real.
- Your pain is valid.
- It is not your fault.
- You are not alone.
- You deserve support.
- You are not unreliable, your health is.
- You are not lazy.
- You are allowed to be angry, but don't become consumed by it.
- Your value is not determined by how much you achieve.
- You are more than your illness.
- Asking for support does not make you weak.

Chapter 7

Endometriosis doesn't discriminate – why do we?

> *'Black women don't have endometriosis. It's more likely to be a sexually transmitted infection.' – GP*

As hard as my journey with endometriosis has been, there are racial, cultural, age, gender, sex and societal obstacles that make many others' journeys even more difficult. These barriers and hurdles were, for the longest time, unknown to me. I assumed endometriosis care was likely pretty poor across the board but, in the midst of my own struggles, never knew just how much these ingrained prejudices persisted.

It would be impossible for me to do justice to the struggles faced by marginalised communities trying to access endometriosis care, both because a single chapter will only scratch the surface and because I have never faced those struggles. I am a White woman, well educated, from a financially comfortable family. I am confident, I am not bound by cultural taboos and I am happy discussing intimate health details. I am a cis woman, meaning I go by the gender I was assigned at birth (female), I am very female presenting and I am heterosexual. Despite having put on 20kg over the last few years, I am still not what society considers 'fat', so I also don't have those stigmas to contend with. The voices and experiences from people who have different lives from mine are featured throughout this book, because I didn't want to relegate them to an isolated chapter. However, I also wanted this chapter to be somewhere their individual struggles can be spotlighted, because, paraphrasing the wonderful Dr Aziza Sesay, GP and women's health advocate, health doesn't discriminate, but its outcomes do.

If I asked you to picture an endometriosis patient, what would you describe? I'm guessing the answer for the majority is a slim, White cis woman huddled over with a hot-water bottle – because that is the image that is nearly always portrayed. But anyone can receive a diagnosis of endometriosis – people of any race, any religion, any socioeconomic status, any gender and, yes, any sex. There are cases of endometriosis in cis men. So, let's hear from these voices. Let's listen to them and amplify them when we are talking about endometriosis care. And if you are a White cis woman like me, remember that no one else's struggle invalidates your own. Talking about these issues does not mean you had it easy, nor do they mean you are a 'bad person' for not knowing about them before. As Dr Sesay explains, 'You don't know what it feels like to be excluded, until you have been.' It just means that you are now recognising the additional hurdles faced by those marginalised by society. Understanding the layers of discrimination through an intersectional lens is absolutely vital to unpick the patriarchal medical system that hurts every single one of us.

Racial disparities

You might be forgiven for thinking that medicine is a subject of science. Of facts, research, curiosity, expanding knowledge, pushing boundaries, experimentation, of lab coats and bleeping machines. But the medical system is not a purely scientific one. It is just as much a socioeconomic-political construct and, as it has evolved throughout the years, it has swallowed and reinforced social conditioning, religion and politics of the day, embedding them deeply into medical practice. Put bluntly, our medical system has gender and race issues that have been baked into it from its origins in Ancient texts, amplified with the passing centuries.

It wasn't until the 1800s that gynaecology as a specialism was established in its earliest form. You might think, finally, women are getting the attention and healthcare that they deserve! But sadly, the birth of gynaecology was not a respectful process. American James Marion Sims is touted as the Father of Gynaecology for his breakthroughs in female reproductive medicine such as the invention of the speculum (he bent a pewter spoon and inserted it into the vagina) and the development of a surgical process for repairing a birth complication called vesicovaginal fistula. But Sims performed his experiments on African-American women, without anaesthesia, because he argued that Black people don't feel pain. Shockingly, this is a bias that still exists in medicine today, as we will see later on. Once Sims perfected his technique, he went on to offer the procedure to White women, sedated, of course. Sims' victims were enslaved on a plantation and had suffered complications during childbirth. This caused frustration to their owner, who leased them to Sims for his experiments. He had complete control over their bodies, and they had no ability to consent to being restrained and operated on, anaesthetised, in front of a room of men who wanted to watch. They underwent procedures for years, as well as being isolated from their families and communities. In his own autobiography, Sims reflected on the advantages of operating on women who were essentially his property – 'There was never a time that I could not, at any day, have had a subject for operation.'

Any advances in gynaecology were made from the pain and exploitation of enslaved, Black women whose names are often relegated to footnotes in medical history. Their names were Lucy, Betsy, and Anarcha. They are the mothers of modern gynaecology.

A speech given by Dr Aziza Sesay, GP and women's health campaigner, at the end of 2024 spotlighted just how current these discussions still are when talking about race in modern healthcare. Black women are three times more likely to die during pregnancy childbirth, and the six weeks following childbirth. They are six times more likely to suffer pregnancy complications. Six times more likely to suffer more serious birth injuries in England. Two times more likely to have a stillborn child. Forty per cent more likely to die of breast cancer. Two times more likely to be diagnosed with late-stage womb cancer and two times more likely to die from that cancer. Less likely to be given pain relief due to a persistent belief that Black skin has fewer nerve endings. More than three times as likely to be sectioned under the Mental Health Act. The health system has a very clear race problem. Dr Sesay says, 'Speaking for myself, as a Black woman, we don't want special treatment. We just want equitable treatment.'

Endometriosis itself has been an issue of race since its discovery. In 1948, during a speech given at the American College of Surgeons and published in *The New York Times*, it was announced that endometriosis would lead to the decline of the White race, 'restricting the propagation of the intelligent class', due to the fertility issues faced by patients. Despite endometriosis being 'discovered' in 1860, by the 1970s it was still being referred to as a disease of White, middle-class, over-ambitious, over-educated and privileged young women who had delayed marriage and childbirth. In 1962, an endometriosis specialist who effectively wrote the guidelines for using hormonal birth control as a 'cure' stated that 'endometriosis is not frequent in the negro'. It was not until 1976 that endometriosis was truly recognised as affecting Black women. Before then, Black patients were typically being diagnosed with sexually transmitted infections or pelvic inflammatory disease (PID).

A study in 1976 found that over 20 per cent of Black women who had been previously diagnosed with PID actually had endometriosis, and I would argue that if the study were repeated today, with the level of knowledge that endometriosis specialists now have, this would be much, much higher. In 2012, researchers in Detroit actually found that Black women can have more severe lesions than their White counterparts. Despite the mounting evidence that Black people not only can and do have endometriosis but that they may also have a higher prevalence and more severe lesions than the wider population, the disease remains underdiagnosed in the Black population. It is thought that, for Black people, diagnosis times can be up to double the average times of eight to 10 years.

Tanya Simon-Hall, founder of The Adeno Gang (*see* pages 148–149), is very clear. 'As a Black woman, my pain is not taken as seriously as a White woman's . . . My medical notes say it all. I had been complaining of pain in my rectum since 2014, but a scan only revealed bowel endometriosis in 2023.' Tanya wasn't even told about her initial indications of endometriosis; she was just expected to deal with the pain. Tanya is now peri-menopausal. 'I had eight periods last year, and six the year before that.' Despite Black women experiencing menopause up to 10 years earlier than their White counterparts, 'I'm still told I can't be peri-menopausal'.

Another patient, who wished to remain anonymous, said that even in 2024, she was told that she was unlikely to have endometriosis as she is Black. 'They said it was probably fibroids, "due to your skin colour". It turned out it was both fibroids and extensive endometriosis. 'Even then, I was told paracetamol would be enough to manage my pain. I remember one time I was in agony, but when I went to A&E they point-blank asked me, "Are you here for drugs. Yes, or no?". The staff wouldn't prescribe anything stronger than paracetamol and, after waiting for eight hours, it was discovered that she had suffered a burst endometrioma and an ovarian torsion, a medical emergency that can, on rare occasions, be fatal.

Despite the volume of statistics featured in this section, the reality is that we know nowhere near enough about how endometriosis affects us based on race. All of the data that we currently have is lumped together as 'patient'

Endometriosis doesn't discriminate – why do we?

data. It desperately needs disaggregating, or splitting up by demographics such as race, so we can build a picture of the needs of marginalised communities. However, the funding for this type of research is not there. Tanya didn't realise just how bad the situation was until she was invited by the charity Bloody Good Period to talk at their parliamentary event about inequalities in menstrual health. 'When it came to researching my speech,' she says, 'I couldn't find concrete data' to back up what we see every day in our communities. 'Because it doesn't exist.'

And it's not just representation in the data that is lacking. Dr Sesay carries around a crocheted prop vulva when she delivers presentations and talks because 'it's the only thing that doesn't instantly offend people'. There have been times when groups to whom Dr Sesay is presenting have asked to see the slides in advance. More than once, she's been 'asked for images featuring gynaecological anatomy to be removed, or replaced with "something less graphic"'. Enter the crocheted vulva, which has become a bit of a mascot and a trademark for Dr Sesay. When I first saw her speak at an event, it was also the first time in my 35 years that I had seen a vulva depicted as brown. 'And that is so important to me,' she says. Traditionally, 'that kind of representation is just not seen in these spaces'. At one point, Dr Sesay could not even find an image on Google of a brown vulva for an awareness video she was making.

In 2024, the charity Endometriosis UK published the results of their study looking into endometriosis diagnosis times in the UK. However, only 6 per cent of the respondents were people of colour. Neelam Heera-Shergil is founder of Cysters, a grass-roots community-led charity that works with marginalised voices. Cysters is now working with Endometriosis UK to gather the much-needed disaggregated data and understand delayed endometriosis diagnosis among people of colour. She says that Cysters had previously applied for funding for this research three times, but each time they were rejected despite heavy support for the proposal. Volunteers are now doing it themselves, for free, because 'otherwise this data simply won't exist. Without that data, there will be no policy change. Without the numbers, the government won't take it seriously.'

Bridget Gorham, former health economics advisor at NHS Confederation, spearheaded a major piece of research titled 'Women's health economics: investing in the 51 per cent', which was published in October 2024. She kindly shared some of her insights with me. The main issue, after funding, was data. 'Finding data disaggregated by sex is hard enough, let alone sex and race, sex and age, sex and socioeconomic status, gender, sexuality, disability . . . We need to do a lot better with the data.' Bridget feels like the NHS could be such a fantastic tool for driving this data-led research, but it's just not happening at the moment. Could this change in the future? 'I think so,' says Bridget. 'The Women's Health Hubs (a government initiative to provide integrated women's healthcare services to communities) would be a great opportunity. Any time you introduce a new service, introducing a data collection service alongside it would be fantastic.' The report places emphasis on the need to conduct further research into health equity, the ability for everyone to attain their full potential for health and wellbeing, particularly when it comes to racial disparities. Whether the money follows to prioritise those recommendations remains to be seen.

Dr Sesay adds that even with the best intentions to increase the participation of marginalised communities in research efforts, some groups can always end up excluded. 'We need to work with the grassroots organisations already in the communities, and we need to remember funding.' Traditionally excluded voices are also some of the communities who have historically been exploited the most. Centuries of systemic racial abuses and biases have created a legacy of distrust. Organisations need to be offering renumeration if they truly value these voices and providing counselling to support the process of repeating their traumas. 'Grass-roots organisations have the trust of their communities and understand their individual requirements. For example, we think of a quick online survey as a simple way to gather data. But how many can actually access the tools you are using to run the study? How many have English as a first language?' It will take some time to build that engagement, but 'representation and education are key'.

Cultural disparities

Neelam Heera-Shergil, who we met earlier in the chapter, first noticed problem periods at around 15–17 years of age. She didn't have debilitating pain at this point; instead, she was experiencing absent, irregular periods. During her first year at Leicester University, she was diagnosed with PCOS and was put on the pill for her symptoms. Her uncles questioned Neelam and her mother about why she was on the pill: 'I was at university to study, not to have sex'.

At this point, she didn't even really understand what PCOS was, having been provided with no information. She just accepted what her doctor told her, as we are taught to do. It was only by doing her own research on internet forums and talking to her mum, a sexual health nurse, afterwards that Neelam started to understand the condition she had been diagnosed with.

Extreme migraines in Neelam's second year at university, caused by the pill she was on, led her to change her medication. Not finding one she was happy with, she came off hormonal medication and tried to self-manage her symptoms. She was living in a house-share with White housemates and, after relentless comments about the smell of her traditional Punjabi cooking (rich in anti-inflammatory ingredients such as turmeric), she acclimatised to eating processed and fast food. She noticed her symptoms worsening and went from a UK size 10 to a size 22 when she graduated.

Her symptoms progressively got worse after university. Neelam went straight into a law firm and had to take a lot of time off, for what she described as 'painful periods'. She really struggled with formalised employment hours due to the constraints on her body. During this time, she was also struggling with declining mental health, suicidal ideation and self-harm.

'I moved to Birmingham, started a new job and collapsed at the office due to pain. I was also suffering from extremely heavy bleeding, although it was just normal to me by then.' In 2014, Neelam went to see a specialist, who ordered an ultrasound and confirmed that she had chocolate cysts or OMAs, which can also be indicative of further, deep disease (*see* page 16). Ten years after that scan, Neelam tells me, 'I have still never had a laparoscopy to remove endometriosis.' Why? 'Because every time I got pregnant, I was removed from the waiting list.' Due to recurrent fertility issues, Neelam never 'made it on to the radar' and surgery never followed.

Neelam is from the Punjabi community, where 'fertility is placed on a pedestal'. When she met her now husband Kal, she was up-front about her conditions and the fact that 'I may not be able to have children . . . I was very conscious that it was going to be make or break for people. I didn't want to get into a relationship and then have it thrown in my face, which has happened before.' She laid all her cards out, and Kal went away, researched Neelam's talks and posts and educated himself. They 'entered the relationship knowing that children might not be possible'. He 'fully accepted it and put no pressure on me, which is practically unheard of in our community'. Their fertility journey has not been an easy or simple one but, as we talk, Neelam and Kal's daughter is on her lap, and Neelam says they are open to growing their family in the future through adoption.

'Even my dress sense has changed because of endo,' explains Neelam. 'I now wear only comfy stuff, I won't wear jeans. I dress according to pain, to bloat. It's amazing how much your life changes around endometriosis without you even realising'.

'If I'm bleeding, and at the Gurdwara (temple), I will only sit down for a maximum of a few minutes in case I leak on the floor. Some people still believe that you shouldn't be in a place of religious worship if you are menstruating, but that is a cultural thing, not a religious one,' she explains. But the cultural nuance around menstruation is deeply entrenched. An ex-partner's mother would not let Neelam come near food while bleeding, 'because if you touch it during menstruation you are considered to spoil it'.

Endometriosis does not even have a direct translation in Punjabi, which is both hard and useful. You might think this would stifle conversations about such a common disease but, instead of focusing on the pelvis and reproductive areas, which would be sexualised and therefore taboo, endometriosis is spoken about as a whole-body condition, 'which makes it more normalised'. Neelam says that while she grew up in an open environment with a mother who taught sexual health, most in the community are still shamed by these issues. They are considered topics to keep to yourself, conversations to keep behind closed doors or not to have at all.

Neelam has been talking about these topics for a while now, stressing cultural nuances and health inequalities. But after talking about periods, vaginas and uteruses, Neelam started to get badly trolled. When she brought up issues around period poverty, her address was doxed (made public), with a message calling her a 'whore' and saying that she was 'encouraging people to be sexually promiscuous'. She has had 10 years of death and rape threats from within her own community. She created Cysters in an attempt to protect herself and add a layer of separation. 'The only way to get rid of cultural misogyny and cultural patriarchy is to challenge it outright.'

Collaboration is the foundation that we need to build up on, says Neelam, with marginalised voices at the centre. 'We need to be collaborating to move forward. We will make more of an impact moving forward together.' We also need to decolonise healthcare, which is not just about race; it's about understanding the history. But in reality, that's not happening. 'The collaboration is sparse, the funding even sparser.' Colonial rule worked on 'divide and conquer', and you can see this playing out daily in charity spaces. 'It's a very Western ideology. We're encouraged to play off each other and compete for funding, rather than to apply collectively and do something together.'

She understands that this conversation is heavily nuanced, and one that some people may not be ready to have. But it's imperative to understand how decolonialism is vital to move us forward. How can you practice this? It is human nature to centralise ourselves in conversations. Understanding and relating to the experiences of others by comparing them to our own is our brain's way of making sense of the world and our place in it. But if we want to understand decolonisation in this conversation, we need to decentre ourselves.

'It's about doing things differently,' Neelam explains. 'We don't have to do things a certain way because that's how it was always done. And I don't always get it right. I don't know what I'm doing . . . no one taught me how to run a charity'. Looking forward, 'when my daughter is my age, I don't want these conversations to still be going on.' Ultimately, Neelam wants to be able to shut down Cysters because it is no longer needed. Until then, she will continue to do the work on the ground, in the communities themselves, until those communities are listened to and supported within the statutory organisations around us. 'Cysters only exists due to the failing of not including marginalised people,' she concludes. 'I'm 34 now, and I've been doing this since I was 24. For the last five years, I have delivered exactly the same speech on International Women's Day. And I will continue to deliberately do so, until I don't have to say those things any more.' In a comment that says it all, she finishes by saying, 'No one has even noticed yet'.

I am so grateful to Neelam for sharing her story and the challenges that she and Cysters face when it comes to the cultural nuances of accessing healthcare. Listening to her opened my eyes to so many issues when it comes to accessing healthcare support that I would never even have imagined, and her thoughts on the decolonisation of not only healthcare but the charity space that exists to fill in the gaps have rarely left my mind since. The theme of collaborating with, and amplifying, marginalised voices is one that I will be carrying through into my own work.

Endometriosis

The cultural nuances in healthcare, particularly surrounding diseases such as endometriosis that have connections to menstrual health, are practically infinite. And they're not just within individual communities themselves. They are also baked into healthcare. Just as the healthcare system, and those that operate within it, have bias and prejudice around women and race, it is also true for cultural differences. Endometriosis patients from around the world kindly shared these experiences with me to help give some context to just how embedded these stereotypical biases are:

- 'You can't have an internal ultrasound. You're not married. You won't be a virgin and no one will want you.'
- 'We can't operate to remove the endometriosis. It could impact your fertility and I know how important that is to your people.'
- 'Oh, I'm surprised to see you here on your period. I thought you all had to hide away during that time.'
- 'He told me he couldn't help me, laughed and said I could try a voodoo doctor instead.'

Dr Nighat Arif, women's health GP, campaigner and author, shared with me another side of cultural nuance, describing a 'handful of cases that have refused a referral because they didn't want endometriosis on their medical records'. She has seen this multiple times, 'particularly in South Asian communities', where the concept of arranged marriages is still commonplace and fertility is placed on a pedestal. She tells me she has encountered mothers saying, 'But I don't want my daughter to be labelled with endometriosis, because how will I marry her off?' Another mother was convinced 'someone had placed a curse on the family'.

'These cultural nuances are likely only to be heard by someone like myself, who looks and sounds like them, and who they know will understand.' While the regularity of this interaction has reduced over the last few years, perhaps due to an increase in awareness and understanding of the disease, it still happens. Dr Arif always tries to reframe the conversation, explaining that an endometriosis diagnosis does not equal infertility and that the early diagnosis means that they can start looking at management. However, these cultural tones permeate through and influence every step of the process.

Gender

No matter what your gender politics are, surely we can all agree that no one should suffer from endometriosis, let alone do so unsupported. However, excluding those who exist outside of the cis-female norm is sentencing them to exactly that. Endometriosis has been a gendered disease since it was discovered, and even now it is referred to as a 'woman's disease' and sits in the realm of gynaecology. But by only focusing on the experiences of cis-gendered women, we are ignoring a large group of people, including trans men and non-binary people, who end up receiving substandard care – if they receive any at all.

Neelam Heera-Shergil, founder of Cysters, is just as passionate about gender inclusivity as she is about any other marginalised group. 'I still get people eye-rolling at me when I jump in and say, "Can we please remember that this also affects the trans and non-binary community".'

So, let's clear this up. You can be a woman and have endometriosis. You can be a trans man and have endometriosis. You can be a non-binary person and have endometriosis. You can even be a cis man and have endometriosis (which we will look at in the section on 'Sex'; *see* pages 242–246). Periods are related to endometriosis for many of us, sure, but not all of us have period symptoms. A uterus is an organ. Having a uterus does not make you a woman, nor does the absence of one preclude you from being a woman. Honestly, after my hysterectomy, I was told at least a dozen times that my lack of a womb meant my womanhood was 'removed', 'revoked' or 'void'. Guess what? Still a woman, still have endometriosis. Ideas about gender are so intrinsically woven into the narrative of endometriosis and, to an extent, I understand. Millennia of medical gaslighting, trauma, dismissal and stigma attached to periods and diseases like endometriosis have made many women protective over that heritage of struggle. However, if it comes with the cost of the neglect and harm of other endometriosis patients, I draw the line. Endometriosis needs a complete 'brand' makeover. Patients and experts are shouting from the rooftops that this is a full-body disease, not a period one. Why can't this area of gender be included in the rebrand?

KJ, a non-binary trans person, has endometriosis and generously agreed to share their story with me. 'Endometriosis care is so heavily gendered,' they said. 'Everything you see', from media articles, photos online and case studies to research findings, is 'focused on affirming cis women'. KJ appreciates that this demographic makes up the majority of cases, but is finding that this blinkered approach makes accessing healthcare extremely difficult.

KJ's gender and endometriosis stories are tightly intertwined. Prior to their periods starting, KJ was diagnosed with 'stomach migraines', debilitating pains that they now believe may have been the starting point for all that followed. They were 10 when they started their period, and it felt like they were 'dying'. 'Each one that I had got worse and worse.' KJ didn't think that there was anything wrong; 'I just thought that it was normal'. Going through their youth 'socialised as a girl', KJ did their best to abide by that and thought painful periods were part of the package. At 15, they went on the pill, which coincided with a relationship that wasn't the healthiest. 'I brushed a lot of my symptoms aside because of the partner I was with'; that partner was prone to gaslighting KJ about their illness. Up until the age of 18, KJ tried numerous pills to manage their symptoms, which they still assumed were normal. They tried the implant for a few weeks, but that caused non-stop bleeding and depleted iron levels. 'My mental health was rubbish too', and that was when 'I started to click that this might be something more'. KJ went back to the doctor.

'I remember finding it incredibly hard to be listened to', and this was exacerbated by the realisation that they were non-binary at the same time. KJ was referred to a gender clinic and an ultrasound during the same appointment. At the ultrasound, KJ was diagnosed with polycystic ovaries, including one cyst 'the size of a clementine'. At the gender clinic three hours away from their home, the clinician whom KJ saw told them, 'I don't know how we can help you'. Everyone that KJ spoke to at that clinic said, 'You can't be non-binary and have endometriosis'.

It took five years for a surgeon to listen to KJ. For those five years, KJ was placed on the GnRH analogue Zoladex, which, as we saw earlier in the book (*see* pages 87–90), should only be used in the short term and with full patient consent. This prescription was for both the pain KJ was in and their gender dysphoria, to stop their cycle. 'But I was just left on it . . . I was meant to have regular bone density scans' to check for adverse impacts, 'but only had three in five years'. KJ is now suffering from spinal issues and bone thinning in their left hip. Eventually, in 2019, KJ had their first laparoscopy, which 'confirmed stage four, deep endometriosis' (*see* pages 15–20) as well as adenomyosis, and in 2021 they underwent a hysterectomy.

Endometriosis doesn't discriminate – why do we?

'I understand that endometriosis care is rooted in gynaecology', but small things like not having to be seen and treated alongside maternity patients would be a big step, says KJ. They believe that 'women's health will always go hand in hand with trans and non-binary healthcare', as well as including intersex individuals. But, KJ adds, 'there has been a breakdown of laws and protection of these groups' recently, with their rights constantly weaponised and used as a 'bargaining chip'. 'People are being medically neglected, not being given the right support and treatment.'

I asked KJ if they felt included in narratives about endometriosis, whether medically, in the media or even within the endometriosis community itself. 'I don't interact' is their reply, and 'I think you probably know the reasons'. I can understand it. I have had my fair share of trolls over the years, particularly when speaking about my hysterectomy. The trolls are reacting to a choice that I made and am happy with. I cannot imagine facing the vitriol experienced by those who speak about their gender experiences, like KJ, or cultural experiences, like Neelam, facing that level of hatred and bile for simply existing as your authentic self. As KJ says, 'If you have an alternative perspective to certain people, especially around gender and fertility, some people can't deal with that.' KJ started an Instagram page to help raise awareness that not all endometriosis patients are women, but they said they had to pull back to protect their mental health. It's the fear of 'trolls, of being visible and exposing yourself to that noise,' they add. 'People have become very comfortable saying the nastiest things . . . I definitely have to be in right head space.'

Currently, accessing healthcare for endometriosis makes KJ feel 'really uncomfortable'. The experience 'pulls me out of the safety that I have built for myself', leaving them vulnerable and distressed. 'It can be really othering,' they say.

Recent analyses of the literature show that the prevalence of endometriosis among trans men could be as high as 25 per cent, two and a half times the accepted one in 10 figure and nearly twice the emerging one in seven statistics. However, the experiences of trans male endometriosis patients suggest they are also be more likely to face increased barriers to accessing care.

Speaking to a trans male endometriosis patient who wishes to remain anonymous, he echoes many of the sentiments shared by KJ. 'I didn't know I had endometriosis until after my transition,' he starts. 'I always had painful periods but thought that was just "part of being a woman", which made me hate the experience even more. I knew I wanted a hysterectomy as soon as possible – for my transition, yes, but to also rid me of that pain.' Once he had transitioned, he noticed he was still suffering from significant pain and numerous other symptoms that we all now recognise as endometriosis. 'Trying to get a doctor to believe me at that point was ridiculous,' he says. 'I was told it was "cateogorically impossible" to have anything like endometriosis as the uterus had been removed and I was now on male hormones.' At work, he was denied time off to manage his symptoms and attend appointments. 'You're a man now, act like one' was the shocking comment from one manager. Eventually, he was forced to leave that job. 'My family ended up all chipping in and I was able to access a private consultant. I'll never forget the look of confusion on their face when I walked in (I present as very masculine), but they did listen and eventually I was scanned and diagnosed with severe endometriosis.'

Weight

As a society, we are fat phobic. Weight gain is seen as inherently negative, and this has come up time and again in discussions with endometriosis patients. My rapid weight gain due to immobility and medications contributed to the decline in my mental health. Neelam Heera-Shergil shared how at one point in her journey, she 'just wanted to lose the weight, to look good again'. KJ revealed that they were put off certain treatments as the discourse at the time was about 'how much weight they would make you put on'. There are constant negative messages around living in a larger body, perpetuated by an inherently anti-fat media. I still can't quite believe the magazines that were available when I was a teen, pointing out celebrities' weight fluctuations, calling them 'fat' and 'lazy' and accusing them of 'letting themselves go'.

The healthcare system is not immune to any bias, including fat phobia. Research has even suggested that many doctors prefer not to treat overweight patients, and that doctors equate higher weights with traits such as laziness and dishonesty: 87 per cent believe obese people are 'indulgent' and 32 per cent believe they 'lack willpower'. This stigma leads to feelings of shame and embarrassment and can result in patients delaying seeking support. In one study, up to 87 per cent of women or AFAB individuals delayed seeking healthcare due to their weight. Even when we do ask for help, inherent bias can hinder diagnosis, leading to conditions going undetected. A 2015 study highlighted that doctors are generally less inclined to examine patients with a higher body mass index (BMI), a tool used to determine whether you're a healthy weight for your height. A study from the previous year showed that two-thirds of medical students had conscious anti-fat biases, and a staggering three-quarters had internalised unconscious biases towards fat patients.

Endometriosis is not excluded from discussions around weight. In fact, the two may be linked. The current data is limited, but there are suggestions that a 'low BMI is reported with increased incidence of endometriosis', while the European Society of Human Reproduction and Embryology (ESHRE), who also produce endometriosis care guidelines, issued a press release stating that 'slim women have a greater risk of developing endometriosis than obese women'. On the flip side, there are also reports that say the 'severity' of disease increases with BMI, potentially up to twice that of 'healthy weight women'. Either way, we can see that weight should not be used to exclude an endometriosis diagnosis or terminate care pathways. Sadly, though, this is the exact scenario many endometriosis patients who have a higher BMI find themselves in, as illustrated by the following experiences:

- 'I was told I was too fat to have endometriosis. That my pain was due to the strain my weight was putting on my body and if I lost weight, I would be fine. I had endometriosis all over my bowels and pelvis.'
- 'They asked why they would spend resources referring me to a specialist if I didn't take my health seriously enough to be a healthy weight.'
- 'My doctor told me that if I lost weight then they would agree to treat me.'
- 'I was denied surgery until I lost weight, apparently due to the limits of the laparoscopic tools. Ironically, one way they suggested I lose weight was to have a laparoscopic surgery.'
- 'I was in so much pain, and bleeding so much, but I've had such terrible experiences at the doctor's and A&E because of my weight. It turned out an endometrioma had ruptured and I just struggled through by myself because I was too scared to the face the judgement.'
- 'The ultrasound tech told me it can't be endometriosis. It must be PCOS, because "that's basically endo for fat women".'
- 'A new GP congratulated me on my pregnancy during our first appointment. I'm not pregnant, I'm overweight. I'm also infertile, thanks to endo and adeno, so that was fun'.

- 'I'm not even sure that I would have considered myself overweight, but I do struggle with endo belly [bloating caused by endometriosis; *see* page 38] quite badly. One doctor laughed and said it was like a "man's beer belly".'
- 'Just eat less. You'll be all right.'
- 'I was told that all of my symptoms were due to excess weight. I was desperate for relief, so I took it to heart and did anything I could to lose the weight. I starved myself and I over-exercised every single day. Guess what? I still had endometriosis, but now I had an eating disorder on top too.'

Neelam Heera-Shergil, who we met earlier in the chapter, tells me, 'I am a fat woman, and endometriosis care for fat women is different. Surgery and surgical recovery is different for fat people, even after a minimally invasive procedure. . . it gives me reservations.' Four months after an emergency C-section, Neelam is still in bandages. She knows that it is an entirely different surgery, but the potentially lengthy, complicated recovery is something that she wishes was spoken about more. It was her combination of being a Brown, fat woman that led Neelam to kick-start her community work, which eventually turned into Cysters. 'I was looking online for these nuanced conversations and just saw the same messaging everywhere': slim White women with laparoscopy scars on flat bellies. She can still picture the images now, with defined hip bones clearly on show. 'There's no way you're finding my hip bones,' she laughs. Neelam remembers thinking, 'None of this relates to me.'

As with any of the systemic disparities mentioned in this chapter, we all have a role to play in calling out weight stigma. If you see someone making jokes at the expense of someone else's body, call it out. If someone is putting off seeking care because of fear of judgement or previous negative experiences, encourage them and ask if you can help advocate for them. Ultimately, the healthcare system needs to address its inherent fat phobia. Medical schools should have specific training for how weight can interact with diseases, as well as the factors that can influence BMI beyond overeating and not getting enough exercise, including medication side effects, genetic disposition or underlying conditions. Sensitivity training should be provided in medical settings, and all hospitals and clinics should have the capability to treat those in heavier bodies. Surgeons need to allow more time to complete surgeries on patients with a higher BMI and put measures in place to account for the increased risk of wound infection. We should also look at the BMI metric, which has long had its critics and controversies, and see if there is a better approach. 'And we need clinical pathways for after-care specifically for fat people,' adds Neelam. All these steps will take resources, but something that can be actioned immediately and for free is for doctors to address their internalised fat phobia, treating all patients, regardless of weight, with respect and empathy.

Socioeconomic status

We saw in chapter 6 that social factors, or our socioeconomic status, have a part to play in our health outcomes. We therefore need to consider these factors when discussing both health and access to healthcare.

Socioeconomic status usually refers to the combination of our education, income and occupation, and is usually considered low, medium or high. Effectively, it refers to our social position and access to resources. Historically, it was thought that endometriosis affected women in upper socioeconomic groups who had delayed childbearing in favour of education and reading. We now know that, just like race, culture, weight and gender, endometriosis does not discriminate based on socioeconomic factors. However, socioeconomic factors can and do massively determine a patient's access to information, care, and treatment.

The 2024 NHS Confederation report that we mentioned earlier in this chapter (*see* page 227) found a 'strong relationship between more severe deprivation and worse health outcomes', including access to women's healthcare services. Looking at the local authorities in the top 20 per cent least deprived areas in the country, 97 per cent scored higher than the national average for health outcomes.

In 2022, a report by Endometriosis UK found that 17 per cent of patients have sought private care for endometriosis due to long NHS waiting times. It is true that, for many of us, our local surgeon may not be an endometriosis expert. So, if we want to access that highly specialised care, we have to find a way to access private clinics. Some of us are fortunate enough to have insurance provided through our jobs. Others use up life savings. Others, myself included, are privileged enough to have families who step in and bear the cost. But only a tiny fraction can comfortably take those hits. I have spoken to patients who have gone into debt, taken out personal loans, put the costs on credit cards and even taken out second mortgages. Every week, I am sent numerous links to patients who are crowdfunding to raise money for private endometriosis surgery, either in the UK or at a global endometriosis centre. Data provided by GoFundMe, the crowdfunding platform, revealed that in the UK, between 2019 and 2023 there was a 69 per cent increase in fundraisers mentioning the word 'endometriosis'. Is it a coincidence that this coincides with the time period when gynaecological waiting lists skyrocketed in the UK? In fact, by 2023, a fundraiser mentioning the word 'endometriosis' was being created every two days, all driven out of a desperation for relief.

But what happens to those who cannot access these options? Should they be resigned to a life of repeated ablation surgeries with general gynaecologists who don't understand the complexity of the disease, purely because that is what is widely available on the NHS?

Endometriosis campaigner Rey @reythewarrior, whom we met earlier in chapter 3 (*see* page 121), is Australian but lives in Scotland. They have noticed something interesting about the way the NHS is positioned in the UK. 'It's like, because it's free, there's a feeling that you should be grateful for it. It's a privilege to be able to access it, and you should be grateful.' Born in a country where the NHS is placed on a high pedestal, but also being a patient who has been caused significant harm by failings in that service, I can see what Rey means. We genuinely are lucky to have this healthcare service, especially when you compare it with other global systems, but that does not mean we cannot challenge its shortcomings, advocate for the best care and expect up-to-date clinical knowledge from our doctors. Unfortunately, the ability to do that often depends on the individual patient and their capacity to deeply educate themselves about their condition.

Access to knowledge, and the ability to confidently assimilate and interpret that knowledge, plays a huge role in the way we navigate the healthcare system, particularly with a disease like endometriosis where we have to do so much self-education and advocacy. 'So many people,' Rey continues, 'will never get the care they need purely because of their situation in life'. That could be 'because of where they live, their access, English might be their second language' – how are they meant to adequately educate themselves to the level that this disease demands? 'The average person doesn't read the NICE guidelines. And to be fair, they shouldn't have to, but to gain access to treatment, that's often the reality.'

Endometriosis doesn't discriminate – why do we?

These issues extend beyond the doctor's room. So many of the symptom management options recommended, by clinicians and those on social media alike, count on access to resources, namely time and money. Fresh, organic diets with grass-fed meat and wild salmon, yoga classes, regular massages, acupuncture, supplements, branded TENS machines, coaches promising to guide you to a new life – all of these cost money. One coaching programme was selling for $2,222 and the messaging in the marketing made me so angry. 'If you're ready to take your illness recovery seriously,' it stated, the insinuation being that if you are un able to afford this course then you are somehow happy suffering and choosing this existence.

Neelam Heera-Shergil finds the rise of the 'endometriosis influencer', who promotes product after product with affiliate links, particularly troubling. 'It's profiting from people's pain,' she says and pretty elitist in its outlook. Most of these options simply are not possible for many endometriosis patients, particularly those in lower socioeconomic groups. Some might have children to look after, jobs to attend, parents to care for. When do they get a spare moment, they are managing life admin, grabbing something to eat and trying their best to get through a flare. Endometriosis is now viewed by some in the wellness and influencer space as a 'niche', a profitable group towards whom marketing can be targeted. This was inevitable, as the wellness industry has long been filling the cavernous holes left by the gender health gap, which are exacerbated by the inequalities we are discussing in this chapter. However, we need to be mindful of the line where it becomes predatory and starts preying on a vulnerable population that is desperate for relief.

Careful consideration needs to be given to socioeconomic nuances when discussing endometriosis diagnosis and management, otherwise we risk leaving increasingly larger chunks of the patient population behind. The types of occupation associated with higher socioeconomic statuses are more likely to have defined equality practices for reasonable adjustment, flexible working and time off for appointments. However, jobs generally associated with lower socioeconomic statuses may mean the opposite. Endometriosis patient Kelly works shifts at her local supermarket. 'It's simply impossible to work from home, and I have to book hospital appointments around my shifts – I'm not allowed to miss work, or it's recorded on my files'. This has meant she has had to turn down appointments, delaying her access to treatment. 'I've tried looking for other work, but there's just nothing here. Even though I can barely get through a shift thanks to pain, it's what pays my bills.'

Socioeconomic status is often layered with other health inequities. For example, we know that areas of high deprivation are often also areas of high diversity, adding further nuance and complications. For example, in 2019, it was revealed that people from all ethnic minority groups other than Indian and Chinese were more likely than White people to live in the most deprived 10 per cent of neighbourhoods in England. People from Pakistani and Bangladeshi communities were over three times more likely than White British people to live in the most income-deprived 10 per cent of neighbourhoods. On the flip side, people from White British, White Irish and White Other ethnic groups were the least likely to live in the most income-deprived 10 per cent of neighbourhoods. Endometriosis care is already a bit of a postcode lottery – you can see that by the distribution of BSGE specialist centres (*see* pages 111–113), but socioeconomic nuances add a whole new layer to the conversation.

Sex

Now, I am not for one minute calling cis men, especially White cis men, a marginalised community. But, believe it or not, endometriosis has been found, and proven through laboratory tests, in this population, so their inclusion here is relevant. Cis-gendered men, who have never had a uterus and never had a period, have been diagnosed with endometriosis. Admittedly, it's rare. The numbers in medical literature range from 16 to 20 cases of confirmed endometriosis in cis male patients, a drop in the ocean relative to the hundreds of millions of women and those assigned female at birth.

However, it's likely not as painstakingly rare as we might think. As endometriosis has historically been viewed as a woman's disease, one of uterine origin and relating to menstruation, of course we have not been looking for it outside of those parameters. For the same reason endometriosis is dismissed in patients post-menopause, post-hysterectomy or with MRKH (*see* pages 45–47), medicine could have been dismissing endometriosis in men. We have no idea. And I'll be honest – even if it is 100 cases, 20 cases or one case, I have witnessed and felt first-hand how destructive and paralysing endometriosis can be. I wouldn't want a single person to go through that. So, cis men should be included in the discourse.

I find the locations where endometriosis has been found fascinating (a weird hobby, I know), and it is equally interesting to see how widespread the lesions are in the cis-male body. Recorded disease locations have included the prostate, the epididymis (the tubes behind the testicles), the testicles, the bladder, within an inguinal hernia, the ureter, the lower abdominal wall and scar tissue from previous hernia repair. The reported ages of these patients range from 27 to 83.

One of the recorded cases of endometriosis in men was that of a 40-year-old man who was diagnosed with endometriosis in his lower genitourinary tract after complaining of abdominal pain. Traditionally, in previous cases of male endometriosis, it had been suggested that prolonged exposure to oestrogen therapy, for certain cancers for example, was a risk factor. These treatments create an environment in which, as we know, endometriosis thrives and that creates spikes in symptoms. However, this 40-year-old man had received no such oestrogen therapy. Instead, it was suggested that the patient's 'hormonal alterations secondary to obesity' were the contributing factor. Adipose tissue, aka body fat, is known to contain and produce oestrogen, so a higher BMI is associated with higher levels of circulating oestrogen. This could account for the more severe endometriosis found in cis women, but also, apparently, for the endometriosis in this cis man.

Critics often cry, 'But they have unusually or artificially high levels of oestrogen, a female hormone; that's the only reason it's possible.' However, just as those assigned female at birth produce testosterone, which has significant benefits to our overall health, those assigned male at birth also produce oestrogen. We don't need to gatekeep hormones; we all have different levels of them anyway. Regardless, no matter what caused this man's symptoms to flare, it does not account for how the endometriosis cells got there in the first place. If we go with the theory of embryological origin, they must have already been there at birth. The literature does not tell us, but I'm risking an assumption here that none of the men who have been diagnosed with endometriosis were on oestrogen therapies or heavily obese at birth. Either way, these cases are further evidence debunking the still widely held belief that retrograde menstruation is the cause of endometriosis (*see* pages 28–30).

And these are not new discoveries either. Reports of endometriosis in cis men reach as far back as 1985. We need to undertake more research into endometriosis in cis men. Hear me out here. I know this is going to elicit some uncomfortable responses. The experience of endometriosis has been a cis-female one for years. We have bonded and united behind a shared experience of misogyny, dismissal, pain and infertility. We have been denied treatments, denied funding, denied new research. We have been kept in harmful treatment pathways for decades, held back by outdated information and influences from outside sources. I understand entirely if you're rolling your eyes and shaking your head at the suggestion we should funnel precious, scarce research funding into the cis-male experience of this disease that has ruined our lives for too long. I get it.

However, researching this book has made me realise that what's currently happening is not working. Things have not changed for decades, arguably longer. And maybe, just maybe, researching cases of endometriosis that simply cannot be caused by retrograde menstruation will finally break us free from the shackles of the idea that this disease is a uterine one. Maybe it will break us out of the confines of the perception that endometriosis is a period issue that we need to manage at home. Maybe it would even help the disease be taken more seriously. As Mr Shaheen Khazali, endometriosis surgeon, tells me, 'Let's face it. If a disease caused a man this much pain with sex', let alone any of the other debilitating symptoms and impacts, 'we would have cured it by now'. When reading the clinical histories of these men, I was infuriated by the fact that each one complained of pain, presented to a doctor or emergency department and was whisked off for immediate investigation, surgical removal of the disease and pathological testing. It shows it can be done. It does not have to take a decade (on average) to receive an answer and then further years of waiting for that same surgical removal. It shows that the system can facilitate it, if it educates our future and current clinicians, listens to and believes patients and follows an effective care pathway.

I don't have the answers. None of us currently do. But the sheer existence of these cases of endometriosis in men show just how nuanced this disease truly is.

Speaking to all of the people in this chapter has really made me question my perspective on endometriosis care. I knew that some of these issues existed, but the generosity of these patients who have shared their experiences and insights highlighted challenges and nuances that I have not considered before now. In all honesty, because of my race, cultural background, socioeconomic status, gender, weight and sex, I have never had to. And there are even more layers to unpick if we are truly to get to grips with looking at healthcare intersectionally, including age, religion, physical and mental disability and sexuality.

The NHS report that came out in 2024, 'Women's Health Economics: Investing in the 51 per cent', did a really good job of showcasing that our healthcare system is built on a White, cis-male, heterosexual model that has permeated everything from research to clinical trials, investment, what we think is important and even what is in the clinical guidelines. It is so deeply entrenched within the system that even our policies are designed around the 'default White male'. The result is that too many patients are left adrift in a system ill-designed to meet their needs. Those who can afford to look for care elsewhere do, but everyone else is left behind.

I asked Bridget Gorham, co-author of the report, if she thinks it is possible for us to tinker around the edges of existing policy enough to make a difference, or if we need a more radical change. 'It depends. It's critical that as we devise new strategies, such as the NHS 10-year plan, that we do so through an intersectional, health equity lens, whether that's gender, race, sexuality, socioeconomic status, disability etc. . . . But our existing policy strategies . . . I would argue there is also justification to start from scratch. We can't just keep adding footnotes that get overlooked. As we learn more about, for example, how race interacts with healthcare outcomes, that needs its own space, its own pathway.'

To achieve health equity, we must decentre ourselves from the conversation, making space for more marginalised voices to be heard. We must challenge the stigmas where we see them and ask, where are the diverse voices? Where are the experiences of Black women? Brown women? Fat women? Non-binary individuals? Trans men? Disabled women? Poor women? Cis men with endometriosis? And all those in between? We must work with the grass-roots communities on the ground who understand the nuances and challenges within each group. There must be continuous, updated professional training for medical students and professionals, not just in diversity but in sensitivity too, and there must be inclusive research with disaggregated data, ideally with financial renumeration for the groups who have historically been taken advantage of. Because, as Bridget concludes, 'accessing healthcare services free from racism, sexism, transphobia, any form of discrimination, is a human right'.

As I said at the start of this chapter, we are only scratching the surface here about the struggles faced by marginalised communities and those traditionally overlooked when it comes to accessing endometriosis care. I deeply encourage you to look at the resources for this chapter at the back of the book and further explore these issues and the work that incredible advocates are doing. We are a quarter of the way through the 21st century and we need to do better. We can no longer keep our heads in the sand and continue to believe that science and healthcare are impartial, balanced. Ignorance is no longer acceptable.

We do not need to gatekeep the experience of endometriosis because, let's face it, no one deserves to deal with everything that comes with this disease. We all need to take stock of our biases and actively listen to the communities that are being left behind. A rising tide lifts all boats, and when we raise the standards of care for the most marginalised in the system, all of us will benefit.

Dr Aziza Sesay's tips for viewing endometriosis intersectionally

- We all have our own biases, including myself. Acknowledge it, admit it and change.
- Educate yourself around the issues faced by those in marginalised communities.
- Don't generalise. One experience is not like another, even within a community. The intersectionality of these inequities makes the nuances even more complex.
- Have humility, and just be a good human.
- Really listen to marginalised voices and give them space.

Chapter 8

This is not the end

*'And what exactly would you like me
to do about that?' – gynaecology surgeon*

I was going to call this final chapter 'The final word' or something similar, then I realised just how disingenuous that would be. This will never be my final word on endometriosis care – not until the statistics we have seen scattered throughout this book are no longer relevant and the experiences shared by the very real human beings underpinning those statistics are no longer being handed down and repeated in future generations.

In their article exploring the ancient history of endometriosis, Drs Camran, Farr and Ceana Nezhat describe the treatment of conditions remarkably similar to endometriosis as one of 'the most colossal mass misdiagnoses in human history' subjecting women to 'murder, madhouses and lives of unremitting physical, social and psychological pain'. They describe examples in medical documents dating back nearly 4000 years of women with endometriosis-like symptoms being subjected to treatments involving 'leeches, straight-jackets, bloodletting, caustic chemical douches, genital mutilation, being hung upside down, surgical fatalities, and even accusations of demonic possession and state-sanctioned executions'. We may not be being hung upside down and executed for our symptoms in the 21st century, but the use of antidepressants and therapy to 'treat' our pain, harsh medications with unknown long-term effects, hysterectomies performed when they needn't be, and organ removals due to inadequate surgical skill are all part of the current endometriosis healthcare landscape. All because our debilitating, but invisible, pain is still so misunderstood and under-prioritised by society and medicine alike.

We have addressed the challenges throughout the book. We have looked at what the current literature tells us and combined that with clinical knowledge from specialists and the lived experiences of a diverse range of patients. In this closing chapter, I want to look at some of the opportunities that we have when it comes to improving endometriosis care. How endometriosis patients are reclaiming purpose through their pain to change outcomes. How technology could alter the future landscape for endometriosis diagnosis and management. Where clinicians think we could harness resources to improve patient outcomes, and what research is on the horizon. Because, as Heather Guidone, Board Certified Patient Advocate and member of the team at The Center for Endometriosis Care, explains, 'It's not all bad'. She's been an advocate for 33 years and in that time, she says 'we have been making progress'. But, she tempers her statement, 'for the amount of effort that we put in, we're not seeing the monumental strides forward that we should be'. There's a lot of work to be done.

Turning pain into purpose

Something that has struck me repeatedly, not only in the process of researching this book but in my own campaigning and advocacy work too, is the sheer number of endometriosis patients who turn their pain into purpose. They take their sometimes harrowing experiences with the disease and healthcare system and turn it into fuel, trying to shift the narrative and improve the lives of current and future patients. Some have started charitable organisations: Neelam, founder of Cysters, friends Anna and Gabz, founders of the Menstrual Health Project, Carla, founder of The Endometriosis Foundation, and Jodie, founder of Endometriosis South Coast, to name a few. Others set up community events focusing on particular aspects of endometriosis management and care. Some dedicate themselves to influencing policy at a local, regional or national level, and others set up companies looking to plug the holes left by millennia of medical misogyny and gender-based pain and health gaps. Dearbhail Ormond, of frendo (*see* pages 186–187), is a great example of a FemTech company (a company that develops software and other tech services that aim to support women's health and healthcare) founded and led as a result of someone's personal story. Others head back to university to undertake research projects to further our knowledge about endometriosis.

This is not the end

Natalie Mitchell found a pretty unique way to turn her personal pain into purpose when the opportunity to write an endometriosis storyline on UK TV drama *Waterloo Road* came up. Natalie became symptomatic at the age of 10. She had 'an amazing family GP' who kept referring her back to gynaecology and paediatrics despite those clinics dismissing her pain as nothing, IBS, in her head, and even 'in her mum's head'. Finally, after two years of back and forth, Natalie had her first ultrasound in 1994 and multiple endometriomas were identified. 'I was 12 when I had my first laparoscopy, and they found endometriosis', but, in a revelation that shocked me despite all the stories I have heard, 'they still refused to put endometriosis on my medical record because they insisted I was too young'. Natalie went on the pill and carried on until she was 23, she had another laparoscopy and endometriosis was confirmed. Again. Except this time, 11 years later, she was allowed to have it on her medical record. Her seventh laparoscopy for endometriosis was in 2023, for which she decided to go privately for the first time. 'I had had enough of multiple surgeries…and was in a really bad way, physically and emotionally. I was a mess.' After her initial appointment with an endometriosis specialist, Natalie says she realised just how much substandard care she had been subjected to in the past. It was a major surgery and the recovery was lengthy, but Natalie says she's now the best she's ever been.

Natalie is a scriptwriter, having previously written for *EastEnders* for 10 years. When the chance came up to pitch possible storylines for *Waterloo Road*, a drama based in a secondary school, she knew she wanted to pitch her story of trying to receive an endometriosis diagnosis so young. At the heart of the storyline is the experience of medical gaslighting 'and the fight that you have to go through'. The producers decided to include the story and asked Natalie to be a part of the ongoing process. The structure of the show was perfect, she explains. 'We didn't have to rush it; we could follow a student for two, three years of dealing with this'. The attention to detail in the storyline is also incredibly powerful.

The reaction to the episodes has been a moment of pride and validation for Natalie. Setting out to reflect the reality endometriosis patients face as truthfully as possible, she told herself, 'If just one person watches this story and it encourages them to go to the doctor and seek help, I've done my job.' Natalie's vulnerability in harnessing her own experiences and combining them with her skillset in storytelling created what is arguably the most faithful depiction of a young person with endometriosis struggling against medical gaslighting that I have seen. It goes to show that endometriosis advocacy can take so many different forms, depending on the strengths, resources, opportunities and connections available to us.

And it's not just endometriosis patients either. We met Dawn Heels and Tanya Simon-Hall, award-winning campaigners for fibroids and adenomyosis, respectively, in chapter 4 (*see* pages 165 and 148).

The ability of patients to harness our experiences, galvanise them and advocate for others is a real testament to our strength and our empathy for others who are also suffering. It shouldn't be up to patients, let's be honest, to fill in the gaps left by a medical system that leaves us confused and debilitated. But it is patients who end up asking me the most, 'what can I do to help?'

How to get involved

I am always being asked, 'How can I get involved in endometriosis advocacy?' First, don't feel like you have to be doing something. You are living with disease and that is enough in itself. Advocate for yourself until you are in a more manageable place – think about the oxygen mask analogy on aeroplanes.

If you do decide you have enough energy and this is something that you would like to do, start small. Look up current organisations or projects and see if you can support them in some way; we have seen throughout this book the importance of collaboration. Share their educational posts. Start normalising conversations around endometriosis with the people in your life. Even the tiniest steps forward are progress. Challenge misinformation and stigmas when you encounter them. Contribute to solid research projects when appropriate opportunities arise. Use your personal strengths and connections. Don't feel like you have to expose your entire health journey and experience on social or traditional media. If you want to, that's great, but be aware that it can also attract unwelcome and frankly ridiculous opinions and trolls, especially if your journey involves periods and/or fertility. You don't have to open yourself up to that if you're not comfortable doing so. Finally, what makes you truly furious about endometriosis care? Start

> there. For me, it's medical school education and medical gaslighting, so I focus my advocacy there. I work with medical schools to improve their endometriosis curriculum, and I set up a project to expose the experiences of medical gaslighting that we are expected to internalise, called They Said What?! @theysaidwhatproject

No one charity, group or individual is going to solve the myriad complex challenges baked into endometriosis care. And it's not going to happen overnight. I don't even know if it will happen in my lifetime, especially when it is thought that it takes on average 17 years for research findings to change clinical practice. And even after those 17 years, only one in five evidence-based interventions actually make it into routine patient care. However, I would like to see strides forward in that time. Working together is the way to make that happen. Not just as patients together, but as patients, researchers, specialists, GPs, policy makers, healthcare bodies, the NHS, employers, media, funding bodies, medical schools – all of us. We need to pool our collective outrage and our collective resources and push towards a common cause. We need to stop the fragmented, repeated conversations and try something new.

Someone who is trying a new approach to the well-established problems is Rey, aka @reythewarrior (*see also* pages 121–124). Rey's corporate career, before they left it behind for a life in Scotland, was 'processing data, recognising patterns and solving problems'. And, as Rey researched endometriosis more deeply, they quickly saw the same repeating patterns across the patient population. It became clear that 'education is the problem, at every single point of the care pathway'. It's not just the GP, or just the gynaecologist; 'it's every discipline that you connect with along the way'. We need more and better clinical education. Not the patient education that is often extolled by policy makers, although, as we've seen, this does still have an important part to play, particularly when addressing health inequities and inequalities. But the knee-jerk reaction shouldn't be to place the burden on the patient.

'I needed to be able to prove, in black and white, that this was a problem.' As has been echoed by many others in this book, we need the data as, without the data, nothing will change. Rey explained that 'I want to prove skills matter, and that's why we need to address the education piece.' How did they achieve that? By gathering 'a significant number of patient stories from those who had had multiple surgeries, who then had to seek expert care and had their life changed for the better'.

It is a massive undertaking, with an 'impact statement, timeline and full medical history required for each patient'. Thousands were whittled down to hundreds and then to 40 to keep the data as clean as possible. 'I don't want this to be an email,' Rey says. Emails are easy to ignore. They want this to be a massive tome, 'slapped on the desk of everyone who needs to see it: heads of royal colleges, heads of NHS departments, whoever needs to see it'. Rey wants them all to see that 'your one lecture on this topic, based on wildly outdated information, is ruining lives. Look at what can be learned from new research, clinical experience and patients.' And the results of Rey's report speak for themselves. Eighty-five per cent of all scans missed endometriosis, and 65 per cent of all surgeries missed disease.

Dr Nighat Arif, women's health GP, advocate and author, supports this. 'As an example, I was taught that peri-menopause stops endometriosis, that a hysterectomy cures it,' she explains. 'I have had to unlearn that outdated information that I was taught as a junior doctor and update it with new research and knowledge.' She explains that while the royal colleges, such as the Royal College of General Practice (RCGP) and the Royal College of Obstetricians and Gynaecologists (RCOG), do try to keep clinicians up to date, it simply 'doesn't happen at the rate of new disease knowledge', especially for a condition as complex as endometriosis. We need to make sure that the initial education, at a medical school level, is robust, consistent and accurate. And currently, it is not.

And Rey knows, as Bridget Gorham did when publishing the NHS Confederation report, 'Women's health economics: Investing in the 51%', that the way to appeal to policy makers and those holding the budgets is to highlight the economic case. 'The lack of efficiency is mind-blowing, the cost to the NHS is astronomical. The number of scans, the number of surgeries... we don't need them. We need one, maybe two,' Rey says. Tanya Simon-Hall made me laugh when we spoke, discussing this very inefficiency. 'Every time the doctors send me for a scan, I get a text telling me it costs the NHS £160 if I don't turn up,' she says. 'But what about the countless times I've been sent for pointless tests and scans? Can I send them an invoice for each of them? I would be a very wealthy woman, that's for sure.'

Rey says, 'The NHS is currently pouring money away, purely because clinical education isn't where it needs to be.' They admit that there are systemic issues to address: 'simple things like operating room access and spaces on wards'. But, they add, 'if we educate the surgeons appropriately, we won't need as much theatre access, because we won't all be having surgeries every year or two!'

Bridget agrees that these economic opportunities might just be the lever we need to prioritise healthcare for women and those assigned female at birth. When she first proposed the study, 'there was a lot of pushback', especially from men. But since seeing the results, some of those who were the biggest critics are now the biggest supporters. Yes, the healthy returns on investment likely converted them (the report found that for every £1 spent on women's health, there would be a return on investment of £11), but Bridget also believes that simultaneously humanising the issue through workplace campaigns and, unusually for a study of this type, focusing on patient voices and experiences has also had a profound impact on getting people to take the issues seriously.

Rey doesn't know if it will work. None of us doing any advocacy or campaigning work really know if our efforts will pay off and actually change endometriosis care for future patients. It will likely take decades to know. But Rey adds, 'I had to try something, and no one has tried this before'.

Technology and endometriosis

AI

Something else that is relatively new to endometriosis care, and health settings more broadly, is the use of AI. When we think of AI and healthcare, lots of us make the connection with its potential to diagnose diseases more efficiently. However, the inherent issue with AI is that it is created and fed by an algorithm that was designed by the status quo we are currently in. That status quo is inherently misogynistic and racist, and it holds biases against all manner of intersectionalities. With the specific case of endometriosis, if we are training AI to spot disease on a scan, for example, how reliable will those results be if the AI inputs do not recognise all disease presentations or how those presentations can vary in adolescent patients? Disease will likely still be missed, and we will be in a similar situation to where we are now. The sensitivity and reliability of AI are reliant on the information we provide it, and we simply don't have enough information about endometriosis right now. Maybe we'll get there soon; progress is being made, but we're not quite there yet.

To give a very flippant example, I asked ChatGPT about endometriosis. To be fair, its answers were better at the end of 2024 than when I first asked it a year earlier. However, it still has issues with its disease knowledge, namely believing that extra-pelvic endometriosis is rare, stating that the only real difference between endometriosis and endometrium is location and relying on the bleed and shed narrative that we know is not how endometriosis behaves.

But that doesn't mean we should discount AI. We saw in an earlier chapter that Mr Mabrouk and his team of global endometriosis specialists envisage AI being a useful tool to eventually underpin their proposed system of vetting for specialist endometriosis clinics and surgeons. And Mr Shaheen Khazali believes that AI can be used to try to help us solve the issues around data collection: 'AI is going to be in every aspect of what we do, but data gathering will be a huge example.' He is working with a team to develop a patient-facing app where you scan in your previous documents, reports, test results, scans and post-surgical findings. The AI system 'reads' them, organises them and summarises your history in a standardised format that you can take to your clinician. It then continues to log and track your experiences and outcomes. On the clinical side, your surgeon would also log all your results, images and surgical findings. Importantly, you, the patient, would have automatic access to these, itself a huge step forward for many. This data could then be monitored by independent organisations to accredit surgeons and their outcomes in a formalised way that doesn't currently exist.

At some point, Mr Khazali says, 'accreditation should no longer be based on 12 cases a year per surgeon'. Instead, it should be based on 'the complexity of your patient group, what your complication rates are and whether your patients are happy with the outcomes of their surgery'. The number of cases a surgeon performs will come into this, but as a way to maintain surgical skills to achieve the above outcomes rather than as an arbitrary number. We've clearly seen that we have an issue with a lack of datasets across endometriosis care. It will be interesting to see if these projects using AI can help us harness the data that already exists but is currently neglected – the surgical outcomes of our endometriosis specialists.

FemTech

Technology doesn't stop with AI. With the rise in awareness and conversations around endometriosis and other associated conditions, FemTech products, apps and solutions are booming. Amelia Isaacs, tech and finance journalist, says this trend is echoed across all of healthcare, but that women's healthcare is seen as a 'captive market' of people desperate to take control of and improve their health. However, is FemTech meeting a genuine need or preying on a vulnerable population? The answer, as is the ever-present theme in this book, is not so simplistic. 'No investment is entirely altruistic; it has to make money,' Amelia explains. Currently, only 2 per cent of available funding goes to female founders like Dearbhail Ormond, who founded frendo and frendo@work (*see* pages 186–187) following her own experiences with endometriosis. Even less funding goes to founders who are women of colour, despite the rising interest in the space in which these companies operate. But if the market sees investment in women's health performing well, it will divert more resources that way. 'Investors will want to be part of that boom and want to put their time, money and energy into it,' Amelia explains. The result could be that more founders, including endometriosis patients like Dearbhail, will receive funding in the future to drive change.

Research

Funding is not just an issue for company boardrooms. We've seen time and again how we desperately need more funding into research about almost every single facet of endometriosis. Only 2 per cent of medical research funding goes towards pregnancy, childbirth and reproductive health (aka 'women's health'. You can only imagine how tiny the slice of pie is for a condition such as endometriosis, despite it being a full body disease, as common as asthma or diabetes. In comparison, a McKinsey analysis found that, in 2019–2023, funding for companies focusing on erectile dysfunction was six times higher than for companies and projects looking at endometriosis, $1.24 billion compared to $44 million.

And when endometriosis, for example, does secure precious funding for research, it is not always in the patients' interest. One staggering example involves an Italian publicly funded study published in 2013. The study chose to investigate attractiveness and breast size in endometriosis patients. The conclusion of this groundbreaking (I hope you can feel my eyes rolling!) piece of research? 'Women with rectovaginal endometriosis were judged to be more attractive than those in the two control groups. Moreover, they had a leaner silhouette, larger breasts, and an earlier coitarche [age of first sexual intercourse]'. Despite this study receiving ethics approval, the women taking part did not give consent to be judged on attractiveness and only white women were selected to be included. This research was, rightfully later retracted, but it still took eight years for that to happen, and no apology was made.

Research is happening, some productive, some not so productive. When funding is so scarce, and organisations are forced to compete and fight against each other in a throwback to the colonial 'divide and conquer' playbook, politics is bound to be brought into the mix. Rey explains how this can dilute the helpfulness of research projects over time, even when they were initiated with the best intentions. 'Such a tiny pool of funding is allocated to women's health research,' they say, which will inevitably lead to some researchers 'bending and adapting proposals as required to access that pool'. Sometimes, the 'perspective of the original aim can be lost', particularly with the issue of funding and the pressure to generate results. That's why we see so many trials still pursuing hormonal interventions, not just for symptom management but as cures or a way to 'shrink' lesions, despite the fact that it's often not what endometriosis patients are asking for. Some of us love the hormonal symptom management options, but others are desperate for alternatives that come without the lengthy and sometimes additionally debilitating side effects.

One interesting research project, still in its infancy, is seeking to make cannabidiol (CBD) and cannabinoid-based options accessible via the NHS. Already known to be effective in reducing inflammation, which can provide symptomatic relief, medical cannabis can already be accessed in the UK for certain conditions, including endometriosis. However, it is only available privately, putting it out of reach for the majority. A symptom management option available on the NHS that does not have the side effects of hormonal interventions, opiates or NSAIDs? Sign me up. But not yet, because the research is still at an exceptionally early stage and only being tested in mouse models, which are not known for their accuracy when extrapolating up to human endometriosis patients.

Most research trials begin on mouse models before moving on to human trials. However, this gets a bit muddy in this study because the results are being measured on displaced endometrium, implanted into the mouse's abdominal cavity. The mice used don't even menstruate, so researchers have to force them to menstruate via human cells that are transplanted into the abdominal cavity of the mouse. Even if mice did menstruate, the results would be staggeringly limited. Why? Because, say it with me, endometriosis is not the endometrium. At one event I attended, an attendee asked, 'Why aren't we researching on endometriosis tissue samples? Why aren't we allowed to donate our tissues post-surgical excision to further endometriosis research?' And the answer, as usual, was funding. 'Not all centres are set up for research, and the funding simply isn't there,' explains Rey, which all feeds back into the education project they are working on. 'The next generation of researchers need updated knowledge so that their research questions are different from what we've been seeing for decades and actually move us forward.'

Dr José Eugenio-Colón, an endometriosis specialist at the US-based Center for Endometriosis Care, is thoughtful when I ask him what he would like to see happen in the future of endometriosis care. He says, 'We've been focusing so much on surgeries, but not on quality research.' He would love to see some form of national patient registry and a system where every doctor has to record their surgery with images and videos, which are also given to the patient. 'We could go back and see that, okay, your original doctor ablated this area, which has now become much worse.' We could compare ablation to excision, or medication to excision, and finally put these debates to rest. 'Because we know it works. But we don't have the time to undertake robust million-dollar studies like pharma companies do. Because I'm needed in the operating room to help my patients.' Using the expertise from specialists and their caseloads is something that has come up time and time again as a way to improve patient outcomes.

Endometriosis in the media

As Heather Guidone, Board Certified Patient Advocate, says, 'Endo is having a bit of a moment right now. Everyone is an expert; everyone is an influencer; everyone has something to say.' This is a double-edged sword. I have seen an increasing number of articles and television reports talking about endometriosis, highlighting patients, their experiences, the challenges that the healthcare system poses and 'new' research findings. I've even been in a few of them. It is, of course, absolutely incredible that endometriosis is getting this coverage, allowing us to normalise conversations and even do something as simple as introduce the word itself to the general public. However, it's important to be careful when navigating these articles, particularly ones promising 'breakthroughs', 'new treatments' or 'hope on the horizon'. 'Don't get too excited when "new research" is in a headline,' cautions Rey. 'We're so hungry for new advances, for good news, for hope . . . but these articles are usually reporting on mice-model stages or talking about drugs that have been around for a while and just been renamed or repurposed.'

The other topic I'm seeing more and more is the celebrity awareness pieces, where well-known names reveal their struggles with endometriosis. But remember, being a celebrity does not automatically mean that they received truly specialist care, even if they flew halfway around the world and paid tens of thousands of dollars.

Dr Nighat Arif, women's health GP and advocate, agrees, saying that 'media outlets are finding that endometriosis is very good clickbait content', finding a ready audience in the millions of sufferers, as well as their loved ones, who inevitably pass the articles on. Take these articles with a pinch of salt; they are good for awareness and destigmatisation, but always remember that any sources referred to in an article may not necessarily be up to date with current disease knowledge.

Social media and endometriosis

Social media is another factor that has contributed to the rise in awareness around endometriosis and its associated issues. Yes, it has its own drawbacks relating to trolls and the unregulated misinformation that exists, but I would argue that the opportunities for social media and health literacy outweigh the cons. To be honest, I feel like I've received just as much misinformation and trolling from doctors anyway.

I, only half-jokingly, say that social media saved my organs. Without endometriosis advocates on Instagram, who taught me the importance of listening to my body and finding a true specialist, I could have suffered kidney failure. Rey, who is actually one of the advocates who first reached out to me when I created my @jen.dometriosis account, can relate to this too. 'I am definitely a case who has benefited from patients online sharing their experiences, who have learned the hard way, after having had multiple failed surgeries.' It still baffles them, though, 'that this information came from an online Facebook group, not a medical or charitable organisation'.

Something that surprised me when speaking to clinicians for this book was how many of them recognised the power and potential of social media. Usually, the topic of social media gets a cold reception in healthcare settings, but time and again it came up in conversation. Mr Francesco Di Chiara, thoracic surgeon, says that if he were to be diagnosed with a 'perceived to be rare' disease tomorrow, the first place he would go would be social media. Not necessarily to take any medical advice, but to understand the context and concepts of the disease and how it affects patients, and to learn from clinicians who share information and resources. Dr Nighat Arif concurs. She thinks that social media, among other factors, is providing younger generations with a sense of validation of their lived experience that just 'never happened for Boomers, Gen X and even Millennials'. 'I love Gen Z and Gen Alpha,' she says. 'This younger group of individuals are kicking back at dogma' and refusing to follow established pathways for the sake of it, 'which should be applauded and amplified'.

Mr Di Chiara doesn't agree with clinicians who berate social media being used for health information. In fact, he thinks that in the future, most departments, specialties and clinics will have their own dedicated social accounts. 'It's a great source of information' that patients can scroll through and then, 'during a consultation, I don't have to spend most of the precious time explaining what thoracic endometriosis is'.

'The NHS loves a leaflet,' Mr Di Chiara adds, but these are slow to update, expensive and often left behind or binned without being read. In news that will shock no endometriosis patient who has used social media to learn about the disease, 'these platforms can provide easy-to-digest, up-to-date information, which is less overwhelming for patients' and that we should be taking advantage of as departments.

What we need

Every March is Endometriosis Awareness Month. It's a month that gives me mixed feelings. On the one hand, dedicated events, talks and media articles are produced to raise the issues endometriosis patients face, and I will always take up those opportunities where I am an appropriate person to do so. On the other hand, the same conversations are had, year after year, and nothing changes, as we have seen reflected in the statistics and in Cysters founder Neelam Heera Shergil's revelation that she deliberately delivers the same speech each International Women's Day (*see* page 231). Awareness is great. But awareness without action is just noise.

We know what we need. We need research into every single facet of this disease. We need data, disaggregated by marginalised voices in particular. We need endometriosis to be considered a separate subspecialty. We need collaboration. We need diverse patient voices included at the tables where new policies are created. Not just to share their trauma or to embellish a report, but from the start and as valued contributors to the direction and scope of change. We need true co-production to break us out of the same cycles that repeat across generations. We need updated clinical education at every single touchpoint. We need to work with the grass-roots organisations already doing the work on the ground in communities who have been ignored for too long – micro-level (community) observations need to inform the macro-level (policy) decisions. We need symptom management options other than hormonal interventions so that we can make informed, better choices. We need transparency around funding and conflicts of interest. We need more endometriosis specialists and multi-disciplinary clinics behind them. We need support for the impacts that endometriosis can have on our entire lives, at school, work and home. We need to be able to access fertility or psychological services if we would like to. We need to address the demoralisation of NHS staff, caused by heavy workloads and resources stretched to breaking point, which has a knock-on effect on the way patients are treated. We need the money and prioritisation to achieve all of these things. We need to repair the broken trust between endometriosis patients and clinical teams. And we need to start listening, and believing, endometriosis patients, the first time they speak up. And, if we're really wishing on a star, we need a cure.

This is not the end

Frankly, we know the problem exists. We patients and those on the front line of endometriosis care have been screaming it for decades. It's time to move past acknowledging the problem and commit the resources needed to fundamentally address it, for every single one of us who suffers from this complex, often cruel, disease.

APPENDIX 1

Letter template for writing a complaint

Earlier in the book, Dr Nighat Arif, GP, women's health advocate and author, reminds us not to be shy about writing a letter of complaint if we received healthcare provision that we were not happy with. But a lot of us struggle with this and aren't sure how to approach it. Use this template as a starting point and remember, if we keep quiet, nothing will change, neither for us nor future generations.

Who you write to will depend on the specific circumstances – for example, if it was a GP, you will write to the practice manager. If you are at all unsure, the best first step is to ask your GP practice, hospital or local trust for their complaints procedure. You may even be able to find this on their individual website.

Dear [insert name]

I am writing to formally express my dissatisfaction with the care I received at [insert location] on [insert date] by [insert doctor's name] with regards to my [suspected/diagnosed] endometriosis. I am concerned about several aspects of my experience and feel it deeply important to bring these to your attention.

[insert description of what happened, for example, were your concerns dismissed? Was incorrect and outdated information provided? Were there any incidences of medical misogyny or gaslighting? You can also add in or attach any later records, scans, surgical reports etc. to support your complaint.]

These experiences have negatively impacted my trust in both [insert Doctor] and [insert practice/clinic/hospital].

In response to this complaint, I would like the following points addressed:

- Use bullet points here and be clear and concise

Put the most important points first
- *Use this section to raise any issues or questions you would like answered – for example, training or education about endometriosis for the doctor and practice in question. If you would like an apology, then say so. If you would like to be seen by a different doctor from now on, then request this.*

I ask that you take these issues seriously and promptly implement the necessary changes to prevent similar experiences for future patients. If you need any further information, then please do not hesitate to contact me.

I look forward to receiving your acknowledgement of this complaint, and the outcomes of your investigation, in line with the NHS Complaints Procedure.

Sincerely,

[insert your name]
[insert your Date of Birth]
[insert your NHS number]

APPENDIX 2

Letter template for writing to a doctor who had dismissed you previously

I am often asked if I have ever written to earlier doctors who told me endometriosis was impossible, to show them my surgical reports. And the answer is yes. The aim here is education, not to 'prove them wrong', as tempting as that may be. We need these medical practitioners to learn and improve their approach for future generations, not to get defensive, so a gentler tone is important. The doctor may or may not get in touch with you, but this approach is the most effective one I've found.

Dear *[insert Doctor's name]*

You recently saw me on *[insert date]* to discuss the symptoms of endometriosis that I had been struggling with. Causing particular issues were *[insert symptoms]*.

Thank you for your efforts to assist me. Unfortunately, my quality of life continued to deteriorate, and I sought additional advice. I am attaching some reports that you may like to see.

Yours sincerely,
[insert name]

APPENDIX 3

Email template to your employer, asking for workplace adjustments

Subject: Request for health-related support

Dear [insert your manager's name]

I'm writing to update you on my health and to make a reasonable adjustment request.

I have been diagnosed with endometriosis, a complex, chronic disease that affects my daily life, including work. Presenting differently for each person, endometriosis for me is characterised by [insert your symptoms here and give details of how your health affects your work and vice versa].

My current role is [insert details]. While I strive to perform to the best of my ability there are times when I experience significant [insert main symptom, e.g. pain] or require medical appointments, which have a knock-on effect on my work. I value my position here and want to ensure that I am contributing effectively while looking after my health and not making my symptoms worse.

To help me manage this balance, I ask that [insert details of what adjustments you would find helpful and why. You can find examples in chapter 3, pages 137–138, but think carefully about your own circumstances and what would make a difference to you]. This would allow me to [insert any benefits your employer].

If you have any questions, then please let me know.

Thank you for your support and understanding in creating a professional environment that allows me to thrive while managing my health.

Kind regards, [or sign off of your choice]
[your name]

REFERENCES

Introduction

characterised by the presence of endometrium-like tissue found outside the uterine cavity: Kennedy, S., Bergqvist, A., Chapron, C., D'Hooghe, T., Dunselman, G., Greb, R., Hummelshoj, L., Prentice, A., Saridogan, E., & ESHRE Special Interest Group for Endometriosis and Endometrium Guideline Development Group. 'ESHRE guideline for the diagnosis and treatment of endometriosis', *Human reproduction (Oxford, England)*, 20(10), 2698–2704 (2005): doi.org/10.1093/humrep/dei135; Klemmt, P.A.B. & Starzinski-Powitz, A. 'Molecular and Cellular Pathogenesis of Endometriosis', *Current Women's Health Reviews*, 14(2), 106–116 (2018): doi.org/10.2174/1573404813666170306163448; Saunders, P.T.K. & Horne, A.W. 'Endometriosis: Etiology, pathobiology, and therapeutic prospects', *Cell*, 184(11), 2807–2824 (2021): doi.org/10.1016/j.cell.2021.04.041; International Working Group of AAGL, ESGE, ESHRE and WES, Tomassetti, C., Johnson, N.P., Petrozza, J., Abrao, M.S., Einarsson, J.I., Horne, A.W., Lee, T.T.M., Missmer, S., Vermeulen, N., Zondervan, K.T., Grimbizis, G. & De Wilde, R.L. 'An International Terminology for Endometriosis, 2021', *Journal of Minimally Invasive Gynecology*, 28(11), 1849–1859 (2021): doi.org/10.1016/j.jmig.2021.08.032

a quarter of a century where nothing has improved: Jones, G., Fisher, V., Musson, D., Budds, K., Jenkinson, C. & Kennedy, S., 'Measuring the Quality of Life of Women & Those Assigned Female at Birth Living with Endometriosis', Endometriosis UK: www.leedsbeckett.ac.uk/news/2024/09/endometriosis-research-pr/-/media/98d32b-6926664ca8955a4453a3555702.ashx

they are actually getting worse: Endometriosis UK, '"Dismissed, ignored and belittled": The long road to endometriosis diagnosis in the UK', March 2024: www.endometriosis-uk.org/sites/default/files/2024-03/Endometriosis%20UK%20diagnosis%20survey%202023%20report%20March.pdf

there are also documented cases of endometriosis in cis men: Extrapelvic Not Rare, 'Endometriosis in Persons AMAB' (n.d.): extrapelvicnotrare.org/endometriosis-in-males/

Chapter 1: What is endometriosis?

the presence of endometrial-like tissue outside the uterus: Kennedy, S., Bergqvist, A., Chapron, C., D'Hooghe, T., Dunselman, G., Greb, R., Hummelshoj, L., Prentice, A., Saridogan, E. & ESHRE Special Interest Group for Endometriosis and Endometrium

Guideline Development Group. 'ESHRE guideline for the diagnosis and treatment of endometriosis', *Human reproduction (Oxford, England)*, 20(10), 2698–2704 (2005): doi.org/10.1093/humrep/dei135; Klemmt, P.A.B. & Starzinski-Powitz, A. 'Molecular and Cellular Pathogenesis of Endometriosis', *Current Women's Health Reviews*, 14(2), 106–116 (2018): doi.org/10.2174/1573404813666170306163448; Saunders, P.T.K. & Horne, A.W. 'Endometriosis: Etiology, pathobiology, and therapeutic prospects', *Cell*, 184(11), 2807–2824 (2021): doi.org/10.1016/j.cell.2021.04.041; International Working Group of AAGL, ESGE, ESHRE and WES, Tomassetti, C., Johnson, N.P., Petrozza, J., Abrao, M.S., Einarsson, J.I., Horne, A.W., Lee, T.T.M., Missmer, S., Vermeulen, N., Zondervan, K.T., Grimbizis, G. & De Wilde, R.L. 'An International Terminology for Endometriosis, 2021', *Journal of Minimally Invasive Gynecology*, 28(11), 1849–1859 (2021): doi.org/10.1016/j.jmig.2021.08.032

Endometriosis creates its own oestrogen: Mori, T., Ito, F., Koshiba, A., Kataoka, H., Takaoka, O., Okimura, H., Khan, K.N. & Kitawaki, J. 'Local estrogen formation and its regulation in endometriosis', *Reproductive Medicine and Biology*, 18(4), 305–311 (2019): doi.org/10.1002/rmb2.12285

at that stage it was referred to as adenomyoma: von Rokitansky, K.F. 'Ueber uterusdrüsen-neubildung in uterus-und ovarial-sarcomen', Druck von Carl Ueberreuter (1860).

causing 'hysterical lumps . . . throughout the body, pain in the bladder, vomiting, diarrhoea, and back pain'.: Nezhat, C., Nezhat, F. & Nezhat, C. 'Endometriosis: ancient disease, ancient treatments', *Fertility and Sterility*, 98(6 Suppl.), S1–S62 (2012): doi.org/10.1016/j.fertnstert.2012.08.001

Endometriosis versus endometrium: Nisolle, M., Casanas-Roux, F. & Donnez, J. 'Immunohistochemical analysis of proliferative activity and steroid receptor expression in peritoneal and ovarian endometriosis', *Fertility and Sterility*, 68(5), 912–919 (1997): doi.org/10.1016/s0015-0282(97)00341-5

different reactions to the hormones oestrogen and progesterone: Chantalat, E., Valera, M.C., Vaysse, C., Noirrit, E., Rusidze, M., Weyl, A., Vergriete, K., Buscail, E., Lluel, P., Fontaine, C., Arnal, J.F. & Lenfant, F. 'Estrogen Receptors and Endometriosis', *International Journal of Molecular Sciences*, 21(8), 2815 (2020): doi.org/10.3390/ijms21082815

can be black, dark brown, red, white, multi-coloured or even clear: Stegmann, B.J., Sinaii, N., Liu, S., Segars, J., Merino, M., Nieman, L.K. & Stratton, P. 'Using location, color, size, and depth to characterize and identify endometriosis lesions in a cohort of 133 women', *Fertility and Sterility*, 89(6), 1632–1636 (2008): doi.org/10.1016/j.fertnstert.2007.05.042

No aromatase enzyme activity: Bulun, S.E., Fang, Z., Imir, G., Gurates, B., Tamura, M., Yilmaz, B., Langoi, D., Amin, S., Yang, S. & Deb, S. 'Aromatase and endometriosis', *Seminars in Reproductive Medicine*, 22(1), 45–50 (2004): doi.org/10.1055/s-2004-823026

inside and around lesions (another reason endometriosis is so painful!): Stegmann, B.J., Sinaii, N., Liu, S., Segars, J., Merino, M., Nieman, L.K. & Stratton, P. 'Using location, color, size, and depth to characterize and identify endometriosis lesions in a cohort of 133 women', *Fertility and Sterility*, 89(6), 1632–1636 (2008). doi.org/10.1016/j.fertnstert.2007.05.042

(a girl aged six recently underwent surgery to remove endometriosis): Takada, L., Kawano, T., Yano, K., Iwamoto, Y., Ogata, M., Kedoin, C., Murakami, M., Sugita, K., Onishi, S., Muto, M., Kirishima, M., Tanimoto, A. & Ieiri, S. 'Ovarian endometrioma: a report of a

References

pediatric case diagnosed prior to menstruation', *Surgical Case Reports*, 10(1), 152 (2024): doi.org/10.1186/s40792-024-01951-5

the incidence is more likely to be one in seven, or 14 per cent: Australian Institute of Health and Welfare 'Endometriosis', 14 December, 2023: www.aihw.gov.au/reports/chronic-disease/endometriosis-in-australia/contents/how-common-is-endometriosis

It is thought that 20–25 per cent of endometriosis patients are asymptomatic (do not experience any symptoms): Bulletti, C., Coccia, M.E., Battistoni, S. & Borini, A. 'Endometriosis and infertility', *Journal of Assisted Reproduction and Genetics*, 27(8), 441–447 (2010): doi.org/10.1007/s10815-010-9436-1

only 18 per cent of those with confirmed endometriosis were diagnosed by scan: Endometriosis UK, "Dismissed, ignored and belittled": The long road to endometriosis diagnosis in the UK', March 2024: www.endometriosis-uk.org/sites/default/files/2024-03/Endometriosis%20UK%20diagnosis%20survey%202023%20report%20March.pdf

have reported a higher incidence of adhesions and the associated problems: Bignardi, T., Khong, S.Y. & Lam, A. 'Excisional versus ablative surgery for peritoneal endometriosis', *The Cochrane Database of Systematic Reviews*, 2019(7), CD008979 (2019): doi.org/10.1002/14651858.CD008979.pub2

is a consequence of inflammation in the pelvis, often seen in endometriosis patients: Maicas, G., Leonardi, M., Avery, J., Panuccio, C., Carneiro, G., Hull, M.L. & Condous, G. 'Deep learning to diagnose pouch of Douglas obliteration with ultrasound sliding sign', *Reproduction and Fertility*, 2(4), 236–243 (2021): doi.org/10.1530/RAF-21-0031

POD obliteration may be suggestive of bowel endometriosis also being present: Khong, S.Y., Bignardi, T., Luscombe, G. & Lam, A. 'Is pouch of Douglas obliteration a marker of bowel endometriosis?', *Journal of Minimally Invasive Gynecology*, 18(3), 333–337 (2011): doi.org/10.1016/j.jmig.2011.01.011

'44 to 80 million of them have endometriosis among one or more body systems other than reproductive'.: Extrapelvic Not Rare, 'Welcome to Extrapelvic Not Rare', n.d.: extrapelvicnotrare.org/

The diaphragm is the most common form of extra-abdominopelvic disease, found in 1–12 per cent of patients: Nezhat C, Lindheim, S.R., Backhus, L., Vu, M., Vang, N., Nezhat, A. & Nezhat, C. 'Thoracic Endometriosis Syndrome: A Review of Diagnosis and Management', JSLS. 2019 Jul-Sep; 23(3):e2019.00029. doi: 10.4293/JSLS.2019.00029. PMID: 31427853; PMCID: PMC6684338.

thoracic endometriosis may occur in up to 12 per cent of those with pelvic disease: British Society for Gynaecological Endoscopy and Royal College of Obstetricians and Gynaecologists, 'BSGE and RCOG joint statement on Thoracic Endometriosis care in the United Kingdom', n.d.: www.rcog.org.uk/media/4iulq0ug/bsge-statement-on-thoracic-endometriosis-care-in-the-uk.pdf; Soares, T., Oliveira, M., Panisset, K., Habib, N., Rahman, S., Klebanoff, J. & Moawad, G. 'Diaphragmatic endometriosis and thoracic endometriosis syndrome: a review on diagnosis and treatment', *Hormone Molecular Biology and Clinical Investigation*, 43(2), 137–143 (2022): doi.org/10.1515/hmbci-2020-0066; Ceccaroni, M., Roviglione, G., Giampaolino, P., Clarizia, R., Bruni, F., Ruffo, G., Patrelli, T.S., De Placido, G. & Minelli, L. 'Laparoscopic surgical treatment of diaphragmatic endometriosis: a

7-year single-institution retrospective review', *Surgical Endoscopy*, 27, 625–632 (2013): doi.org/10.1007/s00464-012-2505-z

These cells then implant and attach themselves to different areas and organs, 'causing' endometriosis: Sampson, J.A. 'Metastatic or Embolic Endometriosis, due to the Menstrual Dissemination of Endometrial Tissue into the Venous Circulation', *The American Journal of Pathology*, 3(2), 93–110 (1927).

They are different in both structure and behaviour: Delbandi, A.A., Mahmoudi, M., Shervin, A., Akbari, E., Jeddi-Tehrani, M., Sankian, M., Kazemnejad, S. & Zarnani, A.H. 'Eutopic and ectopic stromal cells from patients with endometriosis exhibit differential invasive, adhesive, and proliferative behavior', *Fertility and Sterility*, 100(3), 761–769 (2013): doi.org/10.1016/j.fertnstert.2013.04.041

Approximately 90 per cent of people with periods experience retrograde menstruation: Viganò, P., Caprara, F., Giola, F., Di Stefano, G., Somigliana, E. & Vercellini, P. 'Is retrograde menstruation a universal, recurrent, physiological phenomenon? A systematic review of the evidence in humans and non-human primates', *Human Reproduction Open*, 2024(3), hoae045 (2024): doi.org/10.1093/hropen/hoae045

the current endometriosis statistic is that it affects 10 per cent: Endometriosis UK, 'Endometriosis facts and figures', n.d.: www.endometriosis-uk.org/endometriosis-facts-and-figures

there are no photographs of this actually happening: Redwine, D.B. *100 Questions and Answers About Endometriosis*, Jones and Bartlett Publishers, Inc (2009).

Endometriosis has been found in girls who have not yet had their first period, postmenopausal women foetuses: Signorile, P.G., Baldi, F., Bussani, R., Viceconte, R., Bulzomi, P., D'Armiento, M., D'Avino, A. & Baldi, A. 'Embryologic origin of endometriosis: analysis of 101 human female fetuses', *Journal of Cellular Physiology*, 227(4), 1653–1656 (2012): doi.org/10.1002/jcp.22888

a popular theory is Dr Redwine's idea of mülleriosis: Redwine, D.B. 'Mülleriosis instead of endometriosis', *American Journal of Obstetrics and Gynecology*, 156(3), 761 (1987): doi.org/10.1016/0002-9378(87)90093-7

which could help explain the cases in cis men: Duke, C.M. & Taylor, H.S. 'Stem cells and the reproductive system: historical perspective and future directions', *Maturitas*, 76(3), 284–289 (2013): doi.org/10.1016/j.maturitas.2013.08.012

Immunological dysfunction: Maeda, N., Izumiya, C., Taniguchi, K., Matsushima, S. & Fukaya, T. 'Role of NK cells and HLA-G in endometriosis', *Frontiers in Bioscience (Scholar Edition)*, 4(4), 1568–1581 (2012): doi.org/10.2741/s353

Genetics: Nouri, K., Ott, J., Krupitz, B., Huber, J.C. & Wenzl, R. 'Family incidence of endometriosis in first-, second-, and third-degree relatives: case-control study', *Reprod Biol Endocrinol*, 8, 85 (2010): doi.org/10.1186/1477-7827-8-85

Environmental toxins inducing cell changes: Anger, D.L. & Foster, W.G. 'The link between environmental toxicant exposure and endometriosis', *Frontiers in Bioscience*, 13, 1578–1593 (2008): doi.org/10.2741/2782

Lymphatic spread: Escobar, P.F. 'Lymphatic Spread of Endometriosis to Para-Aortic Nodes', *Images in Gynecologic Surgery*, 20(6), 741 (2013): doi.org/10.1016/j.jmig.2013.02.014

References

we're possibly dealing with separate diseases: Khazali, S., speaking at 'The Future of Endometriosis Care' (Endometriosis UK event), October 2024.

the second most frequently reported symptom was fatigue, with 77 per cent suffering from it: Evans, S.F., Brooks, T.A., Esterman, A.J., Hull, M.L. & Rolan, P.E. 'The comorbidities of dysmenorrhea: a clinical survey comparing symptom profile in women with and without endometriosis', *Journal of Pain Research*, 11, 3181–3194 (2018): doi.org/10.2147/JPR.S179409

with endometriosis spotted during another procedure or when the individual is trying to conceive and experiencing difficulties: Ferguson, S. 'What Is Silent Endometriosis?', Healthline (16 October, 2024): www.healthline.com/health/silent-endometriosis

the NHS listed endometriosis as one of the top 20 most painful conditions a human can suffer with: Ritschel, C. 'From shingles to kidney stones: The 20 worst kinds of pain humans can experience', *The Independent* (20 December, 2023): www.independent.co.uk/life-style/pain-body-cause-worst-shingles-gout-b2467514.html

80ml of blood loss across a cycle: BUPA, 'Heavy periods (menorrhagia)' (n.d.): www.bupa.co.uk/health-information/womens-health/menorrhagia

It can also lead to the shortening of the vaginal canal: Imperial College Healthcare NHS Trust. 'Mayer Rokitansky Küster Hauser syndrome (MRKH)', (2019): www.imperial.nhs.uk/-/media/website/patient-information-leaflets/children's-services/disorders-of-sexual-development-and-adolescent-gynaecology/mrkh.pdf

cis men have also been found to have endometriosis: Zámečník, M. & Hoštáková, D. 'Endometriosis in a mesothelial cyst of tunica vaginalis of the testis. Report of a case', *Ceskoslovenska Patologie*, 49(3), 134–136 (2013).

you are around seven times more likely to also suffer from the disease: Macer, M.L. & Taylor, H.S. 'Endometriosis and infertility: a review of the pathogenesis and treatment of endometriosis-associated infertility', *Obstetrics and Gynecology Clinics of North America*, 39(4), 535–549 (2012): doi.org/10.1016/j.ogc.2012.10.002

Endotest: Bendifallah, S., Dabi, Y., Suisse, S., Delbos, L., Spiers, A., Poilblanc, M., Golfier, F., Jornea, L., Bouteiller, D., Fernandez, H., Madar, A., Petit, E., Perotte, F., Fauvet, R., Benjoar, M., Akladios, C., Lavoué, V., Darnaud, T., Merlot, B., Roman, H. & Descamps, P. 'Validation of a Salivary miRNA Signature of Endometriosis – Interim Data', *NEJM Evidence*, 2(7), EVIDoa2200282 (2023): doi.org/10.1056/EVIDoa2200282

infertility can affect 30–50 per cent of endometriosis patients: Macer, M.L. & Taylor, H.S. 'Endometriosis and infertility: a review of the pathogenesis and treatment of endometriosis-associated infertility', *Obstetrics and Gynecology Clinics of North America*, 39(4), 535–549 (2012): doi.org/10.1016/j.ogc.2012.10.002

research is emerging to say their prolonged use may have sustained negativity that we do not yet fully understand: King, R. 'Depo-Provera Brain Tumor Lawsuit – February 2025 Update', King Law (28 January, 2025): www.robertkinglawfirm.com/personal-injury/depo-provera-lawsuit/

those with stage IV is between 50–60%: Center for Endometriosis Care, 'Infertility' (n.d.): centerforendo.com/infertility-1

Despite endometriosis up to doubling the risk of infertility: Prescott, J., Farland, L.V., Tobias, D.K., Gaskins, A.J., Spiegelman, D., Chavarro, J.E., Rich-Edwards, J.W., Barbieri, R.L. & Missmer, S.A. 'A prospective cohort study of endometriosis and subsequent risk of infertility', *Human Reproduction*, 31(7), 1475–1482 (2016): doi.org/10.1093/humrep/dew085

Only 44 per cent of patients were even asked by a medical practitioner if their fertility was important to them: All Party Parliamentary Group on Endometriosis, 'Endometriosis in the UK: time for change' (2020): www.endometriosis-uk.org/sites/endometriosis-uk.org/files/files/Endometriosis%20APPG%20Report%20Oct%202020.pdf

the 'oestrogens stimulate the endometriosis cells to start flourishing': Mohling, S. 'Teenagers get endometriosis. Well, I believe they had it from birth, but when a person goes through menarche, the estrogens...' [Post], Instagram (21 February, 2024): www.instagram.com/p/C3nSy4jLfh-/?hl=en

with 'at least 60% of teens diagnosed with endometriosis presenting with symptoms within 6 months of menarche; 80% within 3 years': Sarıdoğan, E. 'Endometriosis in Teenagers', *Women's Health*, 11(5), 705–709 (2015): doi.org/10.2217/whe.15.58

revealed that 70 per cent of teens suffering from pelvic pain are later diagnosed with the disease: American College of Obstetricians and Gynecologists. 'Committee Opinion on Dysmenorrhea and Endometriosis in the Adolescent' (2018): www.acog.org/clinical/clinical-guidance/committee-opinion/articles/2018/12/dysmenorrhea-and-endometriosis-in-the-adolescent

82 per cent of participants in a 2014 study on the topic had never even heard of endometriosis: Zannoni, L., Giorgi, M., Spagnolo, E., Montanari, G., Villa, G. & Seracchioli, R. 'Dysmenorrhea, absenteeism from school, and symptoms suspicious for endometriosis in adolescents', *Journal of Pediatric and Adolescent Gynecology*, 27(5), 258–265 (2014): doi.org/10.1016/j.jpag.2013.11.008

leading to missed school or reduced performance: Fourquet, J., Gao, X., Zavala, D., Orengo, J.C., Abac, S., Ruiz, A., Laboy, J. & Flores, I. 'Patients' report on how endometriosis affects health, work, and daily life', *Fertility and Sterility*, 93(7), 2424–2428 (2010): doi.org/10.1016/j.fertnstert.2009.09.017

loss of social opportunities: Krsmanovic, A. & Dean, M. ' How Women Suffering from Endometriosis Disclose about their Disorder at Work', *Health Communication*, 37(8), 992–1003 (2022): doi.org/10.1080/10410236.2021.1880053

mental distress caused by living with these symptoms and medical gaslighting: Sims, O.T., Gupta, J., Missmer, S.A. & Aninye, I.O. ' Stigma and Endometriosis: A Brief Overview and Recommendations to Improve Psychosocial Well-Being and Diagnostic Delay', *International Journal of Environmental Research and Public Health*, 18(15), 8210 (2021): doi.org/10.3390/ijerph18158210

Twenty to 40 per cent of adolescents report having to miss school or experiencing a decline in academic performance: Eisenberg, V.H., Decter, D.H., Chodick, G., Shalev, V. & Weil, C. 'Burden of Endometriosis: Infertility, Comorbidities, and Healthcare Resource Utilization', *Journal of Clinical Medicine*, 11(4), 1133 (2022): doi.org/10.3390/jcm11041133

the 82 per cent of teens who had never heard of endometriosis: Zannoni, L., Giorgi, M., Spagnolo, E., Montanari, G., Villa, G. & Seracchioli, R. 'Dysmenorrhea, absenteeism from

References

school, and symptoms suspicious for endometriosis in adolescents', *Journal of Pediatric and Adolescent Gynecology*, 27(5), 258–265 (2014). doi.org/10.1016/j.jpag.2013.11.008

'endometriosis causes scarring and complications much more than the surgery with proper excision': Mohling, S. 'Teenagers get endometriosis. Well, I believe they had it from birth, but when a person goes through menarche, the estrogens...' [Post], Instagram (21 February, 2024): www.instagram.com/p/C3nSy4jLfh-/?hl=en

making them difficult to identify for surgeons unfamiliar with the complexities of the disease: American College of Obstetricians and Gynecologists. 'Committee Opinion on Dysmenorrhea and Endometriosis in the Adolescent' (2018): www.acog.org/clinical/clinical-guidance/committee-opinion/articles/2018/12/dysmenorrhea-and-endometriosis-in-the-adolescent

hundreds of thousands of unnecessary hysterectomies are performed in the United States each year: Center for Endometriosis Care 'Excision of endometriosis' (n.d.): centerforendo.com/lapex-laparoscopic-excision-of-endometriosis

have a lower rate of life-changing surgeries such as stomas and bowel resections, despite handling far higher volumes of these complex cases: Khazali, S., Bachi, A., Mondelli, B., Fleischer, K., Adamczyk, M., Delanerolle, G., Shi, J.Q., Yang, X., Nisar, P. & Bearn, P. 'Intra-operative and post-operative complications of endometriosis excision using the SOSURE approach – A single-surgeon retrospective series of 1116 procedures over 8 years', *Facts, Views & Vision in ObGyn*, 16(3), 325–336 (2024): doi.org/10.52054/FVVO.16.3.030

a staggering 763,694 women: Royal College of Obstetricians and Gynaecologists, 'Waiting for a way forward: Voices of women and healthcare professionals at the centre of the gynaecology care crisis' (n.d.): rcog.shorthandstories.com/waiting-for-a-way-forward/

lungs: Counseller, V.S. & Crenshaw, J.L., Jr. 'A clinical and surgical review of endometriosis', *American Journal of Obstetrics and Gynecology*, 62(4), 930–942 (1851): doi.org/10.1016/0002-9378(51)90180-9

bowel: Maclean, N.J. 'Endometriosis of the Large Bowel', *Canadian Medical Association Journal*, 34(3), 253–258 (1936).

bladder: Henriksen, E. 'Primary endometriosis of the urinary bladder: report of one case', *JAMA*, 104(16), 1401–1403 (1935): doi:10.1001/jama.1935.02760160025008

lymph nodes: Hansmann, G.H. & Schenken, J.R. 'Endometrioses of lymph nodes', *American Journal of Obstetrics and Gynecology*, 25, 572–5 (1933).

cervix: Rushmore, S. 'Endometriosis of the cervix', *New England Journal of Medicine*, 205, 149–50 (1931).

Endometriosis was also reported among teens: Tuthill, C.R. 'Malignant endometriosis of the ovary, resembling arrhenoblastoma: report of a case in a girl aged nineteen', *Archives of Surgery*, 37, 554–61 (1938); Fallon, J. 'Endometriosis in youth', *JAMA*, 131, 1405–6 (1946).

We even knew, in 1957: Chinn, J., Horton, R.K. & Rusche, C. (1957). 'Unilateral ureteral obstruction as sole manifestation of endometriosis', *The Journal of Urology*, 77(2), 144–150 (1957): doi.org/10.1016/S0022-5347(17)66535-2

some of the first to be given this novel treatment were endometriosis patients: Junod, S. W. & Marks, L. 'Women's trials: the approval of the first oral contraceptive pill in the United

States and Great Britain', *Journal of the History of Medicine and Allied Sciences*, 57(2), 117–160 (2002): doi.org/10.1093/jhmas/57.2.117

'the most efficient treatment is radical excision': Weijtlandt, J.A. 'Endometriosis of the Bladder: (Section of Urology)', *Proceedings of the Royal Society of Medicine*, 27(11), 1493–1498 (1934).

'we have excised localised endometrial implants with satisfactory relief and have been gratified to see our patients bear children': Emge, L.A. 'Indications for surgery of the ovary', *California Medicine*, 67(4), 211–216 (1947).

'based on excision...in four fifths of cases...the symptoms entirely disappeared.': Fredrikson, H. 'Pregnancy after conservative surgery for ovarian endometriosis', *Acta Obstetricia et Gynecologica Scandinavica*, 36(4), 468–480 (1957): doi.org/10.3109/00016345709157418

Endometriosis is thought to affect one in 10 women: World Health Organization, 'Endometriosis' (24 March, 2023): www.who.int/news-room/fact-sheets/detail/endometriosis

More recent studies show that this is closer to one in seven: Endometriosis Australia, 'Endometriosis in Australia is now estimated to be 1 in 7 females and those assigned female at birth' (2023): endometriosisaustralia.org/1-in-7-australian-women/

The spleen was the last organ to join the party, having been documented in 2022: Krzeczowski, R.M., Jackson, T.N., Kabbani, W., Grossman Verner, H.M. & Sladek, P. 'Splenic Cysts and the Case of Mistaken Identity', *Cureus*, 14(2), e22012 (2022): doi.org/10.7759/cureus.22012

Chapter 2: Dealing with the system – how to get help

the average diagnosis time is eight to 10 years: Frankel, L.R. 'A 10-Year Journey to Diagnosis With Endometriosis: An Autobiographical Case Report', *Cureus*, 14(1), e21329 (2022): doi.org/10.7759/cureus.21329

Northern Ireland and Wales facing the longest waits of nine years and five months and nine years and 11 months, respectively: Endometriosis UK, '"Dismissed, ignored and belittled": The long road to endometriosis diagnosis in the UK', March 2024: www.endometriosis-uk.org/sites/default/files/2024-03/Endometriosis%20UK%20 diagnosis%20survey%202023%20report%20March.pdf

Black and Hispanic endometriosis sufferers could be waiting double this time: *American Journal of Managed Care*, 'Racial Disparities Associated With Endometriosis Diagnosis [Video]', 'Addressing Health Disparities in Women's Healthcare' Episode 6 (18 May, 2023): www.ajmc.com/view/racial-disparities-associated-with-endometriosis-diagnosis

'the earlier endometriosis is diagnosed and treated properly, the better the outcomes are for those struggling': Center for Endometriosis Care, 'Endo Q&A with Dr. Sinervo [Transcript]' (n.d.): centerforendo.com/endoqa-with-dr-sinervo-transcript

'Delays in the diagnosis of endometriosis are common and are associated with worsened quality of life and greater medical costs': Darbà, J. & Marsà, A. 'Economic Implications of Endometriosis: A Review', *PharmacoEconomics*, 40(12), 1143–1158 (2022): doi.org/10.1007/s40273-022-01211-0

References

This was an increase from 69 per cent just four years earlier: Endometriosis UK, '"Dismissed, ignored and belittled": The long road to endometriosis diagnosis in the UK', March 2024: www.endometriosis-uk.org/sites/default/files/2024-03/Endometriosis%20 UK%20diagnosis%20survey%202023%20report%20March.pdf

... and it can be updated instantly': Di Chiara, F. Interview, 2024.

... driven by a desire to outdo attractive rival women.': Durante, K.M., Griskevicius, V., Hill, S.E., Perilloux, C. & Li, N.P. 'Ovulation, Female Competition, and Product Choice: Hormonal Influences on Consumer Behavior', *Journal of Consumer Research*, 37(6), 921–934 (2011): doi.org/10.1086/656575

to ensure they are meeting all their obligations to be transparent with their users and keep their data safe.': Information Commissioner's Office, 'ICO urges all app developers to prioritise privacy', 8 February, 2024.

A 2024 study by researchers at University College London and King's College London backs these concerns: Malki, L.M., Kaleva, I., Patel, D., Warner, M. & Abu-Salma, R. 'Exploring Privacy Practices of Female mHealth Apps in a Post-Roe World', CHI '24: Proceedings of the 2024 CHI Conference on Human Factors in Computing Systems, 576, 1–24, 11 May, 2024: doi.org/10.1145/3613904.3642521

Mismanaging or leaking reproductive health data can lead to dire consequences, with blackmail, discrimination, and violence being among the worst.': McCullum, S. & Singleton, T. 'Period trackers "coercing" women into sharing risky information', BBC, 15 May, 2024: www.bbc.co.uk/news/articles/cmj6j3d8xjjo

attempts to simplify the scales or adapt them for chronic illness patients who do not quite 'fit' into the traditional scales: Von Korff, M., DeBar, L.L., Krebs, E.E., Kerns, R.D., Deyo, R.A. & Keefe, F.J. 'Graded chronic pain scale revised: mild, bothersome, and high-impact chronic pain', *Pain*, 161(3), 651–661 (2020): doi.org/10.1097/j.pain.0000000000001758

'exclude the possibility of endometriosis if the abdominal or pelvic examination and ultrasound scan are normal and recognise that referral may still be necessary even with a normal scan': National Institute for Health and Care Excellence (NICE). 'Endometriosis: diagnosis and management', 6 September, 2017: www.nice.org.uk/guidance/ng73

usually an indicator that deep pelvic endometriosis is present: Tadisetty, S., Nair, R.T., Heba, E.R. & Dawkins, A. 'I saw the "kissing ovaries" sign: Too close for comfort', *Clinical Imaging*, 100, 7–9 (2023): doi.org/10.1016/j.clinimag.2023.04.012

the chances of having stage IV endometriosis are eight times higher: Kido, A., Himoto, Y., Moribata, Y., Kurata, Y. & Nakamoto, Y. 'MRI in the Diagnosis of Endometriosis and Related Diseases', *Korean Journal of Radiology*, 23(4), 426–445 (2022): doi.org/10.3348/kjr.2021.0405

Kissing ovaries are not only linked to disease severity, but also to fertility issues and increased pain: Williams, J.C., Burnett, T.L., Jones, T., Venkatesh, S.K. & VanBuren, W.M. 'Association between kissing and retropositioned ovaries and severity of endometriosis: MR imaging evaluation', *Abdominal Radiology (New York)*, 45(6), 1637–1644 (2020): doi.org/10.1007/s00261-019-02153-6

Endometriosis

Pain is the most common endometriosis symptom: National Institute of Child Health and Human Development (NICHD). 'What are the symptoms of endometriosis?', 21 February, 2020: www.nichd.nih.gov/health/topics/endometri/conditioninfo/symptoms

NSAIDs can be extremely helpful in reducing inflammation – an environment in which we know endometriosis thrives: Machairiotis, N., Vasilakaki, S. & Thomakos, N. 'Inflammatory Mediators and Pain in Endometriosis: A Systematic Review', *Biomedicines*, 9(1), 54 (2021): doi.org/10.3390/biomedicines9010054

opiates also carry the potential for your body to develop a tolerance to the medication, where you start needing higher doses to offer the same level of pain relief, and are known to be highly addictive: Benyamin, R., Trescot, A.M., Datta, S., Buenaventura, R., Adlaka, R., Sehgal, N., Glaser, S.E. & Vallejo, R. 'Opioid complications and side effects', *Pain Physician*, 11(2 Suppl), S105–S120 (2008).

There is some evidence coming through that hormonal medication may be able to reduce endometriomas (haemorrhagic cysts in the ovaries): Thiel, P.S., Donders, F., Kobylianskii, A., Maheux-Lacroix, S., Matelski, J., Walsh, C. & Murji, A. 'The Effect of Hormonal Treatment on Ovarian Endometriomas: A Systematic Review and Meta-Analysis', *Journal of Minimally Invasive Gynecology*, 31(4), 273–279 (2024): doi.org/10.1016/j.jmig.2024.01.002

guidelines and recommendations for pain relief for IUD fittings: Faculty of Sexual and Reproductive Healthcare (FSRH). 'FSRH Guideline: Intrauterine Contraception', March 2023: www.fsrh.org/Common/Uploaded%20files/documents/fsrh-clinical-guideline-intrauterine-contraception-mar23-amended.pdf

ADAM works 'without affecting sensation or ejaculation'.: Contraline, 'Contraline is inventing the future of male contraception' (n.d.): www.contraline.com/

stating clearly that they only 'treat the symptoms associated with endometriosis': TerSera Therapeutics. 'About Zoladex for Endometriosis', n.d.: www.zoladex.com/endometriosis

aid 'management of endometriosis': AbbVie, Inc. 'Lupron Depot for Endometriosis', n.d.: www.luprongyn.com/lupron-for-endometriosis

these effects may not reverse once the pill is stopped, as was once thought: Hidalgo-Lopez, E., Noachtar, I. & Pletzer, B. 'Hormonal contraceptive exposure relates to changes in resting state functional connectivity of anterior cingulate cortex and amygdala', *Frontiers in Endocrinology*, 14 (2023): doi.org/10.3389/fendo.2023.1131995; Panzer, C., Wise, S., Fantini, G., Kang, D., Munarriz, R., Guay, A. & Goldstein, I. 'Impact of Oral Contraceptives on Sex Hormone-Binding Globulin and Androgen Levels: A Retrospective Study in Women with Sexual Dysfunction', *The Journal of Sexual Medicine*, 3(1), 104–113 (2006): doi.org/10.1111/j.1743-6109.2005.00198.x

projected to grow to US $37.22 billion by 2032: Fortune Business Insights. 'Contraceptive Drugs Market Size, Share & Industry Analysis, By Product (Oral (Combined Contraceptives and Progestin-only Pills), Injectable, and Patches), By Distribution Channel (Hospital Pharmacy, Retail Pharmacy, Clinics, Online Channels, Public Channels & NGOs, and Others), and Regional Forecast, 2024–2032', 16 December, 2024: www.fortunebusinessinsights.com/industry-reports/contraceptive-drugs-market-100063

References

'dramatic worsening of endometriosis symptoms or the appearance of new lesions following the cessation of oral contraceptives, other hormonal suppression treatments or pregnancy.': Vidali, A. [@endometriosis_surgeon], 'Stay tuned for more on rebound Endometriosis !!!!! We discuss a new term called "rebound endometriosis", which refers to a dramatic' [Post], Instagram (3 December, 2024): www.instagram.com/p/DDGSsGpsILv/?hl=en

53 per cent of patients have had to visit A&E due to the severity of their symptoms, while 27 per cent went three or more times: All Party Parliamentary Group on Endometriosis, 'Endometriosis in the UK: time for change' (2020): www.endometriosis-uk.org/sites/endometriosis-uk.org/files/files/Endometriosis%20APPG%20Report%20Oct%202020.pdf

only 2 per cent were investigated for endometriosis during their time there: Endometriosis UK, '"Dismissed, ignored and belittled": The long road to endometriosis diagnosis in the UK', March 2024: www.endometriosis-uk.org/sites/default/files/2024-03/Endometriosis%20UK%20diagnosis%20survey%202023%20report%20March.pdf

'the conscientious, explicit, and judicious use of current best evidence in making decisions about the care of individual patients': Sackett, D.L., Rosenberg, W.M.C., Gray, J.A.M., Haynes, R.B. & Richardson, W.S. 'Evidence based medicine: what it is and what it isn't', *BMJ*, 312, 71 (1996). doi.org/10.1136/bmj.312.7023.71

'dissonance . . . when trying to apply research findings to the clinical encounter often occurs when we abandon the narrative-interpretive paradigm and try to get by on "evidence" alone.': Greenhalgh, T. 'Narrative based medicine: narrative based medicine in an evidence based world', *BMJ (Clinical Research Ed.)*, 318(7179), 323–325 (1999): doi.org/10.1136/bmj.318.7179.323

'thoughtful identification and compassionate use of individual patients' predicaments, rights and preferences': Sackett, D. L. 'Evidence-based medicine', *Seminars in Perinatology*, 21(1), 3–5 (1997): doi.org/10.1016/s0146-0005(97)80013-4

Chapter 3: Understanding endometriosis care and surgery

the BSGE lists 79 centres across the UK: British Society for Gynaecological Endoscopy (BSGE). 'All accredited endometriosis centres', n.d.: www.bsge.org.uk/centre/category/accredited-centres/

79 centres to serve the estimated 2 million endometriosis patients currently in the UK: NHS Digital. 'HES On...Endometriosis', 10 July, 2012: digital.nhs.uk/data-and-information/publications/statistical/hospital-admitted-patient-care-activity/hes-on-endometriosis

of 'laparoscopic excision of severe recto-vaginal endometriosis that required dissection of the pararectal space': British Society for Gynaecological Endoscopy (BSGE). 'Requirements to be a BSGE accredited centre', n.d.: www.bsge.org.uk/requirements-to-be-a-bsge-accredited-centre/

cited 'the surgeon's learning curve, high surgical volume and adherence to a structured approach': Khazali, S., Bachi, A., Mondelli, B., Fleischer, K., Adamczyk,, M., Delanerolle, G., Shi, J.Q., Yang, X., Nisar, P. & Bearn, P. 'Intra-operative and post-operative complications of endometriosis excision using the SOSURE approach – A single-surgeon retrospective series of 1116 procedures over 8 years', *Journal of the European Society for Gynaecological Endoscopy*, 16, 3 (2024): doi.org/10.52054/FVVO.16.3.030

'delaying the proper treatment measures from being applied': Mettler, L., Schollmeyer, T., Lehmann-Willenbrock, E., Schüppler, U., Schmutzler, A., Shukla, D., Zavala, A. & Lewin, A. 'Accuracy of laparoscopic diagnosis of endometriosis', *JSLS: Journal of the Society of Laparoendoscopic Surgeons*, 7(1), 15–18 (2003).

recurrence of endometriomas was observed in 9 per cent of patients who received sclerotherapy and pregnancy occurred in 57 per cent of those desiring to conceive: De Cicco Nardone, A., Carfagna, P., De Cicco Nardone, C., Scambia, G., Marana, R. & De Cicco Nardone, F. 'Laparoscopic Ethanol Sclerotherapy for Ovarian Endometriomas: Preliminary Results', *Journal of Minimally Invasive Gynecology*, 27(6), 1331–1336 (2020): doi.org/10.1016/j.jmig.2019.09.792

40 per cent of those with pregnancy intent conceived post sclerotherapy and 11.8 per cent had disease recurrence: Crestani, A., Merlot, B., Dennis, T., Chanavaz-Lacheray, I. & Roman, H. 'Impact of Laparoscopic Sclerotherapy for Ovarian Endometriomas on Ovarian Reserve', *Journal of Minimally Invasive Gynecology*, 30(1), 32–38 (2023): doi.org/10.1016/j.jmig.2022.10.001

with one 2023 study suggesting rates from 29 to 56 per cent after two years: Atwa, K.A., Ibrahim, Z.M., El Bassuony, E.M. & Taha, O.T. 'Factors associated with recurrent endometriomas after surgical excision', *Middle East Fertility Society Journal*, 28, 21 (2023): doi.org/10.1186/s43043-023-00146-6

participants who underwent ablation indicated either no improvement or worsened symptoms and quality of life: Mackenzie, M. 'Laparoscopic excision vs ablation: "endometriosis facebook" symptom and qol questionnaire results', *American Journal of Obstetrics & Gynecology*, 228(3 Suppl), S901–S902 (2023).

doctors were known to 'dig out the endometriosis nodules with blunt scissors, or even their own fingernails': Nezhat, C., Nezhat, F. & Nezhat, C. 'Endometriosis: ancient disease, ancient treatments', *Fertility and Sterility*, 98(6 Suppl), S1–S62 (2012): doi.org/10.1016/j.fertnstert.2012.08.001

including for the treatment of adhesions and abdominal biopsies: Spaner, S.J. & Warnock, G.L. 'A brief history of endoscopy, laparoscopy, and laparoscopic surgery', *Journal of Laparoendoscopic & Advanced Surgical Techniques. Part A*, 7(6), 369–373 (1997): doi.org/10.1089/lap.1997.7.369

it was reported that 'one should excise ... all evident endometriosis': TeLinde, R.W. & Scott, R.B. 'Diagnosis and treatment of endometriosis', *GP*, 5(6), 61–65 (1952).

the first video laparoscopy excision treatment of advanced endometriosis was reported by Camran Nezhat, MD: Nezhat, C.R. 'My journey with the AAGL', *Journal of Minimally Invasive Gynecology*, 17(3), 271–277 (2010): doi.org/10.1016/j.jmig.2010.01.006

References

global experts report that recurrence rates after expert excision surgery can be as low as seven to 15 per cent depending on disease type and location: Center for Endometriosis Care. 'Endo Q&A With Dr Sinervo [Transcript]', n.d.: centerforendo.com/endoqa-with-dr-sinervo-transcript

recurrence rates are estimated at up to 50 per cent within five years: Guo, S.W. 'Recurrence of endometriosis and its control', *Human Reproduction Update*, 15(4), 441–461 (2009): doi.org/10.1093/humupd/dmp007

Eighty-two per cent of our patients only need one surgery; 2 to 4 per cent need a third': Center for Endometriosis Care. 'Endo Q&A With Dr Sinervo [Transcript]', n.d.: centerforendo.com/endoqa-with-dr-sinervo-transcript

should ensure the GP receives clear written guidance: NHS England. 'Colposcopic diagnosis, treatment and follow up', 27 September, 2024: www.gov.uk/government/publications/cervical-screening-programme-and-colposcopy-management/3-colposcopic-diagnosis-treatment-and-follow-up

a 2024 paper based on over 1000 surgeries at a globally recognised endometriosis centre showed a minor post-operative complication rate of 13.8 per cent and major complication of 1.5 per cent. There were no complications of the most severe kind: Khazali, S., Bachi, A., Mondelli, B., Fleischer, K., Adamczyk, M., Delanerolle, G., Shi, J.Q., Yang, X., Nisar, P. & Bearn, P. 'Intra-operative and post-operative complications of endometriosis excision using the SOSURE approach – A single-surgeon retrospective series of 1116 procedures over 8 years', *Facts, Views & Vision in ObGyn*, 16(3), 325–336 (2024): doi.org/10.52054/FVVO.16.3.030

one globally recognised endometriosis centre reports a 7–15 per cent recurrence rate post excision surgery: Center for Endometriosis Care. 'Endo Q&A With Dr Sinervo [Transcript]', n.d.: centerforendo.com/endoqa-with-dr-sinervo-transcript

Chapter 4: The evil step-sisters – associated conditions

proposing that endometriosis increases the risk of other chronic diseases: Kvaskoff, M., Mu, F., Terry, K.L., Harris, H.R., Poole, E.M., Farland, L. & Missmer, S.A. 'Endometriosis: a high-risk population for major chronic diseases?', *Human Reproduction Update*, 21(4), 500–516 (2015): doi.org/10.1093/humupd/dmv013

characterised by the presence of endometrial stroma and glands within the myometrium tissue of the uterus: Gong, C., Wang, Y., Lv, F., Zhang, L. & Wang, Z. 'Evaluation of high intensity focused ultrasound treatment for different types of adenomyosis based on magnetic resonance imaging classification', *International Journal of Hyperthermia*, 39(1), 530–538 (2022): doi.org/10.1080/02656736.2022.2052366

It was only in 2023 that adenomyosis received its own page on the NHS website: National Health Service (NHS). 'Adenomyosis', 17 July, 2023: www.nhs.uk/conditions/adenomyosis/

the prevalence of adenomyosis ranges from 5 to 70 per cent: Dessouky, R., Gamil, S.A., Nada, M.G., Mousa, R. & Libda, Y. 'Management of uterine adenomyosis: current trends and uterine artery embolization as a potential alternative to hysterectomy', *Insights Imaging*, 10, 48 (2019): doi.org/10.1186/s13244-019-0732-8

most recent reports suggesting around 20 per cent, or one in five: Healthdirect Australia, 'Adenomyosis' (September 2024): www.healthdirect.gov.au/adenomyosis

the incidence of adenomyosis is disproportionately high among Black patients: Yu, O., Schulze-Rath, R., Grafton, J., Hansen, K., Scholes, D. & Reed, S.D. 'Adenomyosis incidence, prevalence and treatment: United States population-based study 2006–2015', *American Journal of Obstetrics and Gynecology*, 223(1), 94.e1–94.e10 (2020): doi.org/10.1016/j.ajog.2020.01.016

adenomyosis can occur in anywhere between 20 and 80 per cent of endometriosis patients: Vannuccini, S. & Petraglia, F. 'Recent advances in understanding and managing adenomyosis', *F1000Research*, 8, F1000 Faculty Rev-283 (2019): doi.org/10.12688/f1000research.17242.1

it is thought that approximately one-third of adenomyosis patients have no symptoms at all: Upson, K. & Missmer, S.A. 'Epidemiology of Adenomyosis', *Seminars in Reproductive Medicine*, 38(2-03), 89–107 (2020): doi.org/10.1055/s-0040-1718920

ranging from 65 to 81 per cent: Vannuccini, S. & Petraglia, F. 'Recent advances in understanding and managing adenomyosis', *F1000Research*, 8, F1000 Faculty Rev-283 (2019): doi.org/10.12688/f1000research.17242.1

if 'clinicians do not know what to look for, they will not find it': Dr Susanne Johnson, expert gynaecology sonographer, speaking at a BSGE endometriosis webinar, March 2024

the prevalence of endometriosis in adenomyosis patients was 80.6 per cent and the prevalence of adenomyosis in endometriosis patients was 91.1 per cent: Leyendecker, G., Bilgicyildirim, A., Inacker, M., Stalf, T., Huppert, P., Mall, G., Böttcher, B. & Wildt, L. 'Adenomyosis and endometriosis. Re-visiting their association and further insights into the mechanisms of auto-traumatisation. An MRI study', *Archives of Gynecology and Obstetrics*, 291(4), 917–932 (2015): doi.org/10.1007/s00404-014-3437-8

some studies have shown symptom improvement: Ma, J., Brown, B. & Liang, E. 'Long-term durability of uterine artery embolisation for treatment of symptomatic adenomyosis', *The Australian & New Zealand Journal Of Obstetrics & Gynaecology*, 61(2), 290–296 (2021): doi.org/10.1111/ajo.13304

recurrence rates appear quite high: Kim, M.D., Kim, S., Kim, N.K., Lee, M.H., Ahn, E.H., Kim, H.J., Cho, J.H. & Cha, S.H. 'Long-Term Results of Uterine Artery Embolization for Symptomatic Adenomyosis', *American Journal of Roentgenology*, 188(1): doi.org/10.2214/AJR.05.1613

'UAE should be offered to women as an alternative to hysterectomy, as many case series (detailed groups of patients undergoing similar treatments) have demonstrated the safety and effectiveness' of the procedure: de Bruijn, A.M., Smink, M., Lohle, P.N.M., Huirne, J.A.F., Twisk, J.W.R., Wong, C., Schoonmade, L. & Hehenkamp, W.J.K. 'Uterine Artery Embolization for the Treatment of Adenomyosis: A Systematic Review and Meta-Analysis', *Journal of Vascular and Interventional Radiology*, 28(12), 1629–1642.e1 (2017): doi.org/10.1016/j.jvir.2017.07.034; Liang, E., Brown, B. & Rachinsky, M. 'A clinical audit

References

on the efficacy and safety of uterine artery embolisation for symptomatic adenomyosis: Results in 117 women', *The Australian & New Zealand Journal of Obstetrics & Gynaecology*, 58(4), 454–459 (2018): doi.org/10.1111/ajo.12767

recognise it as a red flag if this procedure is offered to you: Mengerink, B.B., van der Wurff, A.A., ter Haar, J.F., van Rooij, I.A. & Pijnenborg, J.M. 'Effect of undiagnosed deep adenomyosis after failed NovaSure endometrial ablation', *Journal of Minimally Invasive Gynecology*, 22(2), 239–244 (2015): doi.org/10.1016/j.jmig.2014.10.006

it is not recommended for adenomyosis: Liang, E., Parvez, R., Ng, S. & Brown, B. 'Uterine artery embolisation for adenomyosis in women who failed prior endometrial ablation', *CVIR Endovascular*, 7, 59 (2024): doi.org/10.1186/s42155-024-00471-5

adenomyosis patients can often develop worsening pain after endometrial ablation: Galazis, N., Lazaridis, A. & Disu, S. 'Endometrial ablation in women with adenomyosis; should it be avoided? A case of post-ablation syndrome (PAS)', London North West Healthcare NHS Trust and European Society for Gynaecological Endoscopy (n.d.): esge.covr.be/cmdocumentmanagement/conferencemanager/documents/api/getdocument/5550/cmabstsms/0000186810/0462baffccd0d76a0d16ff527d020640cb69a7d3d913bfe8a83bb-77ba08b4028

This would help counter the negative impact adenomyosis can have on fertility: Moawad, G., Kheil, M.H., Ayoubi, J.M., Klebanoff, J.S., Rahman, S. & Sharara, F.I. 'Adenomyosis and infertility', *Journal of Assisted Reproduction and Genetics*, 39(5), 1027–1031 (2022): doi.org/10.1007/s10815-022-02476-2

some studies show this 'regret rate' to be as low as 2.8 per cent: Bougie, O., Suen, M.W., Pudwell, J., MacGregor, B., Plante, S., Nitsch, R. & Singh, S.S. 'Evaluating the Prevalence of Regret With the Decision to Proceed With a Hysterectomy in Women Younger than Age 35', *Journal of Obstetrics and Gynaecology Canada/Journal d'Obstetrique et Gynecologie du Canada*, 42(3), 262–268.e3 (2020): doi.org/10.1016/j.jogc.2019.08.006

in 2018, doctors in Singapore removed a fibroid from a 53-year-old patient that weighed 28kg: Nierenberg, C. 'Doctors remove "giant" pumpkin-size fibroid from woman's uterus', CBS News, 11 September, 2018: www.cbsnews.com/news/doctors-remove-pumpkin-size-giant-fibroid-from-womans-uterus/

The largest recorded fibroid, which was only discovered upon autopsy, weighed a staggering 63.3kg: Evans, A.T., 3rd, & Pratt, J.H. 'A giant fibroid uterus', *Obstetrics and Gynecology*, 54(3), 385–386 (1979).

around two in three women will develop at least one fibroid at some point in their life: National Health Service (NHS). 'Overview: Fibroids', 9 September, 2022: www.nhs.uk/conditions/fibroids/

more than 80 per cent of Black women will develop fibroids: Giuliani, E., As-Sanie, S. & Marsh, E.E. 'Epidemiology and management of uterine fibroids', *International Journal of Gynaecology and Obstetrics*, 149(1), 3–9 (2020): doi.org/10.1002/ijgo.13102

post-menopause, when levels of these hormones drop, fibroids may shrink and cause fewer symptoms: Ulin, M., Ali, M., Chaudhry, Z.T., Al-Hendy, A. & Yang, Q. 'Uterine fibroids in menopause and perimenopause', *Menopause (New York, N.Y.)*, 27(2), 238–242 (2020): doi.org/10.1097/GME.0000000000001438 in some women, it has been shown to increase fibroid size: Ulin, M., Ali, M., Chaudhry, Z.T., Al-Hendy, A. & Yang, Q. 'Uterine fibroids in menopause and perimenopause', *Menopause (New York, N.Y.)*, 27(2), 238–242 (2020): doi.org/10.1097/GME.0000000000001438

Some fibroids patients have reported more severe or prolonged pain following this procedure: NHS, 'Fibroids: Treatment' (9 September, 2022): www.nhs.uk/conditions/fibroids/treatment/

the data on efficacy and long-term outcomes, especially on fertility, is very limited: NHS, 'Fibroids: Treatment' (9 September, 2022): www.nhs.uk/conditions/fibroids/treatment/

Chapter 5: Living with endometriosis – the art and the science

the All Party Parliamentary Group on Endometriosis released their first major report: All Party Parliamentary Group on Endometriosis, 'Endometriosis in the UK: time for change' (2020): www.endometriosis-uk.org/sites/endometriosis-uk.org/files/files/Endometriosis%20APPG%20Report%20Oct%202020.pdf

one in six of those with confirmed endometriosis have lost their job due to the demands of the disease and its management: Zillman, C. '1 in 6 women have lost their jobs due to managing endometriosis', Sothern Cross University, 26 November, 2021: www.scu.edu.au/news/2021/1-in-6-women-have-lost-their-jobs-due-to-managing-endometriosis.php

20 per cent of endometriosis sufferers 'feel their workplaces are unsupportive of chronic health conditions', and while almost a quarter (24 per cent) of workplaces provide employee support for people experiencing fertility issues, 'there is very little support in the workplace for endometriosis': Ormond, D. 'We need to better support and retain employees with endometriosis', *HR Magazine* (8 March, 2024): www.hrmagazine.co.uk/content/comment/we-need-to-better-support-and-retain-employees-with-endometriosis/

'for the purpose of achieving increased function and participation in meaningful activities': Jamieson-Lega, K., Berry, R. & Brown, C.A. 'Pacing: a concept analysis of the chronic pain intervention', *Pain Research & Management*, 18(4), 207–213 (2013): doi.org/10.1155/2013/686179

difficulty doing certain everyday tasks or getting around because of your condition': UK Government. 'Personal Independence Payment (PIP)', n.d.: www.gov.uk/pip

Chapter 6: Not all endometriosis pain is physical

on top of the physical symptoms of a disease like endometriosis, often result in mental distress: Kocas, H.D., Rubin, L.R. & Lobel, M. 'Stigma and mental health in endometriosis', *European Journal of Obstetrics & Gynecology and Reproductive Biology*, X, 19, 100228 (2023): doi.org/10.1016/j.eurox.2023.100228

95 per cent of endometriosis sufferers said that their wellbeing has been negatively impacted by the disease: All Party Parliamentary Group on Endometriosis, 'Endometriosis

in the UK: time for change' (2020): www.endometriosis-uk.org/sites/endometriosis-uk.org/files/files/Endometriosis%20APPG%20Report%20Oct%202020.pdf

around half of the respondents said that their endometriosis had led to suicidal thoughts: Bevan, G. 'Endometriosis: Thousands share devastating impact of condition', BBC, 6 October, 2019: www.bbc.co.uk/news/health-49897873

90 per cent of endometriosis sufferers were found to have wanted access to psychological support but were not offered any: All Party Parliamentary Group on Endometriosis, 'Endometriosis in the UK: time for change' (2020): www.endometriosis-uk.org/sites/endometriosis-uk.org/files/files/Endometriosis%20APPG%20Report%20Oct%202020.pdf

'psychosocial factors such as stigma also play a role in mental health distress among endometriosis patients': Kocas, H.D., Rubin, L.R. & Lobel, M. 'Stigma and mental health in endometriosis', *European Journal of Obstetrics & Gynecology and Reproductive Biology*, X, 19, 100228 (2023): doi.org/10.1016/j.eurox.2023.100228

They have even been shown to soothe our nervous systems: Linscott, M. 'Glimmers & Triggers: Following Our Neuroceptive Cues', Purdue University Global Academic Success Center (n.d.): purdueglobalwriting.center/2024/05/24/glimmers-triggers-following-our-neuroceptive-cues/

there is a well-documented and clearly understandable link between negative mental health and fertility: Sharma, A. & Shrivastava, D. 'Psychological Problems Related to Infertility', *Cureus*, 14(10), e30320 (2022): doi.org/10.7759/cureus.30320

Chapter 7: Endometriosis doesn't discriminate – why do we?

Black women are three times more likely to die during pregnancy, childbirth and the six weeks following childbirth: Brader, C. 'Maternal mortality rates in the Black community'. House of Lords Library, 12 December, 2023: lordslibrary.parliament.uk/maternal-mortality-rates-in-the-black-community/

he went on to offer the procedure to White women, sedated, of course: Gamble, V.N. 'Under the shadow of Tuskegee: African Americans and health care', *American Journal of Public Health*, 87(11), 1773–1778 (1997): doi.org/10.2105/ajph.87.11.1773

'There was never a time that I could not, at any day, have had a subject for operation.': Sims, J.M. 'The Story of My Life', D. Appleton (1885).

Six times more likely to suffer more serious birth injuries in England: Thomas, T. 'Black women in England suffer more serious birth complications, analysis finds', *Guardian*, 8 April, 2024: www.theguardian.com/society/2024/apr/08/black-women-in-england-suffer-more-serious-birth-complications-analysis-finds

Forty per cent more likely to die of breast cancer: Yedjou, C.G., Sims, J.N., Miele, L., Noubissi, F., Lowe, L., Fonseca, D.D., Alo, R.A., Payton, M. & Tchounwou, P.B. 'Health and Racial Disparity in Breast Cancer', *Advances in Experimental Medicine and Biology*, 1152, 31–49 (2019): doi.org/10.1007/978-3-030-20301-6_3

Two times more likely to be diagnosed with late-stage womb cancer and two times more likely to die from that cancer: Smith, J. 'New analysis reveals Black women in England

Endometriosis

more likely to be diagnosed with late-stage cancer', Cancer Research UK, 27 January, 2023: news.cancerresearchuk.org/2023/01/27/new-analysis-reveals-black-women-in-england-more-likely-to-be-diagnosed-with-late-stage-cancer/

Less likely to be given pain relief due to a persistent belief that Black skin has fewer nerve endings: Weisse, C.S., Sorum, P.C., Sanders, K.N. & Syat, B.L. 'Do gender and race affect decisions about pain management?', *Journal of General Internal Medicine*, 16(4), 211–217 (2001): doi.org/10.1046/j.1525-1497.2001.016004211.x

More than three times as likely to be sectioned under the Mental Health Act: UK Government. 'Detentions under the Mental Health Act', 16 August, 2024: www.ethnicity-facts-figures.service.gov.uk/health/mental-health/detentions-under-the-mental-health-act/latest/

'restricting the propagation of the intelligent class': Hillspecial, G. 'Social Ill Is Laid to Endometriosis; Women's Ailment Restricting the Propagation of Intelligent Class, Says Dr. J. V. Meigs', *The New York Times*, 21 October, 1948: www.nytimes.com/1948/10/21/archives/social-ill-is-laid-to-endometriosis-womens-ailment-restricting-the.html

stated that 'endometriosis is not frequent in the negro': Kistner, R.W. 'Infertility with Endometriosis: A Plan of Therapy', *Fertility and Sterility*, 13(3), 237–245 (1962): www.sciencedirect.com/science/article/pii/S0015028216345034

Black patients were typically being diagnosed with sexually transmitted infections or pelvic inflammatory disease (PID): Chatman, D.L. 'Endometriosis in the black woman', *American Journal of Obstetrics and Gynecology*, 125(7), 987–989 (1976): doi.org/10.1016/0002-9378(76)90502-0

Black women can have more severe lesions than their White counterparts: Shade, G.H., Lane, M. & Diamond, M.P. 'Endometriosis in the African American woman—racially, a different entity?', *Gynecological Surgery*, 9, 59–62 (2012).

for Black people, diagnosis times can be up to double the average times of eight to 10 years: *American Journal of Managed Care*, 'Racial Disparities Associated With Endometriosis Diagnosis [Video]', 'Addressing Health Disparities in Women's Healthcare', Episode 6 (18 May, 2023): www.ajmc.com/view/racial-disparities-associated-with-endometriosis-diagnosis

Despite Black women experiencing menopause up to 10 years earlier than their White counterparts: Velez, A. 'Menopause Is Different for Women of Color', HealthCentral, 10 March, 2021: www.healthcentral.com/condition/menopause/menopause-different-women-color

only 6 per cent of the respondents were people of colour: Endometriosis UK, '"Dismissed, ignored and belittled": The long road to endometriosis diagnosis in the UK', March 2024: www.endometriosis-uk.org/sites/default/files/2024-03/Endometriosis%20UK%20diagnosis%20survey%202023%20report%20March.pdf

'Women's health economics: investing in the 51 per cent': Gorham, B. & Langham, O. 'Women's health economics: investing in the 51 per cent', NHS Confederation, 2 October, 2024: www.nhsconfed.org/publications/womens-health-economics

have created a legacy of distrust: Scharff, D.P., Mathews, K.J., Jackson, P., Hoffsuemmer, J., Martin, E. & Edwards, D. 'More than Tuskegee: understanding mistrust about research participation', *Journal of Health Care for the Poor and Underserved*, 21(3), 879–897 (2010): doi.org/10.1353/hpu.0.0323

References

the prevalence of endometriosis among trans men could be as high as 25 per cent: Carvalho, S.A., Lapa, T. & Pascoal, P.M. 'The Need to Look at Transgender and Gender Diverse People's Health: A Preliminary Descriptive Report on Pain, Sexual Distress, and Health Profile of Five Transmasculine People and One Non-Binary Person with Endometriosis', *Healthcare (Basel, Switzerland)*, 12(12), 1229 (2024): doi.org/10.3390/healthcare12121229

87 per cent believe obese people are 'indulgent' and 32 per cent believe they 'lack willpower': Puhl, R. & Brownell, K.D. 'Bias, discrimination, and obesity', *Obesity Research*, 9(12), 788–805 (2001): doi.org/10.1038/oby.2001.108

can result in patients delaying seeking support: Burke, M.E. 'Stop the Stigma! Eliminating Implicit and Explicit Bias Toward Adult Obese Women Receiving Gynecological Care: A Quality Improvement Project to Cultivate Empathy and Increase Knowledge of Best Practices', University of Amherst Massachusetts, Doctor of Nursing Practice (DNP) Projects, 152 (2018): core.ac.uk/download/pdf/220128486.pdf

up to 87 per cent of women or AFAB individuals delayed seeking healthcare due to their weight: Puhl, R.M. & Heuer, C.A. 'Obesity stigma: important considerations for public health', *American Journal of Public Health*, 100(6), 1019–1028 (2010): doi.org/10.2105/AJPH.2009.159491

inherent bias can hinder diagnosis, leading to conditions going undetected: Tomiyama, A., Carr, D., Granberg, E., Major, B., Robinson, E., Sutin, A.R. & Brewis, A. 'How and why weight stigma drives the obesity "epidemic" and harms health', *BMC Medicine*, 16, 123 (2018): doi.org/10.1186/s12916-018-1116-5

doctors are generally less inclined to examine patients with a higher body mass index (BMI): Phelan, S.M., Burgess, D.J., Yeazel, M.W., Hellerstedt, W.L., Griffin, J.M. & van Ryn, M. 'Impact of weight bias and stigma on quality of care and outcomes for patients with obesity', *Obesity Reviews*, 16(4), 319–326 (2015): doi.org/10.1111/obr.12266

a staggering three-quarters had internalised unconscious biases towards fat patients: Phelan, S.M., Dovidio, J.F., Puhl, R.M., Burgess, D.J., Nelson, D.B., Yeazel, M.W., Hardeman, R., Perry, S. & van Ryn, M. 'Implicit and explicit weight bias in a national sample of 4,732 medical students: the medical student CHANGES study', *Obesity (Silver Spring, Md.)*, 22(4), 1201–1208 (2014): doi.org/10.1002/oby.20687

'low BMI is reported with increased incidence of endometriosis': Hong, J. & Yi, K.W. 'What is the link between endometriosis and adiposity?', *Obstetrics & Gynecology Science*, 65(3), 227–233 (2022): doi.org/10.5468/ogs.21343

'slim women have a greater risk of developing endometriosis than obese women': European Society of Human Reproduction and Embryology (ESHRE). 'Slim women have a greater risk of developing endometriosis than obese women', 15 May, 2023: www.eshre.eu/Press-Room/Press-releases-2013/Slim-women-have-a-greater-risk-of-developing-endometriosis-than-obese-women

potentially up to twice that of 'healthy weight women': Australian Associated Press. 'Endometriosis is more severe for obese women, study finds', *Guardian*, 12 June, 2018: www.theguardian.com/society/2018/jun/12/endometriosis-is-more-painful-for-obese-women-study-finds; Holdsworth-Carson, S.J., Dior, U.P., Colgrave, E.M., Healy, M., Montgomery, G.W., Rogers, P.A.W. & Girling, J.E. 'The association of body mass index with endometriosis and disease severity in women with pain', *Journal of Endometriosis and Pelvic Pain Disorders*, 10(2), 79–87 (2018): doi.org/10.1177/2284026518773939

Surgery and surgical recovery is different for fat people: Plassmeier, L., Hankir, M.K. & Seyfried, F. 'Impact of Excess Body Weight on Postsurgical Complications', *Visceral Medicine*, 37(4), 287–297 (2021): doi.org/10.1159/000517345

Medical schools should have specific training for how weight can interact with diseases, as well as the factors that can influence BMI beyond over-eating and not getting enough exercise: Tomiyama, A., Carr, D., Granberg, E., Major, B., Robinson, E., Sutin, A.R. & Brewis, A. 'How and why weight stigma drives the obesity "epidemic" and harms health', *BMC Medicine*, 16, 123 (2018): doi.org/10.1186/s12916-018-1116-5

Sensitivity training should be provided in medical settings, and all hospitals and clinics should have the capability to treat those in heavier bodies: Lindheim, S.R., Glenn, T.L. & Whigham, L.D. 'Recognizing and eliminating bias in those with elevated body mass index in women's health care', *Fertility and Sterility*, 109, 775–776 (2018): doi:10.1016/j.fertnstert.2018.03.002

Surgeons need to allow more time to complete surgeries on patients with a higher BMI and put measures in place to account for the increased risk of wound infection: McCartney, J. 'Study Clarifies Link between Obesity and Surgical Complications', American College of Surgeons, 11 October, 2023: www.facs.org/for-medical-professionals/news-publications/news-and-articles/bulletin/2023/october-2023-volume-108-issue-10/study-clarifies-link-between-obesity-and-surgical-complications/

Looking at the local authorities in the top 20 per cent least deprived areas in the country, 97 per cent scored higher than the national average for health outcomes: Gorham, B. & Langham, O. 'Women's health economics: investing in the 51 per cent', NHS Confederation, 2 October, 2024: www.nhsconfed.org/publications/womens-health-economics

17 per cent of patients have sought private care for endometriosis due to long NHS waiting times: Endometriosis UK. 'England: Unacceptable care delays for endometriosis', 11 August, 2022: www.endometriosis-uk.org/england-unacceptable-care-delays-endometriosis

people from White British, White Irish and White Other ethnic groups were the least likely to live in the most income-deprived 10 per cent of neighbourhoods: UK Government. 'People living in deprived neighbourhoods', 30 September, 2020: www.ethnicity-facts-figures.service.gov.uk/uk-population-by-ethnicity/demographics/people-living-in-deprived-neighbourhoods/latest/

The numbers in medical literature range from 16 to 20: Rei, C., Williams, T. & Feloney, M. 'Endometriosis in a Man as a Rare Source of Abdominal Pain: A Case Report and Review of the Literature', *Case Reports in Obstetrics and Gynecology*, 2018, 2083121 (2018): doi.org/10.1155/2018/2083121

The reported ages of these patients range from 27 to 83: Rei, C., Williams, T. & Feloney, M. 'Endometriosis in a Man as a Rare Source of Abdominal Pain: A Case Report and Review of the Literature', *Case Reports in Obstetrics and Gynecology*, 2018, 2083121 (2018): doi.org/10.1155/2018/2083121

this 40-year-old man had received no such oestrogen therapy: Rei, C., Williams, T. & Feloney, M. 'Endometriosis in a Man as a Rare Source of Abdominal Pain: A Case Report and Review of the Literature', *Case Reports in Obstetrics and Gynecology*, 2018, 2083121 (2018): doi.org/10.1155/2018/2083121

a higher BMI is associated with higher levels of circulating oestrogen: Mair, K.M., Gaw, R. & MacLean, M.R. 'Obesity, estrogens and adipose tissue dysfunction – implications for pulmonary arterial hypertension', *Pulmonary Circulation*, 10(3), 2045894020952019 (2020): doi.org/10.1177/2045894020952023

Reports of endometriosis in cis men reach as far back as 1985: Beckman, E.N., Pintado, S.O., Leonard, G.L. & Sternberg, W.H. 'Endometriosis of the prostate', *The American Journal of Surgical Pathology*, 9(5), 374–379 (1985): doi.org/10.1097/00000478-198505000-00008

'Women's Health Economics: Investing in the 51 per cent': Gorham, B. & Langham, O. 'Women's health economics: investing in the 51 per cent', NHS Confederation, 2 October, 2024: www.nhsconfed.org/publications/womens-health-economics

Chapter 8: This is not the end

'leeches, straight-jackets, bloodletting, caustic chemical douches, genital mutilation, being hung upside down, surgical fatalities, and even accusations of demonic possession and state-sanctioned executions'.: Nezhat, C. 'History of endometriosis', Carmen Nezhat, Center for Special Minimally Invasive & Robotic Surgery (N.d.): nezhat.org/endometriosis-treatment/history-of-endometriosis/

for every £1 spent on women's health, there would be a return on investment of £11: Gorham, B. & Langham, O. 'Women's health economics: investing in the 51 per cent', NHS Confederation, 2 October, 2024: www.nhsconfed.org/publications/womens-health-economics

only one in five evidence-based interventions actually make it into routine patient care: Rubin, R. 'It Takes an Average of 17 Years for Evidence to Change Practice – the Burgeoning Field of Implementation Science Seeks to Speed Things Up' *JAMA*, 329(16), 1333–1336 (2023): doi.org/10.1001/jama.2023.4387

Eighty-five per cent of all scans missed endometriosis, and 65 per cent of all surgeries missed disease: Endometriosis and the Knowledge Gap, S Harbour, February 2025.

only 2 per cent of available funding goes to female founders: Wood, A. 'Only 2% of VC Funding Goes to Female and Ethnic Minority Founded Businesses', *Startups Magazine*, n.d.: startupsmagazine.co.uk/article-only-2-vc-funding-goes-female-and-ethnic-minority-founded-businesses

$1.24 billion compared to $44 million: World Economic Forum, 'Closing the Women's Health Gap: A $1 Trillion Opportunity to Improve Lives and Economies' (17 January, 2024): www.weforum.org/publications/closing-the-women-s-health-gap-a-1-trillion-opportunity-to-improve-lives-and-economies/

an Italian publicly funded study published in 2013: Vercellini, P., Buggio, L., Somigliana, E., Barbara, G., Viganò, P. & Fedele, L. 'Attractiveness of women with rectovaginal endometriosis: a case-control study', *Fertility and Sterility*, 99(1), 212–218 (2013): doi.org/10.1016/j.fertnstert.2012.08.039 (Retraction published *Fertil Steril*. 2020 Nov;114(5):1123. doi: 10.1016/j.fertnstert.2020.09.001.)

RESOURCES

Individuals worth following

Dr Andrea Vidali, endometriosis surgeon
drvidali.com
@endometriosis_surgeon

Dr Aziza Sesay, GP, speaker and women's health campaigner
@talkswithdrsesay

Clare Bourne, pelvic floor physiotherapy
clare-bourne.com
@clarebournephysio
Strong Foundations (Thorsons, 2023)

Mr Francesco Di Chiara, thoracic endometriosis surgeon
@francesco_thoracic

Dr José D. Eugenio-Colón, endometriosis surgeon
centerforendo.com/drcolon
@drendometriosis

Heather Guidone, BCPA, endometriosis advocate
centerforendo.com

Katie Boyce BCPA, endometriosis advocate
endogirlblog.com
@endogirlsblog

Mr Mikey Adamczyk, endometriosis surgeon
@mikey.adamczyk

Mr Mohammed Mabrouk, endometriosis surgeon and president of European Endometriosis League
euroendometriosis.com

Dr Nighat Arif, GP, author, broadcaster and women's health campaigner
@drnighatarif
The Knowledge (Aster, 2023)

Rey, endometriosis advocate
@reythewarrior

Mr Shaheen Khazali, endometriosis surgeon
@shaheenkhazali

Dr Shanti Mohling, endometriosis surgeon
@shantimohlingmd

Dr Sula Windgassen
healthpsychologist.co.uk
@the health psychologist

Dr Wendaline VanBuren, gynaecological ultrasound specialist
@wendalinevb
eice.ltd

Organisations worth following

The Adeno Gang, adenomyosis and menstrual health support
theadenogang.com
@theadenogang

Cysters charity
cysters.org
@cystersgroup

Endometriosis UK
endometriosis-uk.org

The Endometriosis Foundation
theendometriosisfoundation.org

Endometriosis South Coast
endometriosissouthcoast.com

The Guidance Suite, fibroids support
dawnheels.com/the-guidance-suite
@guidancesuite

Menstrual Health Project
menstrualhealthproject.org.uk

Guidelines and useful websites

BSGE
bsge.org.uk

ESHRE guidelines for endometriosis, published February 2022
eshre.eu/guideline/endometriosis

NICE guidelines for endometriosis, last updated November 2024
nice.org.uk/guidance/ng73

Royal College of Obstetricians and Gynaecologists
rcog.org.uk

Wellbeing of Women, period symptom checker
wellbeingofwomen.org.uk/what-we-do/campaigns/just-a-period/period-symptom-checker

ACKNOWLEDGEMENTS

Just as living with endometriosis is a multidisciplinary process, so is publishing a book. I could never have done it alone, and I have so much gratitude for so many people.

My journey with advocacy started online, and through that work I have met some of the most incredible humans. It would simply be impossible to name every single person who I have had conversations with over the last few years but if you have ever liked, shared or commented on one of my posts, if you have ever sent me a message, or answered questions that I have, then my most heartfelt thanks go out to you. Special thanks to Rey, the first person to reach out to me when everything felt so raw and confusing. Three years ago, I felt alone, that I was just suffering in silence with no one understanding me. Now I know that could not be further from the truth. The power of sharing our stories is immeasurable.

To Sarah Graham, who, over cake in a book shop (fittingly), was the first person outside of my husband that I talked about my ideas for this book; thank you for giving me the encouragement that I needed. Your openness started this whole process of taking a document on my computer and bringing it into the world. To my agent, Julia, thank you for instantly 'getting it'. For understanding the need for this book, for seeing the potential in it, and me. To my editor, Charlotte, I cannot thank you enough for your passion, wisdom, expertise and support. Writing a book while chronically ill, including an unexpected surgery coinciding with a major deadline, is as unpredictable as you might imagine, but the support shown by Charlotte, Caroline, Jess, Gracia and the wider Bloomsbury team is something I shall never take for granted. It is an honour and a joy to publish this book with you. I truly believe that we have created something that will help endometriosis patients and clinicians alike. Thanks to everyone at Bloomsbury who has been part of that process; for seeing our pain and wanting to raise our voices.

I am indebted to the patients and loved ones who spoke to me for this book. Their generosity in sharing such intimate experiences and feelings so vulnerably has made writing this book an experience I will never forget.

Thanks also go to the experts who so kindly shared their time, which they are notoriously short on, and their expertise, which they are anything but short on! Their work is shaping the future of endometriosis care, and I am exceptionally grateful to them for allowing me to collate their knowledge in this book.

I also wanted to thank all the researchers, doctors, medical students, nurses and all other healthcare practitioners who are working every day to improve endometriosis patient outcomes. You give us desperately needed hope, and we need you.

Thank you to my honorary sister, Amber. For the daily messages, check ins, funny videos, encouragement, opinions, and generally just being the type of friend we all dream of. To the friends around me who have been my cheerleaders, encouraging me at every step of the way of this process, never letting me believe the voices of self-doubt, and for sharing my work with anyone and everyone who will listen. Kate, Mak, Helen: thank you for everything.

To my nieces, Ellie and Malina. Thank you for inspiring me every day to create a better world for you.

To my parents, Ann and Steve. Words cannot express my eternal gratitude for you both. For your love, support, generosity and instilling in me my stubbornness to change the world. I love you both so much, and I hope I do you proud.

Perhaps unconventionally, thanks also go to my two cats, Nacho and Simba. Thank you for being the best fluffy little nurses I could ask for. From keeping me company when in pain flares or recovering from operations to attending every online meeting, invited or not, these two have been as part of this journey as anyone else.

Finally, and above all else, I am endlessly thankful to my biggest support and cheerleader, my husband Chris. None of this would be here without you. Not the book, not my work, probably not even myself. Thank you for your tireless love, care, openness, advocacy and self-education. For believing in me when I struggled to believe in myself. For the cwtches when it all felt too much. For the limitless cups of tea and snacks while I was trying to organise my thoughts, write and edit this book. For reminding me that endometriosis is only a tiny part of who I am. And for remembering the human underneath it all. I love you.

INDEX

abdominal ultrasound 49, 78–9
ablation surgery 17–18, 61, 115, 117–18
Adamczyk, Mikey 11, 39–40, 59–60, 110, 121, 127–8, 144–5
adenomyomectomy 158
adenomyosis 4, 38, 84, 147–52
    diagnosing 153–4
    management 155–60
    myth busting 154–5
    surgery 154, 156–9
    symptoms 152–3
adhesions 16–18, 39, 53
advocation in medical appointments, self- 75–7
A&E departments, endometriosis and 103–5
AI technology 253–4
alcohol 179
Arif, Dr Nighat 76, 107–8, 232, 252, 258, 259
aromatase 13

baths, hot 94, 156
belly, endo/adeno 38
Bingham, Dr Wendy 23
bio-psycho-social modeling of endometriosis 204–5
Black women 149, 160, 161, 167, 168, 224–8
bladder/urinary tract endometriosis 34
'bleed' and 'shed' narrative 10, 13, 39
blood clots, passing 42–3
Blue Badge scheme 198–9
body image 209–12
Bourne, Clare 142–4
bowel endometriosis 34
bowel movement 64–5, 136
Boyce, Katie 60
breathing techniques 99
British Society for Gynaecological Endoscopy (BSGE) 111–13, 145

campaigning and activism *see* organisational support
cannabidiol (CBD) medication 256
causes of endometriosis, theoretical 28–30

celebrations/special occasions 191–4
central sensitisation 39–40, 141
chemical menopause 56, 87–8
children and adolescents 54–8, 61, 190–1
cis-gendered men 47, 242–4
clothing 191, 192, 195, 230
cold/ice therapy 195
commonality of endometriosis 14, 22–3, 26–7, 45–7, 55, 61
comparative suffering 208–9, 211
complaints, formal 108, 263–5
constipation 136
contraceptive pill/patches 30–1, 60–1, 85, 90–1, 228–9
see also hormonal management
crotch shooting pain 37
cultural disparities, endometriosis and 228–32
cure for endometriosis, lack of 30–2, 131–2

data security 70–2
decidual casts 42–3
deep infiltrating endometriosis (DIE) 15, 16, 49
Di Chiara, Francesco 24–7, 29, 68, 259
diagnosis, endometriosis 48–50, 63–6, 213–14
diet/nutrition 95–7, 156
discrimination, endometriosis patient 244–6
    cis-gendered men 242–4
    cultural disparities 228–32
    gender politics 233–6
    racial disparities 224–8
    socioeconomic status 239–42
    weight/fat phobia 236–9
dyspareunia 182–5

education, endometriosis and 4–5, 66–70, 190–1
employment *see* work and study, impact on
endometrial ablation 157–8, 164
endometriomas 11, 15, 16, 52, 116–17
endometriosis defined 3, 9–13

endometrium   3, 13, 61
Endotest   50
erythema ab igne/'toasted skin syndrome'   92–3
Eugenio-Colón, Dr José   14, 65–6, 118, 257
European Endometriosis League   130–1
evidence-based medicine   105–7
excision surgery   1, 16, 17, 18, 31–2, 51, 52–3, 57, 61, 116, 117–18, 137, 158
exercise and movement   97–8, 100, 136
experts, finding endometriosis   113–14, 127–8
extra-pelvic and -abdominopelvic   22–7, 66, 139

fatigue *vs* tiredness   35–6
FemTech products and apps   255
fertility   51–4, 62, 175, 217–19, 229–30
fibroids   4, 157, 160–1
  diagnosis   163
  patient's story   165–8
  symptoms   163
  treatment   163–7
  types of   161–2
flare-ups, endometriosis   44–5
  in hot temperatures   194–5
  kits   179, 192
'frozen pelvis'   17
funding, research   255–7

gaslighting, medical *see* misdiagnosis and medical negligence
gender politics and endometriosis   7, 11, 233–6
'glimmers'   214–15
gonadotrophin-releasing hormone (GnRH) treatments   87–9, 156, 234
Gorham, Bridget   227–8, 245–6, 252, 253
Greenhalgh, Professor Trish   106
grief and chronic illness   219–21
Guidone, Heather   12, 130, 168, 248, 257
gynaecology and endometriosis   58–60, 109, 127–8

haemothorax   23
heat and pain management   92–4, 156
heatwaves/hot temperatures   194–5
Heels, Dawn   165–6
Heera-Shergil, Neelam   227, 228–31, 233, 236, 238, 241, 260

historical accounts of endometriosis   12, 117, 247
hobbies and interests   199
hormonal management   10–11, 16, 30–1, 40–1, 51, 57, 60–1, 84–91, 156, 162, 228–9
hormone replacement therapy (HRT)   88, 162
hot-water bottles   92–4
hydration   194
hysterectomy   3, 31, 59, 124–7, 164, 165
hysteroscopic resection   164

'I Love yoU' (ILU) massage   100–1
inflammation   3, 10, 18, 38, 99
inheritability, endometriosis   47–8
iron tablets/infusions   84, 156
Isaacs, Amelia   255
IUDs   85–7, 156
IVF treatment   52–3, 91

Johnson, Dr Susanne   81

Khazali, Shaheen   29, 50, 52, 53, 56–7, 87–8, 106, 112, 119, 244, 254
'kissing ovaries'   81

laparoscopic uterine nerve ablation (LUNA)   157
laparoscopy   48, 49, 115, 134–5, 154
  see also surgery
letter and email templates   263–6
lifestyle changes/homebased management methods   51, 91–102, 146, 156
  see also hobbies and interests; work and study, impact on
lightning crotch/fanny daggers   37
locations of endometriosis   20–1

Mabrouk, Mohamed   109, 130–1, 254
Mallick, Dr Rebecca   118
Mankoski pain scale   74–5
marginalised communities *see* Black women; discrimination, endometriosis patient
massage   100–1
Mayer–Rokitansky–Küster–Hauser syndrome (MRKH)   46–7
media coverage of endometriosis   257–8
medical appointments, advocacy and preparation for   75–7, 107–8, 145, 175–6

Index

medication and management   10–11, 16, 30–1, 40–1, 51, 53, 57, 60–1, 82–107, 193, 194
  see also surgery
menopause   13, 31, 162
  chemical   56, 87–8
mental health   66, 201–8, 221–2
  body image   209–12
  comparative suffering   208–9, 211
  diagnosis times and waiting lists   205–7
  endo emotions   212–15
  and fertility issues   217–18
  'glimmers'   214–15
  grief and chronic illness   219–21
  toxic positivity   215–17
misdiagnosis and medical negligence   4, 5, 7, 11, 19, 24–5, 27, 32–4, 54, 55, 65–6, 119–24, 127–8, 205–7, 263–5
  see also discrimination, endometriosis patient
misinformation, public   68, 69
Mitchell, Natalie   249
mobility aids   211
Mohling, Dr Shanti   57
morcellation   164
MRI scans   15, 49, 79, 81, 154
mülleriosis   29
multi-disciplinary care, need for   109–10
Munchetty, Naga   160
MyChart app, NHS   76
myomectomy   164

Naftalin, Joel   150
Nancy's Nook   113
National Health Service (NHS)   25–6, 39, 68, 76, 108, 113, 118–19, 159–60, 161, 204, 207, 227–8, 239, 240, 245–6, 252–3, 256
nausea   84, 101–2
nervous system   39–40, 141
networking/connecting   200
New York Times   225
NICE guidelines   77–8, 88, 157
NSAIDs   83, 156

oestrogen   10, 13, 31, 85
opiates and codeine   83, 156
organisational support and charities   248, 250–2, 260
  getting involved   250–1
  see also individuals by name
Ormond, Dearbhail   186–7, 255

ovarian endometriomas (OMAs)   15, 16, 49, 53

pacing activity and rest   100, 196–7
pain   4, 16, 17, 19, 32–4, 37, 38–40, 62, 256
  adenomyosis   156
  central sensitisation   39–40, 141
  exercise/movement and pacing   97–8, 100
  heat management   92–4, 156
  maps   75
  medication   83, 156
  'pelvic pain puzzle'   140–1
  post-surgery   136, 137, 140–1, 146
  rating your level of   73–5
pelvic endometriosis   22, 23, 33
pelvic floor physiotherapy   142–5
periods/menstruation   10, 11, 13, 26, 28–9, 36–7, 39, 40–4, 61, 65, 83–4, 97, 136, 230
  tracking apps   70, 71–2
physiotherapy, pelvic floor   142–5
PIP benefits   198
pneumothorax   23, 26
Pouch of Douglas (POD)   21
pre-sacral neurectomy (PSN)   157
pregnancy   31, 52–4, 62, 117
private healthcare, access to   239–40
progesterone   13, 85
progestin-only treatments   85–7, 156

racial disparities and racism, endometriosis and   224–8
  see also Black women; cultural disparities, endometriosis and
rage rooms   214
rebound endometriosis   90–1
recovery from surgery, home   135–8
rectouterine pouch   21
recurrence, post-surgery   118–19
relationships, impact on   170–1
  celebrations/special occasions   191–4
  dating with endometriosis   178–9
  disclosing chronic illness   177–8, 179
  helpful and unhelpful things to say to an endometriosis patient   181–2
  interview with author's partner   171–7
  networking/connecting   200
  sex and endometriosis   182–5
  supporting a loved one with endometriosis   180–1
reproductive rights   70–1
research funding   255–7

retrograde menstruation 28–9
Rey (endometriosis campaigner) 121–4, 134, 163, 240, 251–3, 256, 257, 258, 259
Robbins, Karla 46–7
Rokitansky, Karl Freiherr von 12

Sampson, John 28
scans/medical imaging 15, 49, 55, 78–82, 154
scar protection 195
sclerotherapy 116–17
Sesay, Dr Aziza 77, 224, 225, 227, 228
sex 53, 66, 136, 174–5, 182–5
'silent endometriosis' 36
Simon-Hall, Tanya 148–9, 151–2, 156, 159–60, 226, 252
Sims, James Marion 224–5
Sinervo, Dr Ken 63, 119, 121
sleep 99, 156
social media 26, 68–9, 200, 258–9
socio-economic status, endometriosis 239–42
specialist endometriosis centres 111–13, 139
stages of endometriosis, four 18–20
stress reduction 98–9, 156
stretches/stretching 97–8, 156
studying with endometriosis *see* work and study, impact on
superficial peritoneal endometriosis (SPE) 15, 80
support
  available societal support 197–9
  at home, post-surgery 110, 137–8
  ways to support loved ones 180–1
  workplace 187–90
surgery 25–6, 48, 49, 51, 56–8, 61, 89
  ablation 17–18, 61, 115, 117–18
  ablation *vs* excision comparison 117–18
  adenomyosis 154, 157–9
  diagnostic 114–15
  excision 1, 16, 17, 18, 31–2, 51, 52–3, 57, 61, 116, 117–18, 137, 158
  fibroids 164
  finding an expert 113–14, 127–30
  hysterectomy 3, 31, 59, 124–7
  improving standards 130–1
  multiple procedures 118–19
  need for multi-disciplinary care 109–11
  negative endometriosis outcome 138–9

packing for hospital 133–4
patients' stories 119–20, 121–4
pre-surgery preparation 132–3
questions to ask 128–9, 139
recovery at home 135–8
sclerotherapy 116–17
sex after surgery 136–7, 184
specialist centres 111–13
surgeons' stories 120–1
surgery day – what to expect 134–5
treating heavier people 237, 238–9
symptoms 32–6
  management 51, 82–107
  taboo 64–5
  tracking 70–3, 75–6, 107
systemic/full-body disease, endometriosis 3, 5, 20–1, 58, 61, 62

technological innovations 253–5
TENS machines 95, 156
tests, diagnostic 50
thoracic endometriosis 23–6, 33
toxic positivity 215–16
tracking, symptom 70–3, 75–7, 107
tranexamic acid 83–4, 156
trans and non-binary healthcare, endometriosis 233–6
transvaginal ultrasounds 49, 79, 232
travelling 193–4

ultrasound scans 15, 49, 55, 78–82, 154, 232
urinary tract endometriosis 34
uterine arterial embolisation (UAE) 157, 164

VanBuren, Dr Wendaline 55, 80–1
Vidali, Dr Andea 90–1

Waterloo Road BBC TV drama 249–50
weight stigma/fat phobia 236–40
wellness industry and programmes 102–3, 241
Windgassen, Dr Sula 180, 202–4, 216–17, 219–21
work and study, impact on 185–7
  getting workplace support 187–90, 266
  school and studying 190–1
  self-employment 190